The Army Medical Department
1775–1818

Published by Books Express Publishing
Copyright © Books Express, 2012
ISBN 978-1-78266-094-1

Books Express publications are available from all good retail and online booksellers. For publishing proposals and direct ordering please contact us at: info@books-express.com

The Army Medical Department
1775–1818

Mary C. Gillett

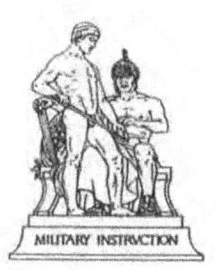

CENTER OF MILITARY HISTORY
UNITED STATES ARMY
WASHINGTON, D.C., 2004

ARMY HISTORICAL SERIES
Maurice Matloff, General Editor

ADVISORY COMMITTEE
(as of February 1979)

Otis A. Singletary (Chairman)
University of Kentucky

Brig. Gen. Robert Arter
Command and General Staff College

Harry L. Coles
Ohio State University

Robert H. Ferrell
Indiana University

Cyrus H. Fraker
Office of The Adjutant General

William H. Goetzmann
University of Texas

Col. Thomas E. Griess
U.S. Military Academy

Maj. Gen. Robert C. Hixon
Training and Doctrine Command

Sara D. Jackson, *National Historical Publications and Records Commission*

Maj. Gen. Enrique Mendez, Jr.
Office of The Surgeon General

James E. O'Neill, *Deputy Archivist of the United States*

Benjamin Quarles
Morgan State College

Brig. Gen. Alfred L. Sanderson
Army War College

Russell F. Weigley
Temple University

U.S. ARMY CENTER OF MILITARY HISTORY
Brig. Gen. James L. Collins, Jr., *Chief of Military History*

Maurice Matloff
Chief Historian

Col. James W. Dunn
Chief, Histories Division

Col. William F. Strobridge
Chief, Historical Services Division

Col. Earl L. Ziebell
Chief, Editorial/Cartographic Division

James E. McSherry
Editor in Chief

Contents

    Foreword   ix

    Preface   xi

1. The State of the Art   1
    Medicine 1/ Surgery 14/ Medical Education and Experience 18

2. Evolution of the Continental Army Medical Department   22
    Creation of the Hospital Department: Church as Director General 22/ Morgan as Director General, 1775 to 1777 29/ New Arrangements for the Hospital Department 35/ Shippen's Controversial Administration 38/ The Hospital Department Under Cochran 44

3. From Siege to Retreat, 1775 to May 1777   50
    The Boston Area, 1775 to 1776 50/ The Northern Department 57/ New York and New Jersey, 1776 to 1777 65/ Hospitals in New York State and New England After the Evacuation of New York City 72

4. Year of Despair and Hope, June 1777 to June 1778   77
    The Middle Department 77/ The Northern Department 92/ The Eastern Department 97

5. From Defeat to Victory, June 1778 to 1783   99
    North of the Potomac: Before the Victory at Yorktown 99/ South of the Potomac: Before the Victory at Yorktown 115/ After the Victory at Yorktown 123

6. Between Wars, 1783 to June 1812   129
    Continental Army Patients Remaining in Hospitals 133/ Campaigns Against the Indians 133/ Forts and Their Garrisons 138/ Wilkinson in the Louisiana Territory, 1809 140/ Management of Supplies 144

7. Administration of Medical Support, June 1812 to January 1815   148
    Opening Months of the War of 1812 148/ Work of the Medical Department 149

Contents

8 Early Campaigns in the North, 1812 to 1813 — 157
   Season of 1812 157/ Season of 1813 164

9 Defeat and Final Victory, 1814 to 1815 — 172
   Campaign in the North 172/ Campaign in the South 178

10 The Lessons of War, 1815 to 1818 — 186
   Indecision and Decision, March 1815 to April 1818 186/ The State of the Art 190

Appendixes

A Some Influential Doctors in the Continental Hospital Department, 1775 to 1783 — 199
B Law of 27 July 1775 — 200
C Law of 17 July 1776 — 200
D Law of 7–8 April 1777 — 201
E Law of 6 February 1778 — 204
F Law of 30 September 1780 — 205
G Hospitals Serving Washington's Army — 210
H An Act to Regulate the Medical Establishment, 2 March 1799 — 211
I Legislation Concerning the U.S. Army Medical Department — 213
J Duties of Members of the Medical Department, 1814 — 213
K Legislation Affecting the Army Medical Department, March 1815 to April 1818 — 214

Notes — 217
Bibliography — 269
Index — 289

Maps

1 Boston Area, 1775–1776 — 50
2 The Northern Department, 1775–1777 — 58
3 Continental Army Hospital Locations, 1776–1777 — 68
4 Continental Army Hospital Locations, June 1777–June 1778 — 78
5 Northern and Eastern Departments, 1777–1778 — 93
6 Hospital Locations, 1778–1783 — 100
7 Sullivan Expedition, 1779 — 107
8 The Southern Theater, 1778–1783 — 116
9 Northwest Territory, 1783–1811 — 132
10 War in the North, 1812–1814 — 158
11 Niagara Frontier, 1812–1814 — 168
12 The Southern Frontier, 1812–1814 — 179

Illustrations

Hermann Boerhaave	1
William Cullen	2
Sir John Pringle	2
Richard Brocklesby	4
Gerhard van Swieten	5
John Hunter	5
Hales's Sketches of Plans for Ventilators	9
John Jones	10
Contrast Between Vaccination and Inoculation	12
Petit's Screw Tourniquet	16
Act Creating Hospital Department	24
Benjamin Church	26
John Morgan	29
Surgeon's Field Case	30
William Shippen, Jr.	34
Benjamin Rush	36
John Cochran	44
John Warren	51
Charles McKnight	51
Return Signed by Charles McKnight	54
Return of the Sick of the Hospital at Fort George	61
James McHenry	62
Brethren's House at Bethlehem	71
William Eustis	73
Bodo Otto	80
Valley Forge Hospital Hut	85
Schoolhouse Used as Hospital at Valley Forge	86
Washington Hall	88
Brethren's House at Lititz	89
Brothers' House at Ephrata	90
James Thacher	94
Philip Turner	98
Hospital Hut Designed by Dr. James Tilton	104
Robinson's House	105
David Oliphant	117
Thomas Tudor Tucker	118
William Read	119
James McClurg	121
College of William and Mary: Wren Building	122
Richard Allison	134
Fort Washington	135
Fort Defiance	136
"Estimate of Medicine, Hospital Stores, etc. for Eighty Men [for] One Year"	145
James Tilton	152
Benjamin Waterhouse	153
William Beaumont	160
Joseph Lovell	161
Fort Niagara	166
"Soldiers Who Died at the Genl. Hospital Greenbush Together With Their Effects"	176
New Orleans in 1815	182
Three Oaks Mansion	183
Statement on Hospital Supplies Sent From New York	189

Tables

1	Authority Within the Continental Army's Medical Services, 1775–83	23
2	Hospital Department Units in the Boston Area With the Status of Patients During Week Preceding 2 December 1775	52
3	Hospital Department Units in the Boston Area With the Status of Patients During Week Preceding 16 December 1775	53
4	Mortality, 16 December 1775–30 March 1776	53
5	Patients in Hospital Department Units, New York City Area, April–June 1776	66
6	Middle Department Hospital Patients, 24 November 1777	80
7	Organization of Medical Support of the Regular Army, 1784–1813	130
8	Pay and Allowances for the Staff of the Medical Department, May 1813	150
9	Admissions and Deaths at the Burlington General Hospital, January 1814–April 1815	173

Foreword

This is the first volume of a history of the U.S. Army Medical Department from the start of the American Revolution to World War I. This book deals with the period when the Medical Department existed only as a wartime expedient and concludes with the passage in April 1818 of the law that finally established the department on a permanent basis. Future volumes will describe all aspects of the medical care of soldiers scattered in small units over the rapidly growing nation and the challenges posed by war in the nineteenth and twentieth centuries. The discipline that governed Army surgeons and their patients enabled them to control treatment and record its results with a precision and regularity impossible in civilian medicine. Thus Army surgeons and the Medical Department played a large role in the progress of medical science, a role not always recognized by the profession, by the scholarly community, or by the public at large.

This new history of the Army Medical Department tells the beginning of that story. It is a significant and long needed contribution to the study of military medicine.

JAMES L. COLLINS, JR.
Brigadier General, USA
Chief of Military History

Washington, D.C.
2 August 1979

Preface

This volume was originally planned as a Bicentennial study of the Medical Department of the Continental Army. Since existing histories of the Army Medical Department were either out of date or based upon antiquated studies, however, the project was expanded to make the present volume the first of a series on Army medicine.

Only the operations of the department are treated here. The activities of surgeons not directly under its authority, such as militia surgeons and, for a short period, regimental surgeons, have not been explored. Coverage of military operations has been limited to that necessary for understanding the demands on the department. And the author has resisted the temptation to condemn the medical men of the period for their unscientific and largely ineffective medicine; they deserve to be judged by the standards of their contemporaries.

Few official records from the period before 1814 exist. People of the era lacked our own devotion to record keeping, and much of their meager accumulation was destroyed by fire in 1800 or lost in 1814 when the British occupied Washington. Most of the documents that survived these two disasters are now held by the National Archives and Records Service in Washington, D.C. The scarcity of official records has made it particularly necessary for the author to explore such unofficial sources as the informal records, diaries, memoirs, and letters of those who were familiar with the work of the Medical Department. This search covered the National Archives, the Library of Congress, the National Library of Medicine, and the Historical Society of Pennsylvania. Many other individuals and institutions have also provided valuable assistance in the form of microfilms or copies of documents, suggestions for further contacts or sources, expert opinions concerning problems encountered as work progressed, or reviews of the manuscript in its entirety or in part.

It is impossible to thank by name all those who have in one way or another contributed to this volume. The author is particularly indebted to Mrs. Dorothy Hanks and the staff of the History of Medicine Division of the National Library of Medicine, including Ms. Lucinda Keister of the Arts Section; Dr. George Chalou and Dr. Elaine C. Everly of the Old Military Records section of the National Archives and Records Service; Mr. Peter J. Parker of the Historical Society of Pennsylvania and Mr. Gary Christopher, formerly of the Historical Society of Pennsylvania; Dr. Richard Blanco of the State University College at Brockport, N.Y.; and Dr. John Duffy of the University of Maryland, who reviewed the first five chapters of the volume. Others who provided especially valuable help were Dr. Whitfield J. Bell, Jr., of the American Philosophical Society Library in Philadelphia; Mr. Francis James Dallett, Archivist of the University of Pennsylvania; Mr. James W. Coleman, Jr., and Ms. Alberta L. Appleby of the Morristown National Historical Park; Mr. William R. Cullison, Curator of Prints and Drawings, Tulane University Library; Miss Margaret Cook of the Library of the College of William and Mary in Virginia; Mr. Vernon H. Nelson, Archivist of the Archives of the Moravian Church in Bethlehem, Pa.; Col. J. E. Henderson, VC, USA, Curator of the Medical Museum of the Armed Forces Institute of Pathology; the staff of the Graphic Arts Branch of Fort Detrick, Md.; and Miss Elizabeth Thomson, who generously shared the fruits of her research on the Doctors Bond.

The author is indebted to Col. Robert J. T. Joy, MC, USA, formerly Director of the Walter Reed Army Institute of Research and now Chairman of the Department of Military Medicine and History at the Uniformed Services University of the Health Sciences, who reviewed the entire manuscript and made many valuable suggestions, including several concerning the true nature of the diseases so unscientifically described by physicians 200 years ago. Dr. Erna Risch, formerly Chief Historian of the U.S. Army Materiel Command, also reviewed the entire manuscript; her comments have contributed significantly to its accuracy and coherence.

Members of the staff of the U.S. Army Center of Military History have also played important roles in the preparation of this volume. Dr. Robert W. Coakley, Deputy Chief Historian, reviewed the entire manuscript and made many helpful suggestions. The maps were prepared under the direction of Mr. Arthur S. Hardyman, Chief of the Cartographic Branch. The author also wishes to acknowledge the support of the successive directors of The Historical Unit of the U.S. Army Medical Department, part of which became the Medical History Branch of the Center of

Military History. The author is especially grateful to Mrs. Mary D. Nelson of the Editorial Branch, who edited the manuscript for publication; the author's historian colleagues, Ms. Pauline B. Vivette and Mr. George W. Garand, who gave freely of their time and expertise; and the late Dr. Rose C. Engelman, Chief Historian of the former Historical Unit, under whose supervision the book was written.

The responsibility for all errors remains entirely that of the author.

MARY C. GILLETT

Washington, D.C.
2 August 1979

1

The State of the Art

The colonial physicians who formed the American Army's Medical Department in 1775 were all civilian practitioners, many without any military experience. A small percentage had earned M.D. degrees, but most were either apprentice or self-trained, and few made any attempt to specialize in the manner customary in Europe, where a choice was usually made among medicine, surgery, and pharmacy. During the second half of the eighteenth century, however, American doctors were growing in stature at home and abroad. Although more of them were receiving a formal medical education, usually in Europe, they were still limited by the general lack of scientific data and by their profession's predilection for reasoning rather than research as a way of discovering better forms of treatment for their patients. The traditional humoral explanation for disease was by this time losing ground to several new and conflicting systems, where fact took second place to theory, in an all-out attempt to reveal one or two basic causes for all disease. Disagreements over therapy gave added intensity to the feuds and controversies which characterized eighteenth century practice, in general, and American medicine, which was not restrained by European guild traditions, in particular. Furthermore, the effort to develop a fundamental theory deemphasized the importance of the diagnosis of specific diseases. Treatment continued to consist largely of bleeding, purging, and blistering, regardless of the symptoms, since surgery alone was based to any significant degree upon experience as a guide in preference to theory.[1]

MEDICINE

The system prevailing in the colonies in the years immediately preceding the American Revolution, that of the great Dutch physician and teacher Hermann Boerhaave, explained disease in terms of chemical and physical qualities, such as acidity and alkalinity, or tension and relaxation, instead of the blood, phlegm, yellow bile, and black bile of the traditional humors, and urged that nature be permitted to aid in any cure. The Boerhaavian system was increasingly challenged in the second half of the century by that of William Cullen, the Scottish physician and teacher so much admired by

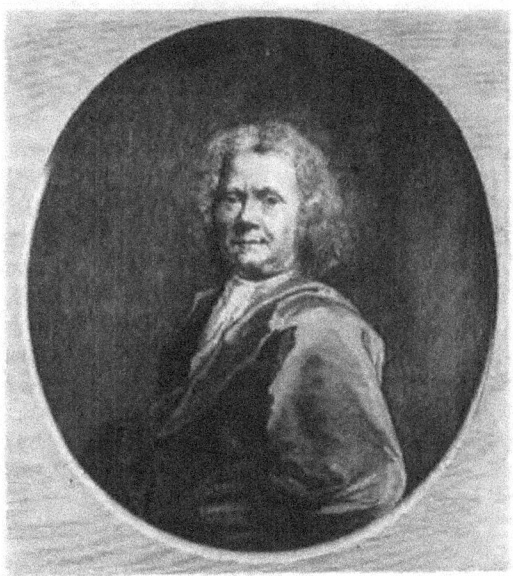

HERMANN BOERHAAVE. *(Courtesy of National Library of Medicine.)*

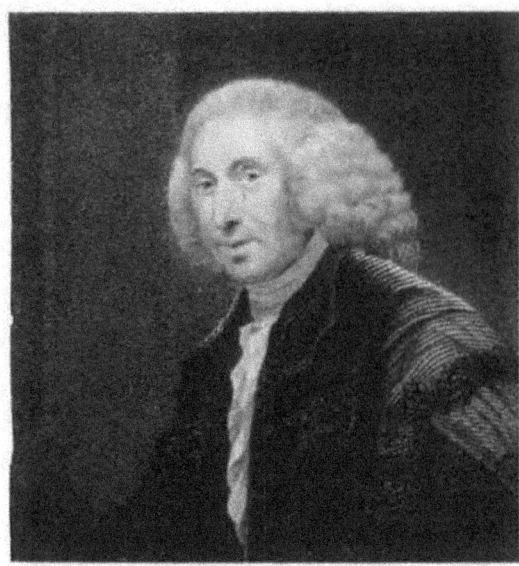

WILLIAM CULLEN. (*Courtesy of National Library of Medicine.*)

Americans studying under him at the University of Edinburgh, many of whom would later be leaders in the Continental Army's Hospital Department. Cullen believed that either an excess or an insufficiency of nervous tension underlaid all disease. Too much tension was often characterized by a fever, to be treated by a depleting regimen including bleeding, a restricted diet, purging, and rest and sedation. A cold or chill, on the other hand, indicated too much relaxation and called for restorative measures. In time, Cullen became so influential that Benjamin Rush, just gaining prominence in American medicine during the Revolution, was able to write his former teacher that the American edition of his work "was read with peculiar attention by the physicians and surgeons of our army, and in a few years regulated in many things the practice in our hospitals." [2]

Despite his doctrine that disordered nervous tension was the cause of all disease, Cullen encouraged the study and classification of specific diseases. Rush, however, eventually modified Cullen's doctrines, which he had originally so much admired, and discouraged the study of separate disease entities by blaming all disease on excessive tension which caused disturbance in the blood vessels. By 1793, he was openly contending that there was but one single disease in existence. The method of treatment upon which Rush insisted with increasing inflexibility called for a low diet, vigorous purges with calomel and jalap, and bleeding until the patient fainted. Rush apparently did not hesitate to remove a quart of blood at a time, or, should unfavorable symptoms continue, to repeat such a bleeding two or three times within a two- to three-day period, it being permissible in his opinion to drain as much as four-fifths of the body's total blood supply. In time, Rush's system and treatment became, in the words of a noted medical historian and physician, "the most popular and also the most dangerous 'system' in America." [3]

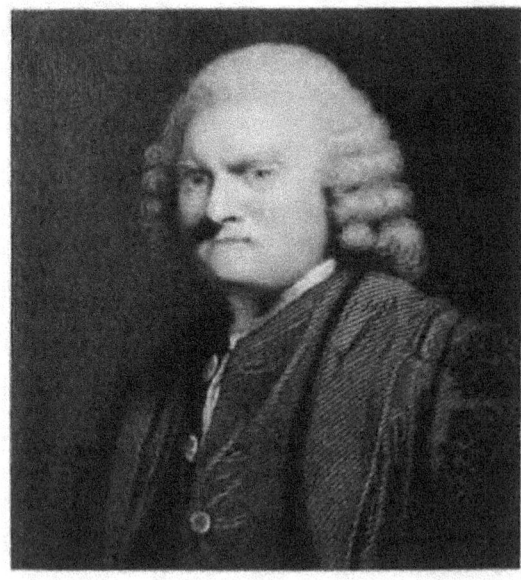

SIR JOHN PRINGLE. (*Courtesy of Library of Congress.*)

Theorists of the eighteenth century did not generally include in their systems an explanation for the outbreak of certain forms of disease among many people in one area within a short period of time. According to his background, training, and experience, therefore, a physician might blame mass outbreaks of disease on climate and season, unhealthy elements in the air, contagion, possibly caused by "animalcules," or God's determination to punish sinful man. There were many discussions of possible sources of disease carried by the air. Rush strongly believed in the danger of bad odors, or miasmas, and Sir John Pringle, a noted British Army surgeon and a Physician General in the British Army from 1745 to 1758, much respected by the many Americans who knew him in their student days, wrote that putrefaction was the greatest cause of fatal illness in armies. He listed corrupted marsh water, human excrement remaining exposed in the hot weather, crowded military hospitals, and straw used for bedding rotting in tents as the four principal sources for putrid air. Although he recognized cold as a predisposing factor in disease, Pringle noted that heat, too, was often a cause of sickness, especially when wet clothes and beds or a very humid atmosphere tended to interfere with normal perspiration, "relaxing the fibers and disposing . . . to putrefaction." He found it "not surprizing [sic] that the dysentery and bilious fever, both putrid diseases, should ensue." The theory of the atmosphere as a cause of many types of fevers was still maintained as late as 1812. David Hosack, a respected American physician, pointed out at that time, however, that disease might also be spread by direct physical contact, as in syphilis and scabies, or through the purest air, as with smallpox. Many authorities at that time also blamed sudden changes in the weather for causing outbreaks of disease.[4]

The average eighteenth century physician had little in the way of either equipment or understanding to aid him in distinguishing one specific disease from another. The concept of a standard body temperature had only been suggested, the body's heat-regulating mechanism was not understood, and Fahrenheit's recently developed mercury thermometer was not commonly used by physicians. The stethoscope was not invented until 1814, and although a "pulse watch" had been developed in 1707, it also was largely ignored by physicians, who preferred describing the pulse to counting it. The use of percussion to aid in diagnosis, however, was beginning to become more widely understood because of the work of the Viennese physician Leopold Auenbrugger. The reasoning underlying some eighteenth century diagnoses, however, may seem strange to us today. When a fever described as yellow fever responded to quinine, for example, rather than concluding that the fever was in reality malaria, the eighteenth century physician assumed that quinine must be effective against yellow fever. Since all fevers were regarded as stemming from the same physical unbalance, such a conclusion was logical. Rashes were not regarded as particularly significant in diagnosis, and differing symptoms appearing in patients believed to have the same disease might be brushed off as indicative merely of the conditions under which the illness was contracted.[5]

In the eighteenth century and, as far as the U.S. Army was concerned, until World War I, disease invariably caused more deaths than wounds. It has been estimated that, during the American Revolution, 90 percent of the deaths occurring among the inexperienced, poorly clothed, poorly fed soldiers of the Continental Army, most of them country boys without previous exposure to communicable diseases, and 84 percent of those among the seasoned, disciplined British regulars were from disease. Under the circumstances, however, it is difficult today to determine from the diagnoses and descriptions of eighteenth century physicians what specific diseases were most common in the army of that period. Respiratory illnesses were most often seen in cold weather and dysenterylike conditions in hot weather, while fevers were always a threat. Venereal disease was common, and smallpox could wreak havoc in the ranks of American armies. Scurvy was a danger on land as on sea, and scabies, otherwise known as the Itch, was a more than ordinary nuisance for military forces. Other diseases, such as diphtheria and scarlet fever, were less common in eighteenth century armies despite their occasionally devastating effects upon the civilian population.[6]

Whatever the eighteenth century diagnoses were, eighteenth century fevers were often in fact malaria, widespread in the colonies and endemic from New England southward. Yellow fever, despite its fearful reputation, was endemic only in the deep South, although rare outbreaks occurred during the summer in a few ports north of Charleston, South Carolina. The incidence of malaria was rising during the Revolution, especially in the South with its long hot summers and undrained swamps, affecting with particular severity, for example, not only Cornwallis's men but also New Englanders participating in the fighting around Yorktown. Although mosquitoes were rarely suspected as carriers of disease, eighteenth century physicians were aware of the relationship of fevers to swamps and undrained areas.[7]

While "intermittent" and "remittent" fevers were probably malaria, those called putrid, malignant, jail, or hospital may have been either typhus or typhoid. Authorities do not agree on the extent to which late eighteenth century physicians could differentiate between these two diseases.[8]

An examination of the writings of the period shows, however, that when British military physician and author Richard Brocklesby made his diagnoses, he did not

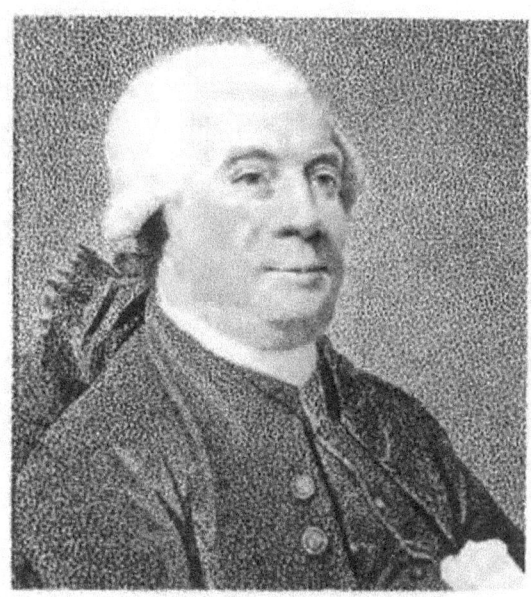

RICHARD BROCKLESBY. *(Courtesy of National Library of Medicine.)*

take into consideration the petechiae which modern physicians believe to be the key to a definite differentiation between the two diseases in the absence of laboratory tests. British surgeon Donald Monro, furthermore, believed that the symptoms manifested by a malignant fever depended upon the conditions prevailing at the time the disease was contracted, and the prominent Austrian military surgeon Gerhard van Swieten considered the appearance of a rash to be an indication of a favorable outcome rather than one of the nature of the disease. A modern authority on the epidemic diseases of pre-Revolutionary America also points out that "Not only was typhus rarely found in the colonial period but even after the Revolution the United States remained relatively free of the infection." He ranks typhus in importance after malaria, dysentery, and typhoid.[9]

Eighteenth century soldiers "often exposed to the putrid Steams of dead Horses, of the Privies, and of other corrupted

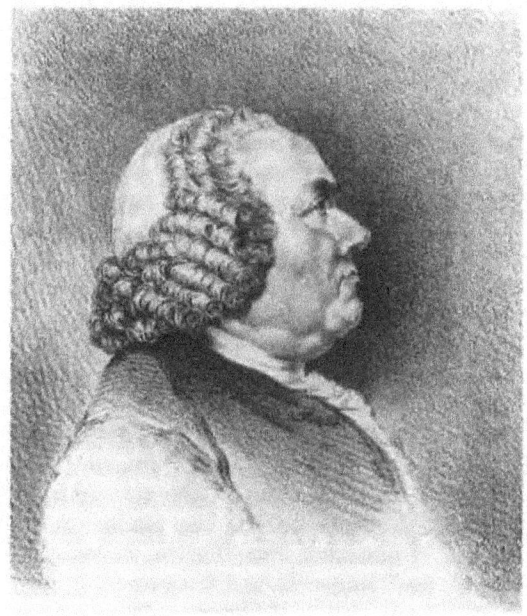

GERHARD VAN SWIETEN. *(Courtesy of National Library of Medicine.)*

very generous doses of purgatives and emetics required by eighteenth century doctrine, or to the blister which would adorn his abdomen should the physician determine that this portion of his anatomy was too tense. It was only after he had survived these remedies that the patient could hope for a dose of opium, which might at least temporarily relieve his agony even if his disease had been misdiagnosed, a distinct possibility, and was actually typhoid or typhus.[13]

Venereal disease was another ever-present threat to the eighteenth century army but one not always reported because of the punishment often administered to its victims. Some modern historians believe that eighteenth century physicians could distinguish between gonorrhea and syphilis, but examination of a number of publications of the time suggests that the distinction was partial at best. The British John Hunter, one of the century's finest surgeons and anatomists, stated that the two were but "different forms of the same disease," gonorrhea

Animal or Vegetable substances, after their juices had been highly exalted by the Heat of Summer"[10] sometimes found themselves afflicted with "A flux of the belly, attended with violent gripings, of very painful strainings for stool."[11] This was blamed on "obstructed Perspiration,"[12] or on "bile grown acrid by the great heats and the fatigue of war" when "the soldier, when hot, suddenly exposes himself to cold air, or sleeps in his cloaths [sic], soaked with rain" as well as on stagnant water and tainted food. Van Swieten, whose work was influential in America, believed that dysentery could be spread through an entire army by the breath of those afflicted with the disease and that ordinary diarrhea could degenerate into dysentery if not promptly treated with a mild purge followed by a dose of opium. In the eighteenth century, however, even dysentery itself often remained untreated. The soldier unlucky enough to be so afflicted might, indeed, prefer neglect to the

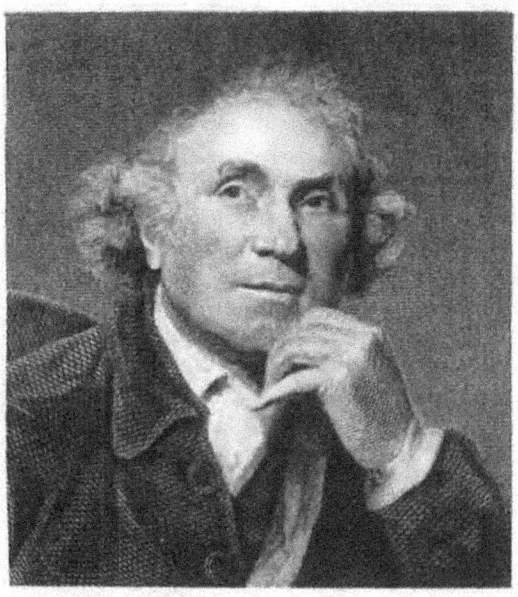

JOHN HUNTER. *(Courtesy of National Library of Medicine.)*

being the form in which the urethra alone was affected and chancre a nonsecreting version of the same disease. Hunter could state this confidently even while he noted with surprise that mercury, which cured chancre, only made gonorrhea worse.[14] Brocklesby, too, considered gonorrhea but one symptom of "lues venera," as did van Swieten and at least one physician as late as 1815.[15]

Although it may not have been fatal, scabies brought more patients to British Army hospitals during the Seven Years' War than any other condition, according to British Army surgeon Donald Monro. Its cause was known to be "Little Insects Lodged in the Skin, which Many Authors Affirm They Have Seen in the Pustules by the Help of a Microscope."[16] The Itch was very common in colonial America, Benjamin Franklin's mother-in-law having advertised a remedy for it in 1731. The condition usually appeared first between the fingers in the form of a "pustule, or two, full of a sort of clear water, which itch extremely: where these pustules are broke by scratching, the water that issues out communicates the disorder to the neighboring parts . . . in its progress the pustules augment both in number and size, and when opened by scratching a disgusting crust is formed." The favorite remedy for the Itch seems to have been sulfur, a remedy still in use today, applied in either an ointment or a soft soap.[17]

Among the respiratory ailments often afflicting armies in the eighteenth century were pneumonia, often called peripneumonia, and pleurisy. Van Swieten suggested treating the former, as soon as diagnosed, by a "large bleeding in the arm" but also urged that the air be kept moist and the patient encouraged to bring up the secretions from his lungs. If the progress of the disease weakened the patient, however, this authority recommended that bleeding, purging, and sweating be avoided. The soldier unfortunate enough to be afflicted with so severe a pleurisy that the pain interfered with his breathing would be treated not only to bleeding but also to blistering, clystering, and, to encourage the pus to drain outward and thus avoid the formation of an abscess, plastering. If the patient could not sleep, he might be dosed with a syrup of white poppies. To soothe his cough, his medicine would be administered while lukewarm, and wine, salt, and acid foods would be denied him.[18]

Specific types of therapy for specific diseases were understandably not too common in the eighteenth century and certain remedies were used for almost all diseased conditions. Bleeding was popular, the amount and frequency varying with the individual physician and the system he followed. A moderate bleeding was considered to be one taking 8 to 12 ounces at a time, a heavy one 16 to 20 ounces. Cleansing the digestive tract was another generalized remedy followed with or without much caution, using such purgatives as rhubarb, manna with tincture of senna, or Rush's favorites, jalap and calomel, emetics such as ipecac and antimony, and enemas of varying formulation.[19]

The following order for medicines and hospital stores for Fort Meigs placed by Brig. Gen. William Henry Harrison during the War of 1812 suggests that the same kinds of medicines remained popular for many decades:

Peruvian bark (in powder)	50 lb.
Opium	10 lb.
Camphor	10 lb.
Calomel	5 lb.
Corrosive sublimate	2 lb.
Tartar emetic	2 lb.
Gambage	2 lb.
Jalap	10 lb.
Ipecuanto	17 lb.
Rhubarb (in powder)	10 lb.
Kino	15 lb.
Colombo (in powder)	20 lb.
Nitre crude	20 lb.
Nitre sweet spirits	40 lb.

Glaubers salts	50 lb.
Prepared chalk	20 lb.
Castor oil	12 gal.
Olive oil	5 gal.
Gum arabic	20 lb.
Allume	5 lb.
Acquous	20 lb.
Adhesive plaster	20 lb.
Barley	2 bbl.
Chocolate	300 lb.
Tapioca	50 lb.
Blistering ointment	20 lb.
Beeswax	20 lb.
Muriated acid	4 lb.
Sulphuric acid	4 lb.
Nitric acid	4 lb.
Vials	5 gross
Instruments	
Amputation	3 sets
Trepanning	3 sets
Pocket	3 sets
Cases scalpels (No. 6)	....
Lancets	3 doz.
Splints	12 sets
Sponge	7 lb.
Muslin	1,000 yd.
Wine	200 gal.
Brandy or rum	100 gal.
Vinegar	200 gal.
Molasses	200 gal.
Coffee	300 lb.
Hyson tea	50 lb.
Rice	5 bbl.
Sugar	5 bbl.
Sago	50 lb.

SOURCE: William Henry Harrison to Secretary of War, 30 Jun 1813, Harrison, *Messages*, 2: 486.

Among the newer ideas in medicine was the belief in the general wholesomeness of fresh air. Benjamin Franklin was among its most ardent supporters. Allied with this was the newly popular "cooling regimen in fevers," involving not only cool fresh air but also the bathing of fever patients in cold water. Yet another generalized remedy of recent origin was mercury, used earlier against venereal disease and as a purgative, but now also used as an alterative to treat many diseases, often in the form of calomel or the reputedly better tasting but more nauseating corrosive sublimate. Its new popularity was, an American physician boasted, "in its origin exclusively American, and ... to our colonial physicians the world is indebted for one of the greatest improvements ever made in practical medicine." Mercury was increasingly prescribed after 1750 for diseases classified as inflammatory, particularly pleurisy, pneumonia, and rheumatism, but it was also eventually used for typhus, yellow fever, dysentery, smallpox, tuberculosis, dropsy, hydrocephalus, and diseases of the liver, with Rush in the forefront of its many enthusiasts.[20] Another noted American physician of the period, David Ramsay, explained the working of mercury by claiming that it set up an artificial illness, "transferring diseases of the head, of the eyes, and of the bowels to the mouth, where they are less dangerous and more manageable,"[21] in line with the principle put forward by John Hunter that "no two fevers can exist in the same constitution, nor two local diseases in the same part at the same time."[22] Others accounted for the action of mercury by its weight, saying that mercury compounds expelled "morbid matter" from the digestive system and cleared out the glands, particularly the salivaries, and the blood vessels, promoting better circulation and eliminating disease.[23]

It is not likely that there were any physicians at that time unaware of the unpleasant side effects of mercury, since even laymen could recognize them and physicians were at times forced to order smaller than usual doses lest the patient realize what he was receiving and refuse to take it. Diarrhea, bleeding gums, nosebleeds, and loosening of the teeth were among the consequences the American physician John Warren described as "frequently troublesome and at times alarming."[24]

A far more pleasant eighteenth century remedy was wine, the use of which was most prevalent from 1700 to 1900. It was used as a stimulant to the appetite, a sedative, a diuretic, and merely as a nutritious addition to the diet. Particular wines might be prescribed to relieve specific symptoms, with or without the addition of spices, fruit juices, and grated rinds. An astringent red wine was recommended for diarrhea, port for anemia and acute fevers, claret and burgundy for anorexia, and champagne for nausea and throat ailments. White wines were thought to make fine diuretics, while fortified wines in general were prescribed for convalescents.[25]

Opium, often in the form of laudanum, came to be used frequently in the late eighteenth century, to the point where it was "generally found in most decent families for domestic prescription." Samuel Bard, a noted colonial physician, had studied the effects of opium on the human body and recorded that it acted on the nervous system rather than the blood, slowed bowel action, suppressed urine, lessened pain and spasms, and brought sleep.[26]

Quite aside from the state of the art of diagnosis and treatment, the hospital in which he found himself played an important role in the fate of the sick or wounded soldier and, indeed, in the long run, in the fate of the army itself. The wars of the eighteenth century and particularly the Seven Years' War between France and Britain, therefore, inspired much writing by experienced army surgeons of both nations on the military hospital and its management. Considerable emphasis was placed upon the need for planning ahead for the number and types of hospitals required. The Frenchman Hugues Ravaton, considering this problem in 1768, wrote that one could assume that three of every 100 soldiers would be ill at the beginning of a European campaign. Halfway through the campaign, a probable five or six of 100 would be out of combat because of disease, and by the end of a campaign, if the victims of venereal disease and nonbattle injuries were counted, ten to twelve of 100 would be unable to fight because of illness. A day's battle would produce, he estimated, ten wounded per 100 combatants, but this percentage would drop as the number involved approached 100,000.[27]

Armed with this type of information, an army medical department could predict the number of general and regimental hospitals needed for the predictable number of patients. The general hospital remained in one place and was staffed by the physicians and surgeons of the medical department, as was the flying hospital in the British Army, which accompanied an army as it moved about. The regimental hospital was directed by the regiment's surgeon and mates, and its patients could be sent back to the general hospital, as were those of the flying hospital when it had to move. Considerable controversy raged at times between the proponents of the general hospital and those of the small regimental one. The infection and bad air of the general hospital caused many authorities to favor the smaller facility or at least to urge that the general hospital be divided among several locations. Locating hospitals so that the sick or wounded soldier would have to be moved for any great distance was also considered inadvisable.[28]

In the management of the individual hospital, eighteenth century military experts emphasized the necessity for good order, good air, and careful sanitation, as well as for the proper staff, which should include physicians, surgeons, mates who functioned as assistants to either physicians or surgeons, apothecaries, nurses, and a purveyor to handle supplies. Although the principle was not always observed in the British Army, Monro in particular emphasized that the direction and the purveying for a hospital should never be assigned to the same man, "as the Temptation of Accumulating Wealth has at all Times, and in all Services, Given Rise to the Grossest Abuses," a truth of

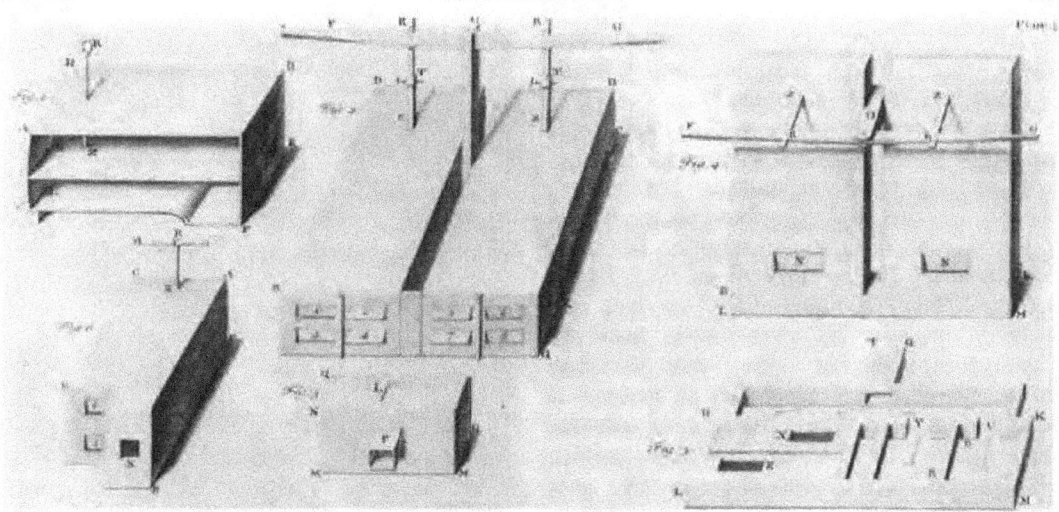

HALES'S SKETCHES OF PLANS FOR VENTILATORS. *(Courtesy of National Library of Medicine.)*

which the organizers of the Continental Army's first medical department should have been more conscious. Also required was a guard to keep order and to see that patients obeyed the orders of the physicians, particularly in regard to such matters as drinking and receiving visitors. An inspector general should be assigned to visit each hospital at least once a week to ensure proper care and discipline.[29]

Good air supply could be achieved by using large rooms with high ceilings, by avoiding overcrowding, and even by using the newly developed, manually operated Hales ventilators, by means of which "foul air may be removed from hospitals," by burning frankincense, juniper wood and berries, or sulfur, or by using the steam from vinegar. Good sanitation also required proper care of privies, frequent scrubbing of walls, floors, and bed frames, and thorough airing or even impregnating woolen clothing and blankets with the fumes of muriatic or nitric acid or of burning sulfur. Straw rather than feathers was preferred for filling mattresses because of the difficulty of cleaning feather beds.[30]

Contagion could also be prevented by putting surgical and venereal disease patients into a separate room or even a separate hospital, away from those ill with fevers and dysentery, who should have their own well-aired wards and, hopefully, their own nearby privies. As much as possible, those with similar diseases should be kept together. Each patient should, in any case, be bathed and dressed in clean clothing before being admitted to a ward, and his hands and face washed routinely every morning. The physician visiting patients should wear clothing especially set aside for the purpose plus a "waxed linen coat to wear above them in going round to wards" and should never visit a hospital with an empty stomach if he wished to avoid becoming ill himself. When visiting patients with infectious diseases, furthermore, the physician should take tincture of bark before entering the room, put rolls of lint impregnated with camphorated spirits in his nose, place a bowl of camphorated vinegar near the patient he was visiting, and hold his breath while physically examining the patient, standing back from the bed when it was necessary to ask a question. Peter Middleton, another prominent American physician, suggested that the doctor in such instances might even hold tobacco in his mouth to guarantee that he did not swallow saliva which might have become infected while he was in the sickroom.[31]

Preventive medicine played an extremely important role not only within the military hospital but also throughout the entire eighteenth century army. Increasing attention was now also being paid to the idea of being sure that the soldier was reasonably healthy before he entered the service, especially since it was recognized that the stress of entering the army made the new recruit particularly susceptible to disease. It had long been realized that, since disease was caused by "changes in the sensible qualities of the air, excesses in dirt, and irregularities in exercise," effective prevention of disease also required the close regulating of the soldier's everyday life and environment once he had officially joined the army. The choice of a campsite was of the greatest importance, with damp areas being particularly undesirable. Thick forests were also to be avoided because of the restricted circulation of air there. Where the army was living in tents, the straw used for bedding must be quickly changed should it become damp, while officers should spread waxed cloth on the damp ground under their beds to keep out the moisture. When it was raining, the tents should be tightly drawn to lessen water penetration and drainage ditches should be made around them. Campsites and barracks should, of course, be kept clean and free of accumulated garbage. Privies should be built near the camp, preferably over running streams. Even after exercising all these precautions, however, the army should avoid camping too long in one place, especially "when bloody flux prevails."[32]

Concern about the soldier and the weather extended to the soldier's clothing. Since sudden temperature changes, as occurred when the soldier left a warm hut to go outside in the winter, were considered particularly dangerous, it was considered wiser in cold

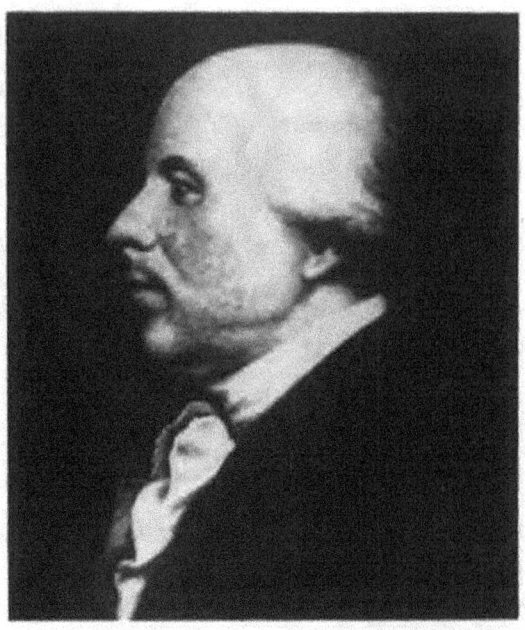

JOHN JONES. *(From Steven T. Charles, "John Jones, American Surgeon and Conservative Patriot,"* Bulletin of the History of Medicine *39 (1965): 437. Courtesy of Johns Hopkins University Press.)*

weather to keep the men warm with extra garments and blankets than with the creation of great heat by stoves or fires. Flannel rather than linen, some authorities said, should be worn next to the skin, especially, of course, in the winter. At least one American authority strongly favored wearing flannel underclothing even in the summer, since it would prevent chilling if the temperature were to drop markedly during the night. John Jones, one of America's foremost army surgeons, however, believed that lighter clothing should be worn in hot weather and that linen, washable and cheaper to buy, was preferable to flannel.[33]

Concern went beyond the soldier's camp and clothing to his personal hygiene. It should be required that "no soldier be permitted to ease himself anywhere about the camp except in the privies." He should bathe frequently, in the running water of a warm stream when possible, and wash his clothes as often as he could. He should keep his hair short or at least greased and combed daily to avoid the buildup of dirt and perspiration on his head.[34] Pringle believed that even the amount of sleep the soldier received should be regulated, since "when soldiers are off duty, they sleep too much, which enervates the body, and renders it more subject to diseases." Adequate exercise was also most important.[35]

Close supervision of what the soldier ate and drank was necessary. Ideally he should drink only from the center of a moving stream or from wells giving pure water. When this was impossible, impure water should be mixed with vinegar or with chalk or alum and then filtered. By the early 1800's, the presence of "animalcules" in swamp water was recognized and boiling as well as straining of questionable water was urged. For hot weather use, Jones suggested adding vinegar, highly regarded by many for its supposed ability to preserve the health in the summer. This mixture would "serve to correct in some measure, the natural tendency of the humans to corruption, at that season." The drinking of beverages stronger than water, however, caused considerable discussion. Monro recommended diluted spirits for soldiers scheduled for night duty in cold weather, and Jones agreed that something stronger than water or "small beer" was necessary for men long exposed to the cold and damp. The American Army surgeon Edward Cutbush, however, warned against giving out undiluted spirits to soldiers and suggested that beer be substituted for stronger liquors.[36]

Defective diet was not classified as among the most important causes of illness. Many believed that, by having to contribute his food allowance to a mess and thus being unable to squander it on liquor, the soldier was guaranteed an adequate diet. Some concern was shown, however, that too much meat was being eaten in proportion to fruits and vegetables in the diet. Sugar was recommended as a method of making vegetables taste better, so as to lower the consumption of meat. Others speculated as to whether fresh fruit caused dysentery, Pringle believing it did not. Because of the concern for the possibly harmful effect of meat, the proportion of it given to hospital patients was restricted for those on "low" and "middle" diets. By the early years of the nineteenth century, concern was also being shown by Americans for the health of the meat animals the Army used for its messhalls.[37]

The only important deficiency disease generally recognized at this time was scurvy. By mid-century, James Lind had conducted experiments which showed to his satisfaction that oranges, lemons, and limes cured even the severest scurvy. By the time of the American Revolution, van Swieten had recognized that the eating of plenty of ripe fruits and vegetables could prevent this condition, but he and a surprising number of authorities, including even Lind himself, continued to assume that additional factors were also involved. Lind noted the importance of "warm, dry, pure air, with a diet of easy digestion, consisting chiefly of a due mixture of animal and vegetable substances," adding that "a glass of good sound beer, cyder, wine, or the like fermented liquor" would be advisable.[38] Van Swieten, as late as 1776, blamed scurvy on "Noisome vapours, arising from marshy grounds, and stagnating waters, inaction, drinking of corrupted and stagnating waters, . . . damp and low lodging" as well as "scarcity of green vegetables, . . . the use of salted and smoaked [sic] flesh and fish, and of cheese too old and acrid." A number of others writing in the period immediately preceding the Revolution expressed themselves along similar lines.[39] Nevertheless, Lind urged that the army plant "antiscorbutic plants" where it was garrisoned, suggesting, among others,

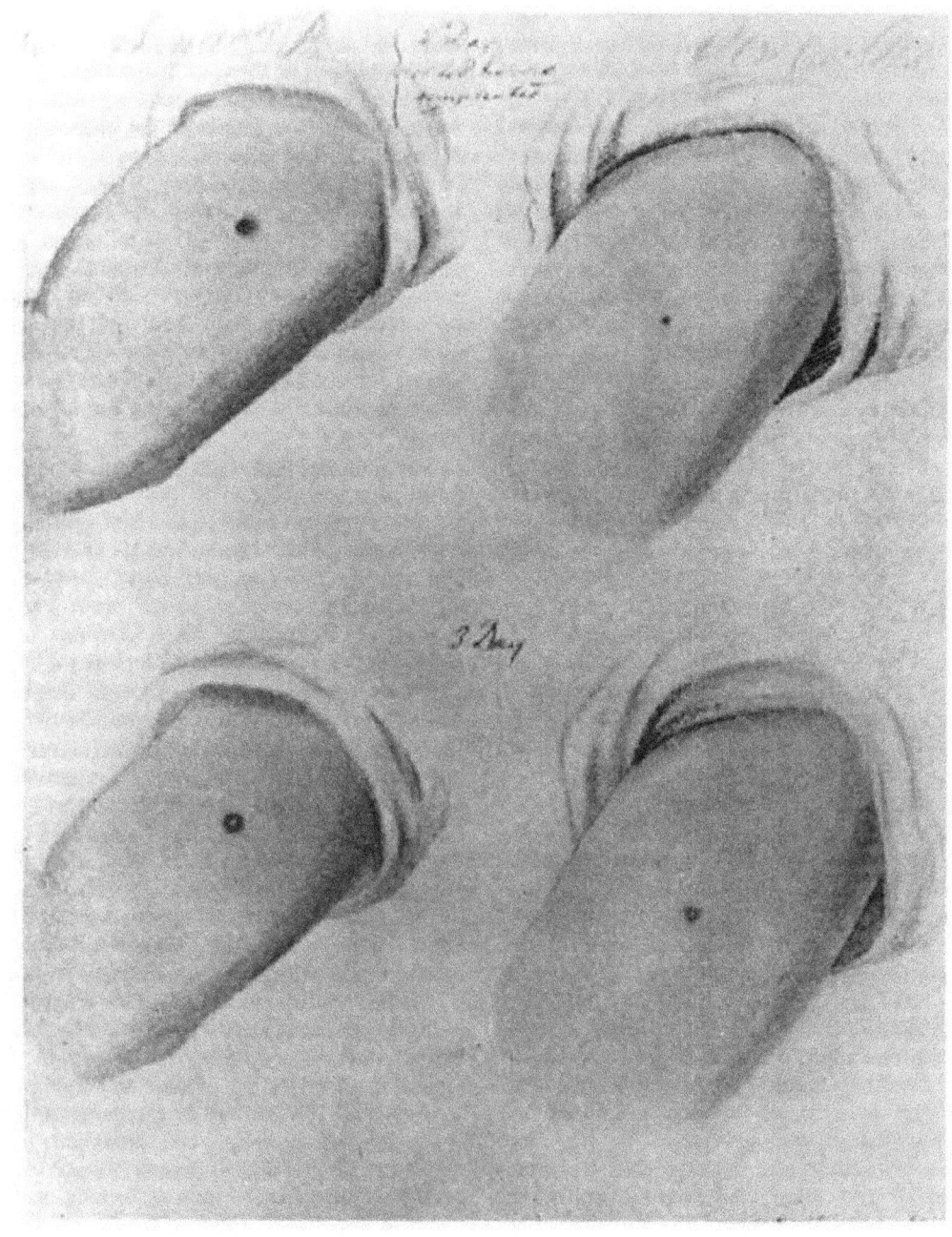

CONTRAST BETWEEN VACCINATION AND INOCULATION. *Left, inoculation; right, vaccination. Second and third days. (From Cecil Kent Drinker,* Not So Long Ago *(New York: Oxford University Press, 1937.)*

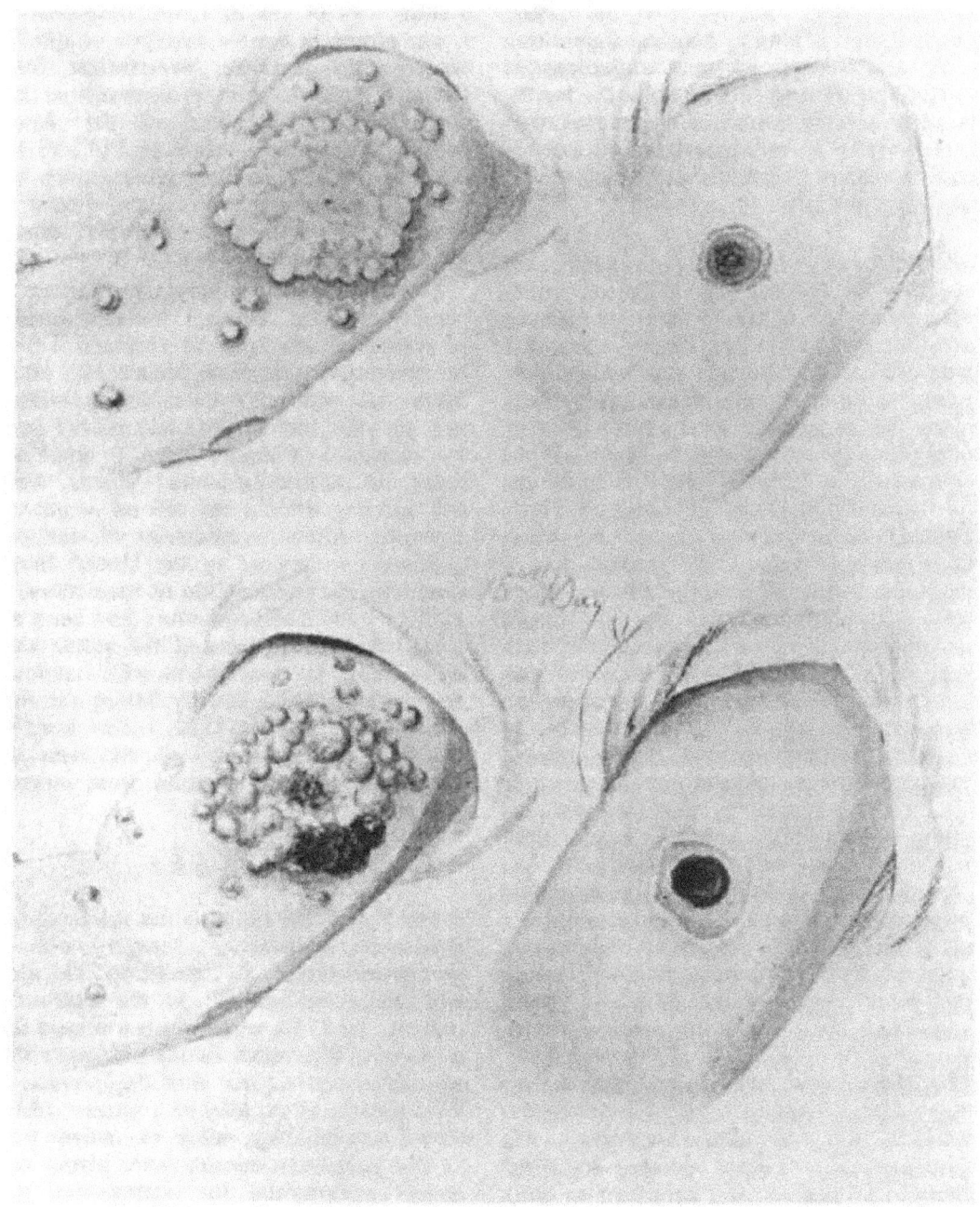

CONTRAST BETWEEN VACCINATION AND INOCULATION. *Left, inoculation; right, vaccination. Fourteenth and fifteenth days. (From Cecil Kent Drinker,* Not So Long Ago *(New York: Oxford University Press, 1937.)*

"garden cresses," and in 1776, the Continental Congress told its Medical Committee to be sure to have sufficient antiscorbutics on hand for the army operating in the North. In 1808, an army physician commented that if fresh fruits were impractical, an essence could be made of oranges and lemons to be used as a preventive for scurvy.[40]

The only disease for which prevention in the form of immunization was available was smallpox. Inoculation, the deliberate introduction into the body of material infected with the smallpox virus, thereby causing a mild case of that disease, was widely used during wartime by the British Army even before the American Revolution, after its initial introduction in both England and the colonies in the 1720's. The procedure ran into much opposition, especially in New England, in part because the person inoculated became a source of infection for all those with whom he came in contact. Many areas, particularly in New England, hoped to avoid smallpox merely because of their isolation, yet the ultimate result of this attitude was the appearance in the American Revolutionary Army of a large number of men who were not immune to the disease. The method of inoculation most commonly used in the colonies at this time was the Sutton or Dimsdale method, named after the Englishmen who developed it. As adopted in the colonies, this method required a two-week preparation period before inoculation, during which the patient was put on a diet of light and nonstimulating foods, dosed with mercury and antimony, bled, and purged. The inoculation itself was done by means of puncture rather than incision, as had been customary earlier, and on the leg, so that it would be as far as possible from the head and other vital areas. The patients were put on a "cooling regimen," exposed to cool air, and permitted to drink cool water while suffering from the disease which, acquired in this manner, was reputed to have become "an innocent disease" with a death rate of one in 1,000, compared to a rate of one in ten for smallpox caught by unintentional exposure. Nevertheless, John Cochran, soon to gain prominence as the fourth Director General of the Army Medical Department, wrote in 1772 of his concern that the mercury given during the smallpox inoculation process could lead to other diseases once the patient had recovered from the smallpox itself.[41]

It was not until the very early nineteenth century that Dr. Edward Jenner's method of preventing smallpox by vaccination with the cowpox virus became popular. By 1800, Jenner had vaccinated about 6,000 patients, and by 1804, his method had proved itself by causing a dramatic drop in smallpox deaths in both London and Vienna, without bringing with it the risk of a general epidemic. Although epidemics of smallpox continued to appear in the United States even after the introduction of vaccination in 1800, by 1812 the procedure had been accepted throughout most of the nation as a replacement for inoculation with smallpox, and in May 1812, shortly before the outbreak of the War of 1812, orders were issued to Army surgeons to vaccinate the entire Army using material from cowpox vesicles.[42]

SURGERY

While "Medicine ran into the cul de sac of therapeutic nihilism . . . , surgery, with all its imperfections . . . , could and did cure with some confidence" in the eighteenth century. By 1750, surgery was a respectable profession. The work of John Hunter, who was described as the first Englishman to raise surgery to the level of a science, added to its respectability, while the many wars of the eighteenth century were giving surgeons opportunities for observations and study which they otherwise would never have had. American John Jones urged that surgeons acquire as much learning and training as possible [43] and took particular exception to the idea he had heard suggested that surgeons should operate only under the direction of physicians, becoming merely "surgical machines ... under the direction of their medical masters." Jones also preferred that medicine and surgery be combined, as it was to such a great extent in the colonies.[44]

A surprising variety of surgical procedures was occasionally performed by a few eighteenth century surgeons, but such procedures as lithotomy, or cutting for bladder stones, setting of fractures, reduction of dislocations, and amputations were very common. The skill with which Jones was able to perform lithotomies when he returned from his training abroad removed from this operation the bad name it had acquired in the colonies. Jones was reported to be able to perform a lithotomy in three minutes and at times in one and a half, using a lateral perineal approach. Other surgeons of the time wrote of dealing successfully with torn tendons, hydrocele, various types of hernias, and fistula lachrymalis, or abnormal openings in the tear duct. In France, Louis XIV's successful surgery in 1686 for anal fistula had inspired confidence both in French surgeons and in this operation, while the British surgeon William Cheselden had attracted attention with, among other accomplishments, his successful operations for cataract.[45]

Isolated reports of successful gynecological and obstetrical surgery began to appear in this period, proof that abdominal surgery was not always undertaken in vain. American John Bard reported in 1760 on surgery performed ten years earlier in which the patient survived when he removed a dead fetus resulting from an abdominal pregnancy. In the following years there were other scattered reports in the colonies of successful surgery performed for ectopic pregnancies, and in 1809, the Edinburgh-trained American physician Ephraim McDowell performed his famed ovariotomy. By the time of the American Revolution, Jones could write of the proper handling of penetrating wounds of the abdomen with enough confidence and in sufficient detail to make it obvious that he believed survival from such wounds to be possible. He described the type of suture he used for wounds in the intestine and discussed the removal of sutures when the injury had healed, as if the patient's survival to this point were not a total surprise. Among other achievements in eighteenth century surgery was the work of William and John Hunter, with whom a number of the Continental Army's surgeons studied, in developing a new surgical technique for handling aneurysms, one soon followed by others. There were also rumors in the 1760's of a splenectomy so well executed that the soldier-patient was able to return to duty. A successful appendectomy was performed in 1759, although apparently little notice was taken of it. Furthermore, before the end of the century, the indomitable John Hunter was experimenting with organ transplants in chickens, moving the testicles and spurs of cocks from one bird to another. He also noted that "Teeth, after having been drawn and inserted into the sockets of another person, united to the new socket which is called transplanting." [46]

Regardless of the nature of the injury, the medical care the surgical patient was likely to receive ran along familiar lines: "moderate evacuation, by bleeding, and gentle purging, together with a low diet." [47] In addition, "when the wounded person has not suffered any great loss of blood, it will be advisable to open a vein immediately and take from the arm a very large quantity, and to repeat bleeding, as circumstances require, the second, and even the third day." To be considered in the making of decisions on bleeding the surgical patient, Hunter believed, was the violence of the inflammation, the power of the patient's body to make

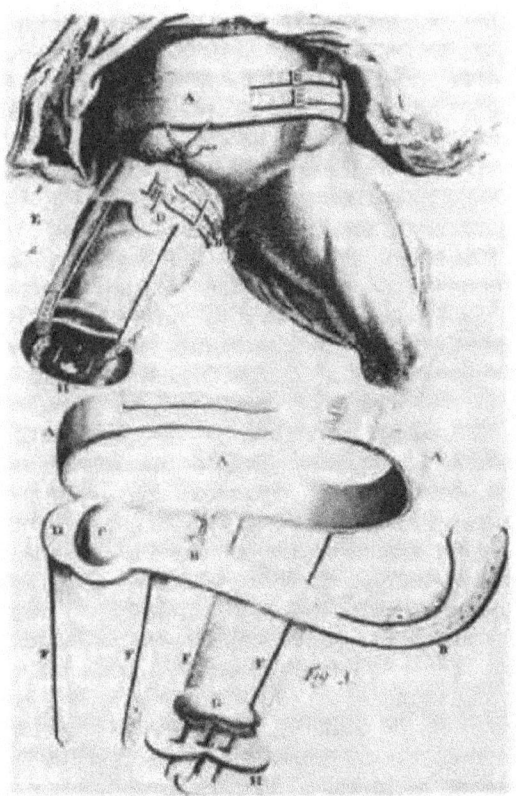

PETIT'S SCREW TOURNIQUET. *(From Owen H. Wangensteen, Jacqueline Smith, and Sarah D. Wangensteen, "Some Highlights in the History of Amputation Reflecting Lessons in Wound Healing," Bulletin of the History of Medicine 41 (1967): 115. Courtesy of Johns Hopkins University Press.)*

blood, the distance of the injury from the sources of circulation, the nature of the part injured, and the duration of the inflammation.[48]

Among the potions most highly regarded by military surgeons were opium and bark, usually peruvian or cinchona bark, the source of quinine, praised in almost identical terms by both Jones and British Army surgeon John Ranby, who extolled "the sovereign and almost divine power of opium; next to this I likewise add bark, a medium which no human eloquence can extol with panegyric proportioned to its inestimable victories." Of bark he added, "I have known it to procure rest, if given in large doses, when even opium had been taken without any manner of effect."[49] Van Swieten regarded the bark as the best available remedy against gangrene, and John Jones maintained that it contracted the blood vessels, "restoring their due action upon the blood, when too great a quantity of that necessary fluid is lost by profuse haemorrhage, provided the larger wounded vessels are secured by a proper ligature from future bleeding." On the other hand, "where there is a great fulness, or too much strength and contractile powers in the solids, and an inflammatory state of the system . . . the bark is not advisable."[50]

Excess bleeding from a wound was one of a number of problems with which eighteenth century surgeons wrestled. Although crude tourniquets were used as early as the sixteenth century to arrest hemorrhage before and during surgery, a new type of tourniquet, developed by French surgeon Jean Louis Petit in 1718 and tightened by means of a screw, was now being employed. The importance of proper ligation of major arteries was well recognized. The use of ligatures did not become popular for almost a century after their initial appearance, however, partially because amputation above the knee was not often performed, surgeons being well aware of the fact that the danger to the patient increased with the level of the amputation, and because the cautery was sufficient to control bleeding from small-caliber vessels. Closure of the wound was achieved with a variety of sutures. John Hunter preferred to use, wherever possible, the dry suture, since otherwise additional points of infection could appear at the site of each stitch, but he pointed out that the dry suture was not appropriate for penetrating wounds. Four other types of suture were also used after mid-century: the twisted, then used in harelip repair and for wounds presenting similar problems, and the interrupted, quilled, and glovers' sutures, this last almost entirely for wounds of the intestines or stomach. Both interrupted and quilled sutures were used with abdominal wounds, with the latter preferred. Jones recommended the removal of sutures "as soon as the union is complete, which generally happens either the second, or third day, often in twenty-four hours." The double-flap technique for amputations had already been developed, but the promotion of healing by the first intention was considered to require great care and forethought.[51] It was suggested by Hunter for "wherever a clean wound is made in sound parts and where the surfaces can be brought into contact, or where there is sufficient skin to cover the part." On the other hand, wounds involving lacerations might be impossible to handle by the first intention, while wounds which might contain foreign matter should be left open so that pus could bring any debris to the surface.[52]

The care of the patient after surgery was carefully supervised both to ensure appropriate care of the wound itself and to note and treat possible complications. Hunter believed that dry lint should not be used as a dressing. Poultices were called for when it was desired that the wound suppurate. Where poultices were not appropriate, he maintained that dry lint was likewise inappropriate. He suggested in these cases that oil and wax or some other "unctuous matter" be used, or that it might even at times be better not to use ointments. Jones praised this British conservatism and added that, if an ointment had to be used, it should at least be very mild. The use of wine and alcohol as a remedy against putrefaction, however, was recommended by van Swieten, while turpentine, used in the eighteenth century to combat minor bleeding, now appears to have real value against bacteria.[53]

The appearance of "laudable pus" was regarded as a good sign, since suppuration was considered to be the body's attempt to rid itself of harmful materials. Pus caused a "very happy effect, by separating the lacerated vessels and extravasated fluids from the sound parts which then grow up a-fresh. Hence laudable pus is esteemed by surgeons as one of the best signs." Redness and heat around a wound were seen as inevitable, as was fever in serious wounds.[54] It was expected that the various healing processes might bring on a condition called "the hectic," the result of the body's trying unsuccessfully to heal itself and characterized by "debility, a small, quick, and sharp pulse; the blood forsaking the skin; loss of appetite; often rejection of all aliment by the stomach; wasting; a great readiness to be thrown into sweats; sweating spontaneously when in bed; frequently a constitutional purging; the water clear."[55] Once "digestion of the wound" had taken place, fever, inflammation, and pain could be expected to lessen. The average eighteenth century surgeon was so unaware of the causes and effects of infection that, when a colleague achieved an unusually low mortality rate, the explanation was sought in his surgical techniques and not in his standards of cleanliness.[56]

Among other possible complications arising in the wounded soldier was tetanus. Thomas, in 1815, admitted the difficulty of bringing a patient through tetanus and stressed instead attempts to prevent it. He cited among these efforts the Navy's custom of using a wound dressing containing tincture of opium and the use by a Dr. James Clark of calomel before and after surgery as a preventive. Rush noted in 1787 the vast quantities of opium then routinely used to treat tetanus, but stated that he personally had effected a gradual but complete cure by administering two to three ounces of bark and up to three pints a day of wine and raising a blister between the patient's shoulder blades to which he applied a mercurial ointment.⁵⁷

The types of surgery most commonly performed in the Army involved, of course, gunshot wounds and their consequences. By the late seventeenth century, when it was realized that the ball was not poisonous, surgeons were urged not to probe deeply but rather to let the ball remain if it could not be located easily. Jones preferred to dilate wounds to facilitate drainage or to aid in the reduction of fractures, but Hunter, believing that the edges of a wound were quite elastic, concluded that enlarging the opening was not required unless there were severe hemorrhaging, a suspected skull fracture, or debris or bone fragments to be removed. Many surgeons now believed that the caustic dressings once popular for gunshot wounds were no longer necessary.⁵⁸

When battle injuries involved fractures, the question of amputation arose, many surgeons favoring immediate amputation in compound fractures. Such injuries, when treated in crowded hospitals, were all too frequently followed by infection, making amputation eventually necessary even though similar fractures, treated in a rural environment, might never require such drastic measures. Van Swieten and John Hunter preferred to postpone amputation until it was obvious in each instance that it would be required. Amputation did not necessarily save the patient's life, however. The mortality rate was often 45 to 65 percent where the leg was removed at mid-thigh, although some surgeons lost markedly fewer patients than this. Jones believed that immediate amputation was definitely advisable when the heads of bones were broken or capsular ligaments were torn. When the fracture involved the skull, the danger posed to the brain by excessive pressure was well recognized and the eighteenth century surgeon was prepared to trephine. The patient would be fortified against these ordeals by the administration of opium and, perhaps, rum and his ears filled with lamb's wool to deaden the sound.⁵⁹

Although they were at times willing to attempt a wide range of surgery, eighteenth century surgeons generally acknowledged their inability to save patients with wounds involving the heart, aorta, cerebellum or medulla of the brain, or the cisterna chyli. Wounds of the spinal cord, major blood vessels, or the principal organs of the chest or abdomen were considered very dangerous. Amputation at the shoulder was generally avoided because of the danger of hemorrhage. And, of course, anyone could become fatally infected, a fact of which army surgeons in particular were only too well aware.⁶⁰

MEDICAL EDUCATION AND EXPERIENCE

Increasing numbers of young American medical students were studying abroad; their training added to the prestige of their profession in the colonies, although specialization in the European manner was rendered impractical by the generally scattered population of the colonies which required the physician to become a medical jack-of-all-trades, physician, surgeon, and apothecary all in one. The medicine practiced by some of these men carried purging and bleeding beyond the extent customary in Europe, and although physicians with European training were at times most outspoken in their criticism of the poor quality of American medicine, it was often they who, like Rush, went to those extremes which we today so deplore. The social status of physicians at this time could be great; they were found in colonial legislatures and local assemblies, on college boards, and among the wealthy merchants and landed proprietors so influential in colonial society.⁶¹

It has been estimated that by 1775 approximately 3,500 physicians were practicing in the colonies, caring for a population of three million, but that only 400 had M.D. degrees from medical colleges. By 1776, the two medical schools then functioning in America had conferred only 51 M.D. degrees. A majority of colonial physicians were either self-taught or taught through apprenticeships; and of the approximately 1,200 medical practitioners serving with the Continental Army in the Revolution, only an estimated 100 had M.D. degrees. Among the leaders of the Army's Hospital Department, however, were some of the best trained physicians in the colonies.[62] (See Appendix A.)

Training by apprenticeship was a highly individualized process which varied with the preceptor. Some required their apprentices to have a knowledge of Latin, natural history, mathematics, and grammar, but others were less demanding. Some apprentices might spend a large part of the traditional seven-year training period doing menial and semimenial tasks, receiving at the end of that time a certificate which was almost meaningless.[63]

As the colonies became increasingly prosperous, greater numbers of young Americans, including many future leaders in the Continental Army's Hospital Department, went abroad for their medical education. Proper preparation for such study was considered to include a college education followed by three years of apprenticeship to a physician who himself was well educated. The British schools, which were at the height of their popularity before the American Revolution, included Edinburgh, where clinical instruction was emphasized. Paris, where surgery was increasingly respected, became more popular with Americans after the French Revolution. Colonial students at this time usually studied in Paris only after having received their M.D.'s, as did John Morgan, William Shippen, Jr., and Benjamin Rush after receiving their degrees from Edinburgh. John Jones earned his M.D. at Rheims before moving on to Paris to study under eminent French surgeons. A few individual European practitioners were especially influential, among them, of course, Cullen of Edinburgh. In London, the Hunter brothers, William and John, also played important roles in the lives of many American medical students, including not only Rush and Jones but also Morgan and Shippen, both of whom were later Director Generals of the American Army Medical Department during the Revolution. John Pringle was another strong influence upon young American students of surgery.[64]

The first form of organized classes in medicine in the colonies was a system of lectures and demonstrations, often managed by a physician whose training abroad led him to feel acutely the need for better medical education in the colonies. Classes in human anatomy, however, were highly unpopular among ordinary citizens, who associated dissection with body snatching and regarded it as a desecration of the human body. Even postmortem examinations were infrequent and their purpose was limited to determining cause of death when murder was suspected. Nevertheless, in 1762, Shippen began a series of anatomy classes involving both a human body and a series of anatomical plates and casts donated by a prominent London physician. His first class held only ten students and triggered a minor riot, Shippen being accused, despite his denials, of grave robbing. The popular assumption that dissection of the human body implied body snatching lasted at least until the 1788 Doctors' Mob riot in New York City when three days of violence, put down only by military force, inspired the first practical laws regulating such matters.[65]

The first American medical school was established in Philadelphia in 1765 by Morgan. His failure to consult Shippen, with whom he had formulated the early plans for the school while both men were studying at Edinburgh, added fuel to the fire of the enmity already growing between the two men. Morgan was given the first appointment as professor at the new school where Shippen, who had been teaching for several years in Philadelphia, and later Rush, among others, joined him. Students at this school were required to have studied Latin, Greek, mathematics, and philosophy, and Morgan strongly recommended a familiarity with French as well. By the turn of the century, three more medical schools were in operation in the United States, at Kings College, Harvard, and Dartmouth, all with faculties in which foreign-trained physicians predominated.[66]

By the time the Revolution broke out, American physicians were no longer isolated from the thought of their colleagues, either those in their own communities or those in Europe. Books and journals were available to them, and scientific societies in the more populous areas gave them a forum where they were encouraged to present their own ideas. Here again, however, the shadow of things to come was cast by the formation in Philadelphia of rival societies by groups led on the one hand by Morgan and on the other by Shippen. Few of the medical publications in circulation in the eighteenth century were of American origin, but a number of public and private libraries were being created and foreign authors became very influential, among them not only the British Pringle and Brocklesby but also the Austrian van Swieten, French surgeons such as Jean Louis Petit and Henri François Le Dran, and many others. The influence of French military medicine also appeared in the form of translations of the French *Journal de Médecine Militaire* which were circulated in the United States from 1783 to 1790.[67]

Some of the men who were to join the American Army Medical Department had gained limited experience in military medicine during the French and Indian War. Morgan, for example, was an army surgeon with the Pennsylvania militia at that time and John Jones had taken part in the British attack on Canada. Experience with the British exposed some of the apprentice-trained colonial physicians to a higher level of practice than they had known before and familiarized them with the lower level operations of an army medical department. During the Revolution, even such men as Benjamin Rush, who had no previous military experience, expressed a wish to see the American Army Medical Department modeled more closely upon its British counterpart.[68]

During this period, the British Army's medical department was headed by a council of three civilians, usually prominent London practitioners, functioning as Physician General, Surgeon General, and Inspector General. Under them an inspector general was assigned to every twenty- to thirty-thousand-man army, where yet another inspector general served each division of four to five thousand men. The principal, or general, hospital for such an army might have 400 beds and a staff of six medical officers (including a physician and two assistants, a surgeon and one assistant, and an apothecary) and fifty other workers. The need for a sergeant to keep order among hospital patients was first recognized during the French and Indian War, and two orderlies were appointed who could assist in maintaining discipline. The British also emphasized hospital sanitation, good air and ventilation, and the prevention of overcrowding. It was intended that each regiment have its own surgeon and, in wartime, two assistants, and its own hospital in a house or tent. Fairly high standards were used in the selection of physicians, but regimental surgeons bought their commissions without showing any qualifications except that of experience, although in this instance, after the French and Indian War, higher standards were being urged. Regimental surgeons serving the Americans during that war tended to be poorly trained. The sick and wounded at times went untended for days, no efficient system of evacuation was developed until the Napoleonic Wars, and supplies and food were inadequate. The troops occasionally suffered from jaundice, and there was no evidence that the problem of typhus was handled any better by the British then than by the Americans during the Revolution.[69]

The practice of military medicine in the eighteenth century by nations experienced with the demands of war left much to be desired, even by the standards of the time. It could not, therefore, logically be expected that the newly created Continental Army Medical Department, directed by relatively inexperienced men whose personal antipathies toward one another were rapidly growing, could, in the early years of the Revolution, function in a manner we would find acceptable today.

2

Evolution of the Continental Army Medical Department

The Continental Army's Medical Department, established in July 1775, was assigned an almost impossible task by the Continental Congress. A staff for the most part totally unfamiliar with military medicine, handicapped by a serious and chronic shortage of drugs and by confused and inadequate legislation, was expected to provide uniformly competent care for an untrained army whose health was jeopardized by poor hygiene and frequently inadequate food and clothing. Medicines and supplies were in many instances imported and, even before the war, often in very short supply. The chain of command was confused because the legislation establishing the department did not recognize the existence of regimental surgeons and regimental hospitals and, when the scope of the medical service's activities broadened to cover operations beyond Massachusetts, did not define the relationship of the heads of the hospitals in other areas to the original Director General. (*Table 1*) In an era when violent quarrels between ambitious men were common, these legislative omissions fueled disagreements and even feuds which would threaten the Medical Department with paralysis. Thus the medical service was all too frequently unable to provide adequate and compassionate care, even by eighteenth century standards, for the Army's ill and wounded.[1]

CREATION OF THE HOSPITAL DEPARTMENT: CHURCH AS DIRECTOR GENERAL

When George Washington arrived at Cambridge, Massachusetts, on 3 July 1775 to take command of the Continental Army, the hospitalized sick and wounded, most of whom were from Massachusetts, were being cared for by Massachusetts regimental surgeons in Massachusetts facilities. It was obvious to all concerned, however, that this approach would be inadequate when units from other colonies became involved and when the fighting spread beyond the confines of that colony. Washington pointed out that already "Disputes and Contentions have arisen and must continue until it is reduced to some system."[2]

On 27 July, the Continental Congress, in a brief resolution, created for a Continental Army of approximately twenty thousand men what was termed in the language of the day "an Hospital" or, in modern terms, a hospital system or medical department, whose physicians were not, however, given military rank. This piece of legislation, like others to follow, was a source of considerable confusion, but the major problem at this time was caused by the failure to outline the relationship of the new department and its director to the existing regimental system, organized by each individual colony for the benefit of the regiments from that colony.[3] (*See Appendix B.*)

The legislation creating the Hospital Department also failed to discuss its relationship to the Congress. In September 1775, however, in response to the increasing seriousness of the drug shortage, the Continental Congress created a Medical Committee "to devise ways and means for supplying the Continental Army with Medicines." This new committee, to which a

TABLE 1—AUTHORITY WITHIN THE CONTINENTAL ARMY'S MEDICAL SERVICES, 1775–83

Date	Highest Authorities Within Hospital Department		Highest Authorities Within Regimental System
	Highest Independent Authority	Major Subordinates	
July 1775	Director General and Chief Physician	Surgeons, apothecaries	Regimental surgeons
September 1775	Director General and Chief Physician; Director General and Chief Physician in the North [a]	Surgeons, apothecaries, mates	As above
June 1776	As above, Director General and Chief Physician in the South [a]	As above	As above
July 1776	As above	As above, including surgeons functioning as hospital directors	Regimental surgeons: must submit medicine chests for inspection to Hospital Department's hospital directors
September 1776	As above	As above	Regimental surgeons responsible to heads of Hospital Department
April 1777	Director General	Deputy Directors of each district [b]	Physician and Surgeon General for each army; reports to Deputy Director for his district [c]
August 1777	Director General; Director of the hospitals in the South	As above	As above
September 1780	Director General; Deputy Director General for area south of Virginia	Three chief hospital physicians	Chief surgeon and physician for each army
March 1781 [d]	Director General	As above, Deputy Director in the South	As above

NOTE: Only the legislation of April 1777 and March 1781 gave the Director General supreme authority over all medical services.
[a] His relationship to the Director General and Chief Physician was obscure.
[b] The Director General functioned as the Deputy Director in the middle district.
[c] The regimental system from this point onward was a part of the Hospital Department.
[d] No further changes in command structure occurred during the Revolution after this date.

physician, Benjamin Rush, was first appointed in August 1776, was but one of several which were to concern themselves with the Hospital Department at one time or another during the course of the Revolution. Its authority gradually grew, and by early 1777, it had become involved in such matters as the hiring and firing of Hospital Department personnel, smallpox inoculation policies, and the resolution of the internal disputes of the Hospital Department.[4]

Rush failed of reelection to the Continental Congress in February 1777, and the new Medical Committee which was formed after the elections contained no holdovers from its predecessor. Its responsibilities were broadly outlined from the outset; it was "to devise ways and means for preserving the health of the troops, and for introducing better discipline into the army." Some type of Medical Committee appears to have been in existence from this time until its functions were assumed by the Board of War in May 1781.[5]

ACT CREATING HOSPITAL DEPARTMENT. *(Courtesy of National Archives.)*

70

Storekeeper To receive & deliver the bedding & other necessaries by order of the director

On Motion, Resolved, That the sum of twenty five thousand dollars be paid by the continental treasurers to Reese Meredith, George Clymer, Samuel Meredith & Samuel Mifflin Merch[an]ts of the city of Philad[elphi]a and that the like sum of twenty five thousand dollars be paid by the S[aid] Treasurers to Philip Livingston, John Alsop & Francis Lewis Merch[an]ts of New York to be by them apply'd to the purpose of importing gunpowder for the continental armies & that they be allowed out of the same five p[er] cent. for their trouble & expences therein, that they keep all their proceedings as much as possible a secret from every other person but the congress & the general of the continental forces for the time being that they keep up a correspondence with the s[ai]d General and make such dispositions of the powder they may import as he shall order. ——

The Congress then proceeded to the choice of officers for the Hospital when

Benjamin Church was unanimously elected as director & chief physician in the hospital and the apothecary

Resolved, that the appointment of the four surgeons be left to Doct[o]r Church.

That the mates be appointed by the surgeons; that their number do not exceed twenty; & that the number be not kept in constant pay, unless the sick & wounded should be so numerous as to require the attendance of twenty & to be diminished as circumstances will admit to ____

That one clerk & two storekeepers be appointed by the Director

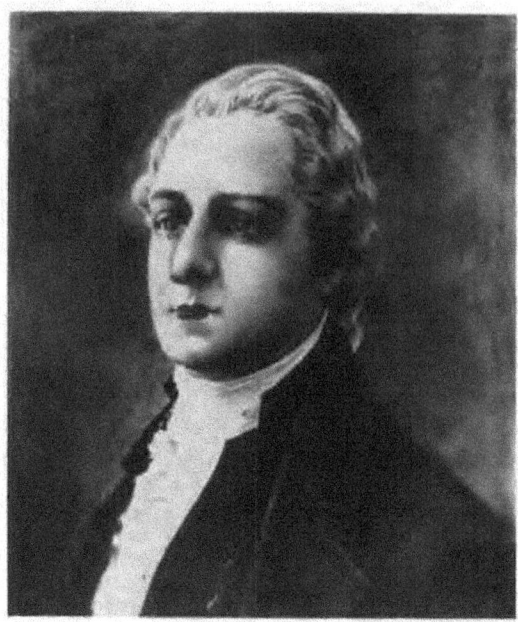

BENJAMIN CHURCH. *Apparently no picture of Church taken from life exists. This portrait was based on "contemporary description" (James Evelyn Pilcher, "Benjamin Church, Director General and Chief Physician of the Hospital of the Army, 1775," Journal of the Association of Military Surgeons 13 (1903): 324). (Courtesy of National Library of Medicine).*

Despite the existence of the Medical Committee, the Congress continued to involve itself directly in the operations of the Hospital Department. The shortage of drugs eventually became so critical, however, that even Committees of Safety from various states joined the attempts to relieve it and the search for medicines was expanded to include France, Holland, and the West Indies.[6]

To head the newly created Hospital Department, the Continental Congress unanimously elected Dr. Benjamin Church of Massachusetts as the first Director General and Chief Physician.[7] Church was known not only as a talented and well-educated physician and surgeon but also as an enthusiastic poet-patriot, an author of Liberty songs who played an active role in the operation of the hospital system for Massachusetts military units and in the examination of candidates for positions as surgeons for those units. He had received his medical training in London, practiced in Boston, and served Massachusetts as a member of both the Provincial Congress and the Boston Committee of Correspondence.

When Church assumed office, colonial soldiers were being cared for in about thirty hospitals, some of which were in wretched condition under the management of surgeons who had little understanding of the problems which faced them. He continued within the new department the same policy of examining candidates for medical positions which was originally followed in the appointment of surgeons for Massachusetts units and moved to consolidate hospitals, ordering regimental surgeons to send their patients, whenever possible, unless their complaints were very minor, to the general hospitals. Massachusetts surgeons generally cooperated with Church's efforts, but those from the regiments of other colonies generally did not.[8]

Many believed that the smaller hospital intended for the care of the ill and wounded of a four-hundred- to five-hundred-man regiment was less hazardous to the health of its patients than the large general hospital. It was also true that soldiers felt more secure when cared for by their own doctors among the men of their own units. General hospitals, however, were reputed to be more efficient and to have better staffs, since regimental surgeons and mates were a motley crew named by their respective colonels and their competence was not necessarily tested before appointment.[9]

Church found that the costs of running the regimental hospitals were extremely high and believed that this indicated the existence of "inexcusable neglect" on the part of the regimental surgeons managing them. He wished to have patients moved to general hospitals rather than to have medicines issued to regimental surgeons to permit them to continue to care for their patients. By the end of August, although he acknowledged organized resistance to his plans, Church believed that he was making progress in his fight against the supporters of the regimental hospital. He was sure that the soldiers themselves appreciated the advantages of the hospitals he had established and claimed that regimental surgeons had begun to seek out mates' berths in the general hospital.[10] In early September, Washington expressed support for the general hospital concept, commenting, "there is no need of regimental Hospitals without the Camp when there is a general Hospital so near and so well appointed."[11]

The opposition continued, however. Regimental surgeons complained to their officers whenever the general hospital denied them the drugs they demanded. Brig. Gen. John Sullivan protested that his wounded were being moved three to four miles to Cambridge to have their wounds dressed while his regimental surgeons stood virtually idle. His officers continued to bring pressure upon him: "Are the Dolorous Groans of the Disconsolate, agreeable to any human Ear— That they should be still Increas'd by Dragging our sick . . . In Waggon Loads to Cambridge? Humanity shudders at the Prospect." General Sullivan insisted that fully half of the patients ordered by Church to the general hospitals refused to go, "Declaring they would rather Die where they were and under the care of those Physicians they were acquainted with." The period of enlistment for the Continental Army at this time was for one year, making it necessary to raise a new army at the end of the soldiers' terms. Consequently the effects of the controversy over medical service on the morale of the average soldier were of great concern. General Sullivan commented, "I greatly fear that if it does not Ruin the present Army [it will] prevent another being raised in America."[12]

Although a second problem which plagued the Continental Medical Department, that of the Director General's authority within the expanding Continental medical establishment, did not appear in its ultimate dimensions under the Church administration, its foundations were laid in September 1775 when Dr. Samuel Stringer was appointed "director of the Hospital, and chief Physician and surgeon for the Army in the northern department." Stringer was to be paid a salary equal to Church's and had the right to appoint four men to serve under him. These men, however, were to be surgeon's mates, not surgeons, implying that Stringer's position was comparable not to Church's but to that of a surgeon. Although Church was clearly supreme within the establishment centered at Cambridge, Congress had failed to define either the relationship of the new system in the north to the one in Massachusetts or Stringer's position in the chain of command and had thus created fertile ground for future quarrels.[13]

It was in the midst of his struggle with the advocates of the regimental hospital that Church fell from power. By September, the quarrel between the two factions was so intense that Washington ordered that an investigation be conducted within each brigade. He required each brigadier general to sit with his officers as a court of inquiry into the various complaints, talking to both the Director General and the regimental surgeons. On 20 September, after three such hearings, Church attempted to resign, but Washington urgently requested the doctor to consider the matter at greater length. The final hearing was planned for 30 September, but on that day Washington announced the postponement of this last inquiry because "of the Indisposition of Dr. Church."[14]

The true reason for the postponement, however, was the discovery of a letter from Church to a British officer within British-occupied Boston. It had been suspected for some time that someone in the Provincial Congress of Massachusetts was informing to the British, but Church had explained his own suspicious friendliness with an enemy officer as an effort to keep himself informed of enemy activities. Washington now learned of a letter written the preceding July which had been left with a patriot by the "infamous hussy" who had been asked to deliver it. His suspicions aroused by her obvious anxiety, the patriot had offered to take the message into Boston for her. Although written in cipher, the letter was easily decoded and the woman, questioned by Washington himself, finally confessed that Church was the author. An immediate search of the doctor's papers, however, revealed nothing incriminating, leading the general to conclude that a protégé of Church's had removed anything suspicious.[15]

The letter was, according to John Adams, "the oddest Thing imaginable. There are so many lies in it, calculated to give the enemy an high Idea of our Power and Importance, as well as so many Truths tending to do us good that one knows not how to think him treacherous: Yet there are several strokes, which cannot be accounted for at least by me, without the Supposition of Iniquity." Indeed, it was only in the period immediately preceding World War II that the discovery of Church's letters to the British General Gage definitely proved that he had been sending secret military and political information to the British for six weeks before the battle of Lexington. Until that time, many others shared Adams's uncertainty. Church himself claimed that the letter was intended for his Tory brother-in-law in Boston and was designed to bring about a delay in the British attack which was anticipated when their momentarily expected reinforcements arrived, since colonial forces were still weak. James Warren and Samuel Adams, however, noted as significant the fact that Church had apparently never mentioned the correspondence to George Washington or, indeed, to any of the patriots.[16]

While Washington laid the question of how to proceed before his generals on 3 October 1775, Dr. Isaac Foster (also spelled Forster), head of the Massachusetts military hospital system before the creation of the Continental system, was appointed acting Director in Church's place. The next day, Washington's Council of War unanimously decided that Church had been caught in "criminal correspondence with the enemy." Close examination of the Articles of the Continental Army revealed, however, that the only punishment which the Army could legally inflict upon Church for this treason was cashiering and either the loss of two months' pay or thirty-nine lashes. Further legal problems arose from the fact that the alleged crime was committed before Church's appointment to the Army post and that the letter, the only evidence then available of his treason, was never actually delivered.[17]

Washington turned to the Continental Congress for a way out of this dilemma, but with the decision of that body on 14 October 1775 to elect a new Director General, Church passed beyond the scope of this history. It might be added, however, that although the Continental Congress and both Massachusetts and Connecticut attempted to find some satisfactory way to dispose of this case, none was ever found. Commented John Adams in June 1776, "Nobody knows what to do with him. There is no law to try him upon, and no court to try him. I am afraid he deserves more punishment than he will ever meet." Church's health began to fail, however, and he was permitted to board a ship bound for the West Indies. Neither he nor the ship was ever heard from again. His widow successfully applied to the king for a pension as the widow of a loyalist, claiming that her husband had been imprisoned for services rendered the British crown.[18]

MORGAN AS DIRECTOR GENERAL, 1775 TO 1777

On 17 October 1775, Dr. John Morgan was selected by the Continental Congress over three other official nominees to be Director General. Morgan was not Washington's first choice, however, since the general wished to see his young friend, Dr. William Shippen, already Morgan's rival in their home town of Philadelphia, take the post.[19]

Although the quality of Morgan's mind and training was undeniable, the honors he had received were many, and his "moral character" was deemed "very good" by John Adams at the time of his selection,[20] none other than James Boswell, Samuel Johnson's famous biographer, who joined the youthful Morgan for a tour of Holland in August 1763, called him "un fat bonhomme," translated by Morgan biographer, Whitfield Jenks Bell, Jr., as "a conceited fool."[21] Several years after Morgan's dismissal from the department, Dr. Barnabas Binney called him "the most implacable, revengeful man under the Heavens."[22] Morgan, Bell has stated, always suffered from "the same tension between the ideal and the possible, the same conflict between what he knew ought to be and what in the actual circumstances could be, and the same inability to understand the difference." Unable "to see anything touching himself in normal perspective,"[23] Morgan was driven by the demands and disappointments he experienced as Director General of the Continental Hospital Department to the point where vengeance upon the man he eventually blamed for his every frustration became his main goal in life.

Morgan was appointed Director General in October, but before actually reporting for duty, he took a month to put his personal affairs in order and to collect drugs and instruments. Washington was sufficiently distressed by the delay to point out that

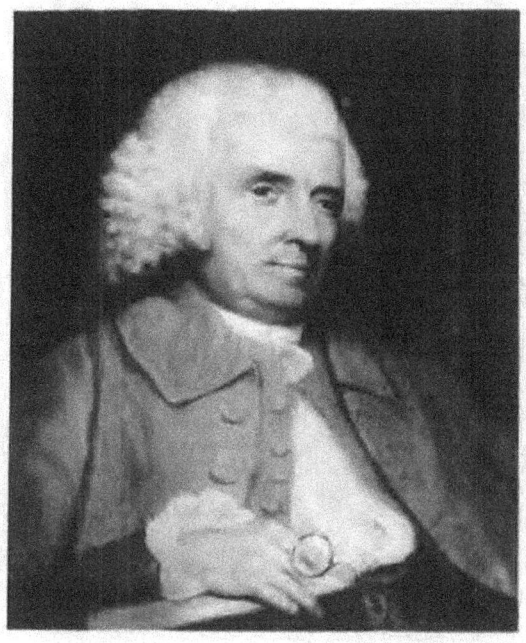

JOHN MORGAN. *(Courtesy of Historical Society of Pennsylvania.)*

Morgan's presence was most urgently required at camp and that the Director "ought not to delay his departure for the camp a moment, many regulations being delayed, and accounts postponed, till his arrival." When he finally did arrive in Cambridge, Morgan was confronted with hospitals crowded with the victims of various diseases, Army officers inexperienced with the maintenance of the health of large numbers of men, and a department already experiencing increasing difficulties keeping up with the demand for supplies. The problems posed by two parallel and conflicting medical systems were by no means diminishing, while those posed by conflicting authorities within the department were just beginning.[24]

Seemingly undaunted, Morgan inspected the entire department and its operations. The stock of medicines and hospital supplies on hand proved to be totally inadequate. There were almost no blankets, for example, although there were more than 500 mattress

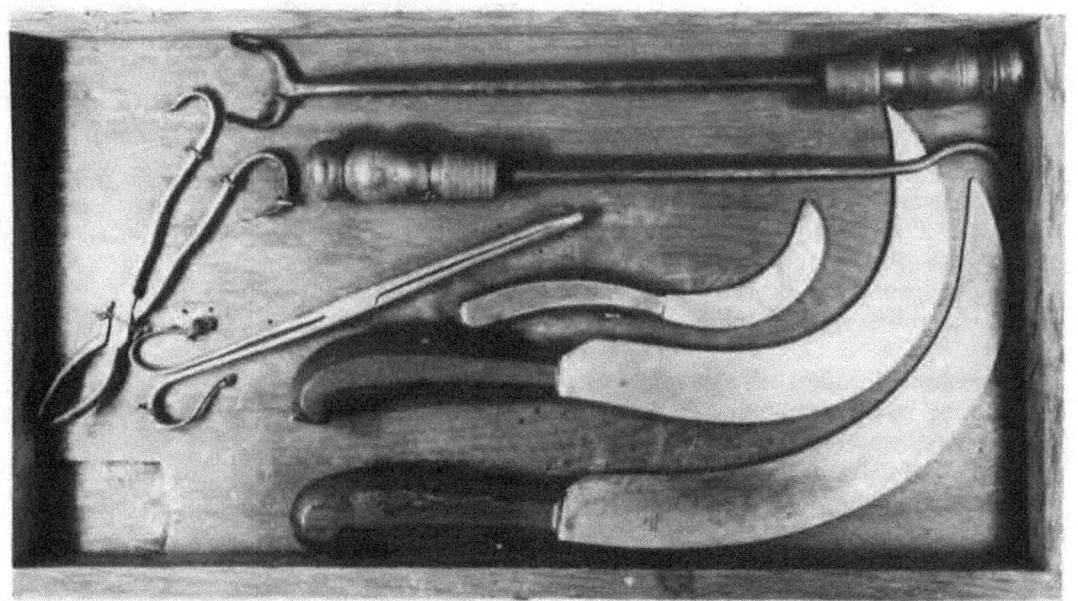

SURGEON'S FIELD CASE. *(Courtesy of Armed Forces Institute of Pathology.)*

ticks. There were only 200 bandages and little in the way of materials from which to make more. The report on drugs from the apothecary revealed that, although 120 different items were on hand, the supply of some of the most highly regarded medicines was very limited.[25]

Medicines were being brought in from Philadelphia, but they came in slowly while the number of soldiers in the area increased rapidly. Morgan's position required him to deal with the supply crisis directly. Instruments were so difficult to obtain that he was reduced to suggesting to one surgeon that he use a razor blade as an incision knife. He succeeded, nevertheless, in equipping chests for regiments both in Boston and elsewhere. The wool and woolen cloth so highly valued by many eighteenth century military physicians were hard to obtain, although some was purchased on credit in France. The general shortage of textiles meant that even tent materials were in short supply. Congress rarely voted enough money to meet the department's needs, and Washington further complicated the problem in December 1775 by underestimating the costs of supporting the hospitals required by the Army.[26]

The conflict between the Hospital Department and the regimental medical system which caused so many difficulties under Church also continued under Morgan and was intensified by the shortage of medicines and hospital supplies. Morgan's necessarily meager release of supplies from the general hospital to regimental surgeons, which was in part caused by his desire to stockpile stores against future need, only served to heighten the tensions already existing between the two systems. Regimental surgeons assumed that they had a right to draw on the general hospital's stores and blamed hospital surgeons for the shortages which they experienced, but Morgan maintained that he had no orders to supply regimental needs. Since he was unable to account for the way in which regimental surgeons used what they drew, he believed it necessary to limit carefully what they were issued. Morgan did think, however, that the regimental hospital served a useful purpose and was even reasonably confident of his own ability to handle the situation if Congress would clarify the legal relationship between the two systems. Morgan believed it was essential that the regimental surgeons, whose number was increasing as new regiments were formed, be "placed in some subordination." He asked Congress to inform him whether regimental surgeons were subject to any rule "that may be devised for the government of the Hospital, and the good of the service."[27]

Morgan was expected to participate in the preparation and issuance of medicine chests and the instruments and drugs in them to regimental surgeons. Since new regiments were being formed rapidly at this time and supplies were running short, finding the items necessary for these chests was quite difficult. Morgan realized, however, the potential threat to the general hospital which would arise should regimental surgeons choose to alleviate the strain on their system by turning all their patients over to the Hospital Department. He predicted to Washington that the population of the general hospital might be increased by such an approach from the approximately 300 there at that time to 2,000 and therefore suggested, with Washington's concurrence, that regimental and general hospitals be brought into harmony. On 17 July 1776, however, Congress itself finally passed legislation which, while to some degree officially clarifying the relationship of the two medical systems as far as supplies were concerned, failed to eliminate ill feeling. (*See Appendix C.*) The resolve stated that regimental surgeons were not to be permitted to draw anything but medicine and instruments from the Hospital Department and that patients whose treatment required anything more were to be sent into the general hospital. The directors of individual hospitals were entitled to inspect the regimental chests and surgical instruments; if regiments were reduced in size, instruments and medicines not being used were to be turned over to the Director General who would report on their number to Congress. Regimental surgeons also were required to submit returns on the number of sick under their care to the Hospital Department.[28]

This new act also permitted an increase in the number of Hospital Department surgeons and mates up to one surgeon and five mates for every 5,000 men and the hiring of as many storekeepers, stewards, nurses, and other hospital employees as deemed necessary, to be appointed by individual hospital directors. The suggestion, favored by Morgan, that hospital expenses be met at least in part by a deduction from the pay of each soldier did not pass, but some economies were achieved by stopping the regular rations of the sick as long as they were in the hospital. Hospital directors were required to give the names of the sick and dates of their hospitalization to the commissary and to the Board of Treasury to ensure accurate accounting.[29]

Unfortunately, neither Morgan's efforts nor those of the Continental Congress had much alleviated the conflict between the two systems. Complaints against the general hospital continued, and at least one colonel, Maryland's Smallwood, removed his men from the general hospital and refused to have others enter it, commenting that they were better off housed "in a comfortable house in the country, and supplied with only common rations." The Continental Congress forbade the placing of regimental hospitals near general hospitals and ordered commanding officers to send an officer once a week to check on the condition of their men in department hospitals.[30]

Many thoroughly distrusted regimental surgeons. Washington had been disillusioned by the facts brought out at the hearings of the preceding September and called regimental surgeons "very great Rascals" willing to certify as sick those who were perfectly healthy. These surgeons were "aiming, I am persuaded, to break up the Genl. Hospital." Their bickering was endangering the entire army and their insistent demands for furniture and accommodations were resented by Morgan, who could not legally accede to their wishes. Washington now believed that only the subordination of regimental surgeons to the Director General would resolve the problem, but others maintained that the controversy could be ended by a firm decision either to take everyone who was too ill to perform his duties into the general hospital or to have the general hospital provide regimental surgeons all they needed to care for their patients. Unfortunately, however, because of the shortage of medicine and hospital supplies, the Hospital Department was in no position to undertake either alternative.[31]

Regimental surgeons were also dissatisfied because, while they received only $25 a month, a sum raised in June 1776 to $33⅓, and regimental mates were paid but $18 a month, hospital surgeons received $40 a month from the outset and hospital mates $20. (*See Appendix B.*) Appeals to Congress resulting from the conflict between the two systems poured in even as a tendency to partisanship among the members of Congress grew and medical policy became highly controversial. The tension was increased by suggestions that it might not be possible to raise more troops unless the medical service was reformed. Congress's resolution of 30 September 1776 subordinating regimental surgeons to the heads of the divisions of the Hospital Department did not end the controversy.[32] (*See Table 1.*)

Meanwhile, the confusion about the Director General's authority over the Director of the Hospital in the Northern Department had come to a head. Dr. Samuel Stringer took his post in the North in September 1775, a month before Morgan's official appointment. He apparently set to work at once to carve out an independent niche for himself among the troops under Maj. Gen. Philip Schuyler gathering for an invasion attempt against Canada. Saying that the four mates allowed him earlier were not enough, Stringer asked Congress in late October 1775 to assign him surgeons and more mates. Were surgeons assigned to work under him, his own position would, of course, be strengthened.

By 1776, an all-out three-way power struggle was developing, with Stringer attempting to maintain his own independence, Morgan attempting to "subordinate" Stringer, both physicians scheming to receive the support of Congress for their own ambitions, and Congress refusing to be pushed or manipulated by anyone into clarifying the situation. Washington himself urged that Congress set one single head over the entire Hospital Department. Stringer's request in May 1776 for an increase in his staff to a total of four surgeons, twelve mates, and other lesser figures was granted by Congress on 22 May in terms which did not make clear who was to name these men. Stringer now also informed Washington that his supply of medicines was totally inadequate for his predictable needs, but Washington referred the request for supplies to Morgan, implying by so doing that Stringer's position was subordinate to Morgan's.[33]

By June, Morgan was demanding that Congress clarify the situation. "From all I am able to learn," he commented, "everything in the Medical Department in Canada displays one scene of confusion and anarchy; nor have the Congress taken upon itself to establish . . . any person whatever with a power sufficient to establish a General Hospital in Canada." The positions of Stringer and Dr. Jonathan Potts, recently sent north, were unclear. Morgan warned that the surgeons in Canada were spreading smallpox through unwisely handled inoculation, something which did not happen, he insisted, where he was in control. Help was badly needed everywhere in the North, furthermore, and he recommended that he be given permission to appoint more surgeons, mates, and apothecaries so that he did not have to send men already on duty and needed in the New York City area. Stringer, however, although he admitted the difficulty of finding surgeons and mates, refused to accept the officers sent by Morgan in response to his stated need.[34]

The solution Morgan proposed to problems in the North was the establishment of a general hospital in Canada and the placing of all Hospital Department operations in the North under his own authority. The department as a whole would operate more smoothly if he, as Director, chose all surgeons, since unhappy effects would result from any undermining of "that idea of subordination so necessary in an Army." He boldly stated that "some resolves of Congress have been incautiously entered into . . . or titles of rank and distinction given, which have a tendency to interfere with mine." The public, however, not understanding the situation, tended to blame only Morgan for conditions existing under Stringer's command. Stringer and Morgan continued to importune Congress, and Stringer even left his post in the guise of seeking a supply of medicines to pursue the matter personally with Congress. The response of Congress, however, was to state rather vaguely that Stringer had been appointed "director general and physician for the hospital in the northern department only" and to add that each hospital director was entitled to appoint his own subordinates unless Congress directed otherwise.[35]

Congress, indeed, was so little impressed with its own share of the responsibility for the conflicts among the medical officers serving the Continental Army that in June 1776, on the urging of the Virginia Convention, it created yet another hospital system, this time in Virginia, headquartered at Williamsburg, where Dr. William Rickman was appointed Physician and Director General.[36]

In September, one of Morgan's friends and supporters in the Continental Congress, Thomas Heyward, Jr., returned to South Carolina, after informing Morgan that he would not be able to continue to help him. Congress, meanwhile, was harried and harassed by the number and seriousness of the problems with which it had to deal and by late 1776 was apparently running out of patience with both Stringer and Morgan. In November 1776, Oliver Wolcott of the Continental Congress ominously commented that he hoped that "the Medical Department will undergo a Reform of Men at least, if not of Measures, that not so much Complaint which I fear has been too well grounded, may be heard respecting the Conduct of that Department."[37]

Morgan's position was further undermined in the last six months of 1776 by a quarrel with another Hospital Department physician. His opponent in this instance was more dangerous to him than Stringer, for Dr. William Shippen was talented, charming, superbly trained, highly regarded, and well connected by reason of both his own Philadelphia family and his marriage to a member of Virginia's influential Lee family. Despite Washington's desire to see him become Church's successor, Shippen had not joined the Hospital Department until the summer of 1776, when he became chief physician to the flying camp under the command of Gen. Hugh Mercer, himself a physician. This organization was composed of militia and state troops called in on short enlistments to form a strategic reserve in the emergency created by the impending British attack on New York, but it apparently never reached its 10,000-man goal.

The appointment of a man he already regarded as a dangerous rival alarmed Morgan, who later maintained that Shippen's

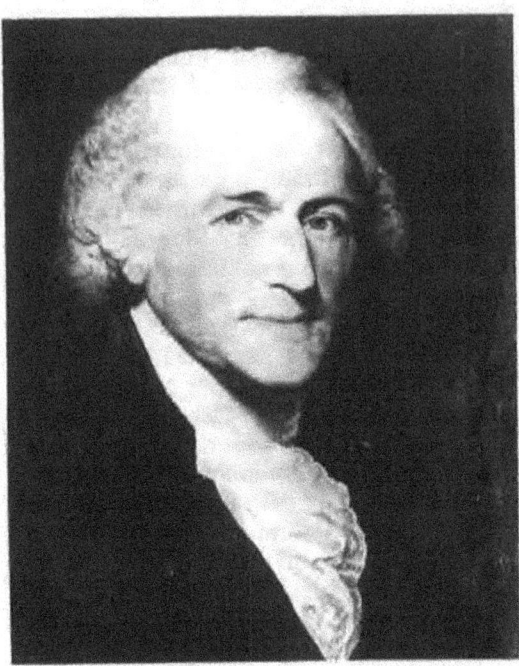

WILLIAM SHIPPEN, JR. *(Courtesy of National Library of Medicine.)*

assumption of the post was part of a plot to take his place. The wording of the notification sent to Shippen, however, casts some doubt on Morgan's theory, since the phrase "should you accept the appointment" implies uncertainty as to Shippen's acceptance. By the fall of 1776, however, Shippen may have been thinking in different terms, since he let it be known that he was available should there be changes in the structure of the Hospital Department.[38]

On 9 October 1776, and apparently without consulting Washington, the Continental Congress once more produced a confusing resolve. Shippen was directed to "provide and superintend an hospital for the army, in the state of New Jersey" and Morgan one "for the army posted on the east side of Hudson's river." There was, in this instance, again no definition of the relationship of the two men, even though the Congress did detail carefully how the hospitals were to be managed.

The month was not over before Shippen wrote Washington that, although Congress had assigned him all army patients on the New Jersey side, Morgan had told all medical officers to follow only the Director's orders until either he or Washington told them otherwise. The basic issue, in Shippen's opinion, was whether he was to give orders only for patients of the flying camp, as Morgan seemed to think, or for all sick and wounded in New Jersey, as Congress, in Shippen's opinion, intended.

Washington apparently assumed that those of his men who retreated from New York to New Jersey nevertheless remained the responsibility of Morgan, as chief physician for the main army; he stated that he interpreted the resolution to mean that Morgan should hospitalize and care for patients of the main army wherever he found it to be most convenient, on either side of the river, and that Shippen should restrict his care to the men of the flying camp. He noted that the problem would in time probably solve itself, since wounded soldiers were now beginning to return to the army and Morgan would soon no longer need facilities on the Jersey side.

Shippen, declaring his own confusion, turned to General Mercer, who suggested that Shippen appeal for clarification to Congress. This Shippen did, commenting that Washington seemed to make no distinction between Shippen's original appointment in July and Congress's newer directive of October. The response of that body to his appeal was to state that all the sick in New Jersey were Shippen's responsibility.[39]

Morgan's position by December 1776 was very weak, and he blamed Congress for tying his hands by undermining his authority. Congress ordered investigations into the department and there were calls for reform. Shippen, in writing to his brother-in-law in the Continental Congress, Richard Henry Lee, referred to directors who were not directing and noted that the care of the sick was being delegated to ignorant mates while surgeons and physicians found other things to do. Shippen presented a detailed plan to reform the Hospital Department, one which, he maintained, would have among its virtues the elimination of any need for regimental hospitals. Washington pointed out, however, that the clash between Morgan and Shippen greatly increased the sufferings of the sick in 1776.[40]

On 9 January 1777, without warning, the Continental Congress passed this brief resolve: "Resolved, That Dr. John Morgan, director general, and Dr. Samuel Stringer, director of the hospital in the northern department of the army of the United States, be, and they are hereby, dismissed from any farther service in said offices." [41] Washington, in his letter of 18 January notifying Morgan of his dismissal, noted "What occasioned the above Resolve I cannot say, I can only assure you, it has not been owing to any representations of mine." The general confessed that he was "amazed to hear Complaints of the Hospital on the East Side of Hudson's River; Doctr. Morgan, with most of his Mates has been Constantly there, since I left with the main body of the Army" and stated his belief that Morgan had also done his best to keep costs down.[42] Samuel Adams, however, writing to his cousin John Adams the day the resolve was passed, commented that both men were "dismissed without any reason assigned" and added that Congress had a perfect right to proceed in this manner. Echoing earlier comments by critics of Church's administration, Samuel Adams added, "The true reason, as I take it, was the general disgust, and the danger of the loss of any army arising therefrom," since "Great and heavy complaints" had been expressed concerning "abuse in the Director-General's department in both our armies; some, I suppose, without grounds, others with too much reason." [43]

Because of the abrupt nature of Morgan's dismissal, neither the charges against him nor his defense initially received an airing. Morgan, however, spent many long months working first to clear his own name and then to bring about the disgrace of his successor. His pride had been severely hurt and he made no secret of his bitterness. He explained:

. . . to be stripped of the rank of Director General, of the power of my station, and to be left but the shadow of a Director, and yet to be accountable for every accident, or misconduct of others, as well as my own department, and, from the highest post, to be rendered the mere dependent of a junior and subordinate officer, was what I would never submit to.

The source of all his miseries, the "junior and subordinate officer," was William Shippen, Jr.[44]

Morgan was not officially cleared of all charges of wrongdoing in office until June 1779, in part because of his attacks on others. In his *Vindication* of himself, he furiously attacked Shippen rather than limiting himself strictly to the matter at hand. One of Morgan's supporters in Congress drew censure from its President for altering Morgan's official appeal after its formal presentation to Congress in an attempt to make the document less vitriolic. It was, therefore, only on 12 June 1779 that Congress resolved that Morgan "did conduct himself ably and faithfully in the discharge of the duties of his office." He was never reinstated.[45]

NEW ARRANGEMENTS FOR THE HOSPITAL DEPARTMENT

Benjamin Rush, who was still a member of the Medical Committee, reacted quickly to the dismissal of Morgan, writing on 14 January to Richard Henry Lee to urge that the appointment of a new Director General be held in abeyance until the two men could

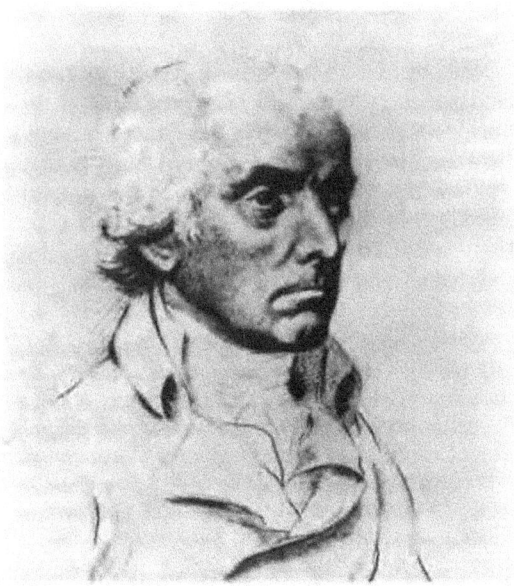

BENJAMIN RUSH. *(Courtesy of the University of Pennsylvania.)*

discuss the matter. He stated that he wished to give Lee the names of men who, like John Cochran, were so able that they should be appointed at once to high positions on the department's medical staff. He also wished to advise Lee on the reform of the Hospital Department, which, he believed, should be designed more along British lines in order, for example, to further remove the responsibility for obtaining supplies for the department from the office of the Director, so as to minimize the possibility for corruption.[46]

Shippen, also impressed by the British system, continued to work on his plan for hospital reform, at Washington's request with the aid of the same Dr. Cochran whom Rush so much admired. This plan suggested the appointment of purveyors to manage supplies received by the Hospital Department and of an Inspector General to inspect hospitals and apothecary shops. The general, who made it plain that he still wished to see Shippen become Director, was not sure that the higher salaries recommended by Shippen would be granted, although he himself felt them necessary, and pointed out that the Shippen-Cochran plan did not differ fundamentally from the ideas favored by Morgan himself.[47]

In response to Washington's urging, a special committee was appointed by Congress on 22 March 1777 to study the health problems of the Army. The report they issued was repeatedly brought up for consideration in late March and early April, but its consideration was also repeatedly postponed, often with suggestions for minor alterations. The absence of a Director General and the uncertain nature of future organization gave cause for concern to those who held responsible positions under the old system. Washington found it necessary in at least one instance to reassure an anxious medical officer that those who had been performing their duties faithfully had nothing to fear.[48]

At last, on 7–8 April 1777, legislation changing the organization of the Hospital Department, much along the lines suggested in the Shippen-Cochran plan, was passed by the Continental Congress. *(See Appendix D.)* Nothing in the new resolve suggested that the Director was not the head of the entire department. Among his many duties was to be the personal supervision of the hospitals of the Middle Department, between the Hudson and Potomac Rivers. The Eastern and Northern Departments, separated geographically by the Hudson River, were each to be managed by a Deputy Director General; a third Deputy Director would supervise hospitals south of the Potomac River if the military situation seemed to require the establishment of a formal organization in this part of the country. The new law implied that the relationship of this last deputy to the Director General would be identical with that of his counterparts to the north. Assistant Deputy Directors, with the hospital surgeons and attendants who would serve under them, an apothecary general with his mates, and a commissary with his assistants were to work under each Deputy Director General.

In each geographical division (casually referred to as either a department or a district), the practice of medicine was to be supervised by a Physician General and the practice of surgery by a Surgeon General. In addition, a Physician and Surgeon General would be attached to the army in the Champlain area of the Northern Department, a second to the units in New England, in the Eastern Department, and a third to the army personally commanded by General Washington, for the specific purpose of supervising the work of the regimental surgeons and their mates and the management of regimental hospitals. These officers would be responsible to the Director General and to the Deputy Directors General of the districts in which they were serving.

Among the features of the original Shippen-Cochran plan not found in the new legislation were the positions of the Purveyor, whose office was so important in the thinking of Benjamin Rush, and of the Inspector General. As a result of the elimination of these positions, the management of the department's supplies, as well as the responsibility for the condition of the department's facilities, remained entirely in the hands of the Director General, although the Medical Committee was empowered to inspect any aspect of the Hospital Department at any time.[49]

The reaction to the new plan for the Hospital Department seems to have been one of general satisfaction. John Adams considered it "A most ample, generous, liberal provision. . . . The expense will be great, but humanity overcame avarice." The pay scale was indeed high, since it gave the senior surgeon, for example, approximately a dollar a day more than a colonel of the Continental Army earned. The fundamental problem lay not with the pay scale but rather with the late payment of the assigned salaries, which ran months, if not years, late.[50]

Modifications and additions to the legislation as originally passed began to appear before a week had passed, partially as a result of an apparent trend away from the British custom which separated the function of the surgeon from that of the physician and toward a tacit recognition of the actual practice in the colonies. The Shippen-Cochran plan in the form it took on 14 February 1777 mentioned both senior surgeons and senior physicians and although the desirability of keeping the wounded and the sick physically separated was reiterated, the requirement of the 7–8 April legislation for separate positions of Surgeon General and Physician General was partially removed on 12 April when Congress gave both identical duties; each should function in the capacity of Physician and Surgeon General. The complete elimination of any distinction between the duties of the physician and the surgeon at all levels was not officially achieved until September 1780.[51]

On 22 April 1777, Congress issued still further additions to the new regulations. Concerned with providing care for military patients as quickly as possible, the legislation ordered that the Director and Deputy Directors publish frequently in the local newspapers the locations of military hospitals so that men unable to continue their march could be sent to the one closest to them. Officers were authorized to send patients to the nearest private physician for care if no military hospital were at hand, but were required to send them as soon as possible thereafter to a military facility.[52]

Shippen was not formally elected Director General until 11 April when the other high offices of the department were also filled, although his election was by the unanimous vote of the states. His Surgeon General in the Middle Department was Benjamin Rush, who had first worked with the department as a volunteer in December 1776, and others of his staff were also experienced physicians; it was hoped that the reorganization would result in an influx of well-trained doctors to the Hospital Department.

The complete list of officers of the Hospital Department elected on 11 April 1777 is as follows:

Director General, William Shippen, Jr.
Physician General of the hospital in the Middle Department, Walter Jones
Surgeon General of the hospital in the Middle Department, Benjamin Rush
Physician and Surgeon General of the army in the Middle Department, John Cochran
Deputy Director General in the Eastern Department, Isaac Foster
Physician General of the hospital in the Eastern Department, Ammi Ruhamah Cutter
Surgeon General of the hospital in the Eastern Department, Philip Turner
Physician and Surgeon General of the army in the Eastern Department, William Burnet
Deputy Director General of the hospital in the Northern Department, Jonathan Potts
Physician General of the hospital in the Northern Department, Malachi Treat
Surgeon General of the hospital in the Northern Department, Francis Forgue
Physician and Surgeon General of the army in the Northern Department, John Bartlett

SOURCES: Ford, *Journals of the Continental Congress*, 7: 253; Francis Bernard Heitman, *Historical Register of Officers of the Continental Army During the War of the Revolution, April 1775 to December 1783* (Washington: 1892-93).

On 5 June, in a further attempt to enhance the department's image, a notice signed by Shippen and Cochran in their official capacities was placed in the *Pennsylvania Evening Post*, publicizing the new appointments and stating that "all the military hospitals of the United States are in excellent order, and that the Army enjoy [sic] a degree of health, seldom to be seen or read of." The significance of this announcement becomes apparent when it is considered in the light of the fact that Washington believed that the condition of the Army's hospitals had contributed to the melting away of his entire army in the winter of 1776-77.[53]

SHIPPEN'S CONTROVERSIAL ADMINISTRATION

Shippen, like Morgan, was trained at Edinburgh and London after receiving his undergraduate degree in the colonies and serving there as an apprentice. Although he gained distinction as a physician who was genuinely concerned for his patients, it was as a teacher and as a social animal that he especially shone. "Nature had been uncommonly bountiful in his form and aspect," wrote a fellow physician, "his manners were extremely elegant . . . he belonged to a family proverbial for good temper . . . he was . . . particularly agreeable to young people." It was said that before the enmity arose between the two Philadelphia doctors, "there was no one who did not wish him well" and that at his death in 1808, "he left the world without an enemy." [54]

Shippen was immediately faced with the problems which had haunted both Church and Morgan. Supplies were disastrously short, rivalries were flourishing, the department's organization was still far from perfect, and Congress was still contributing as much to the problems as to their solutions. It is also possible that the new Director General himself to some degree added to the department's problems since, except for his first two winters in the Army, he continued to teach anatomy as he had before the war, and thus did not devote his entire time to the Hospital Department. It is also possible that he was unwilling to endure prolonged personal hardship and deprivation, although the matter is open to question.[55]

The number of sick, which was high even before the campaign of 1777 began, grew even higher as the cold weather came on. "The extreme fatigue and hardship which the Soldiers underwent in the course of the Winter, added to the want of Cloath [sic], and, I may add, Provisions, have rendered them very sickly," Washington believed.[56]

This same lack of food and clothing also helped to make the sick in the hospitals even sicker. John Adams, noting that disease killed ten soldiers for one killed in battle, added that "Discipline, discipline is the great thing wanted. There can be no order nor cleanliness in an army without discipline." [57]

Supplies of almost any description were very hard to find and the problems experienced in this regard by the Hospital Department were but a reflection of the overall situation, although the larger budget allowed by Congress for drugs kept the situation from becoming in this respect as desperate as it was in 1776.[58] Food, especially vegetables, vinegar, soap, and clothing were particularly hard to obtain for Army patients, although in August 1777, the Continental Congress gave the Hospital Department permission to draw upon the issuing commissaries. Many patients otherwise ready to rejoin their units were unable to do so because they were literally naked. By late October, Shippen was begging Congress for clothing but it was not until 19 November that this body granted Army hospitals a share of the Army's clothing supply and permission to install stoves to keep the unclothed patients warm.[59]

While Washington admitted that "It is but too melancholy a truth, that our Hospital Stores are exceedingly scanty and deficient in every instance, and I fear there is no prospect of their being better shortly," [60] many did not understand the nature of these shortages and blamed the sufferings of the Army's patients upon the Hospital Department and its Director, as they had under Morgan. By the end of 1777, for example, Rush was attacking Shippen with increasing vigor, citing as causes of patient wretchedness both the "want of checks upon the lower officers of the hospitals" and also what he maintained was Shippen's refusal to deal with these officers and to join him in appealing to Washington and to Congress. Rush was certain that Shippen's influence among politicians could produce action which would cure the problem. Congress, in response to the spiraling costs, resolved in early January 1778 that every officer hospitalized with venereal disease should be fined ten dollars and every soldier four, the sums so collected to be used to buy blankets and shirts for hospital patients.[61]

Congress was increasingly displeased about the operations of the Hospital Department and complained that for a lengthy period of time it had been forced to assume the role of Director General of the hospitals in addition to that of the other Army department heads. Great hopes were held out, however, for a reform plan adopted in February 1778, partly as a result of the urgent complaints of Rush, who showed little awareness of the inevitable effects of the universal shortage of supplies and sought to solve the department's problems by reorganization. (*See Appendix E.*)

Under the new plan, the Director was relieved of all supply responsibilities. The new position of Deputy Director for the Middle Department was created and Jonathan Potts was named to fill it. Although he was not given the title of purveyor, the new Deputy Director would assume all purveying functions. He would pay salaries and incidental expenses and buy medicines and supplies, distributing them with the aid of assistant deputy directors to be specifically assigned responsibility for such matters in each district. Accounting procedures were tightened. The staff which would in the years to come assist the officer functioning as purveyor generally included not only clerks and storekeepers but also purchasing agents and assistants to help with the distribution of supplies. Estimates of need were routinely sent to the purveyor, who then turned to such agencies as might reasonably be expected to provide the requested items. Among these possible sources were state agencies, the Commissary General, the Quartermaster General, the Clothier General, the Continental Druggist, and the various contractors serving the Army. When the purveyor attempted to buy privately, however, he was forced to bid against other governmental representatives, a situation which resulted in artificially inflated prices for all. Congress through its committees looked as far as Europe and the West Indies for drugs which, when received, were turned over to the Apothecary General by the purveyor. The new organization was, of course, unable to keep inflation and inadequate funding from interfering with the department's ability to supply its needs.[62]

The new legislation also reduced the responsibilities of the office of the Deputy Director General in the Eastern and Northern Departments, where there was little action after Burgoyne's defeat in the fall of 1777. The number of hospitals in each district, for example, would be determined by the district's Physician General and Surgeon General, who would also consult directly with the Director General concerning supply needs rather than work through the Deputy Director. In the absence of the Director General, these two officers would also appoint the wardmasters of their district. Reports from the Physician General and the Surgeon General would no longer be routed through their Deputy Director but would be submitted directly to the Director General. (*See Appendix E.*)

It was also in February 1778 that the French entered the war against Great Britain. Although this development was crucial to the eventual winning of the war, initially it only added to the supply problems faced by the Americans, since the French handled their own supply and paid higher prices than the Americans to be sure of obtaining what they needed, which raised the prices the Americans had to pay.

Following the appointment of Jonathan Potts as Deputy Director for the Middle Department, Congress was for a time financially more generous to the Hospital Department, and both morale and hospital conditions seem to have improved. By the fall of 1778, the clothing situation appears to have improved as well. As time went on, however, congressional generosity no longer sufficed. The Treasury did not have enough money to give the Hospital Department that which Congress assigned to it, and increasing inflation was severely undercutting the purchasing power of such sums as the department did receive. By the end of 1779, inflation was so great that $30 in Continental money was not worth $1 in specie, and food was again short everywhere, although appeals to the local populace at times produced good results. By the summer of 1780, the department was "destitute of those necessaries which are indispensable for the sick," and suggestions were even being made that Potts might be profiting from his position. In attempting to defend himself, Potts accurately pointed out that a number of men including other physicians within the department and assistant Directors General, such as Thomas Bond and James Craik, commissaries, assistant commissaries, and stewards handled purchasing at one time or another.[63] John Cochran, soon to become the fourth Director General, had little hope for improvement in the supply situation and blamed Congress and its Medical Committee "who will probably pow-wow over it awhile and nothing more be heard of it." [64]

Although the legislation of April 1777 ended the regimental medical system as a separate entity, the enmity between regimental and hospital surgeons also continued to plague the department for a time and their "continual jealousies and altercations" in January 1778 "had a very pernicious influence," in Washington's opinion. His efforts to have regimental surgeons submit regular weekly reports to the officers of the local division of the Hospital Department on the number and condition of their patients apparently met with limited success, since he found it necessary to repeat them from time to time. Eventually, however, general distrust of regimental surgeons began to wane, and Washington himself noted his desire to see the regimental surgeon given more leeway, since being moved to a general hospital could harm many patients.[65]

The confusion about the extent of the authority of the Director General, however, did not disappear under Shippen. Although the April 1777 legislation placed no geographical restrictions on Shippen's authority, in August 1777 the Continental Congress stated that the April reform plan was not to be applied to the division of the Hospital Department operating in Virginia under Rickman and, furthermore, that Shippen must withdraw any doctors whom he, assuming that he was Rickman's supervisor, may have sent into the South.[66]

Presumably already damaged by the confusion within the department, morale was further damaged by the fact that in the early years of the war the men of the Continental Hospital Department had neither military rank nor the privileges of the military officer.[67] They appealed to Washington in April 1779 for permission at least to draw clothing from Army stores, but Washington did not have the authority to permit this. In November 1779, after Congress passed and then rescinded one resolution on the matter, a clothing allowance was finally voted, to be granted on the same basis as it had been in 1777 to line officers. When additional regulations governing the drawing of clothing were passed for line officers a few days later, physicians were again omitted, and the oversight was not remedied until September 1780. It should be noted, however, that as late as March 1780, even line officers were apparently not in actual practice receiving clothing from the Army. The members of Congress also agreed in November 1779 upon legislation assigning Army physicians a monetary subsistence allowance to replace the rations assigned them in 1777 and to be based on a formula derived from the pay scale of line officers, the Director General receiving a colonel's share.[68]

Army doctors resented, however, the fact that they still had not been granted retirement half pay for a seven-year period as had line officers in 1778. To force Congress to assign them half pay, they threatened in December 1779 to resign en masse the following January 1780. An attempt to put through the desired measure on 3 January 1780 failed of passage, but the men of the Hospital Department did not, despite their disappointment, desert their patients by carrying out their threat of mass resignations, even when line officers were given half pay for life in October 1780. Not until 17 January 1781 and only after strong urging by Washington were medical officers included under half-pay provisions passed earlier for line officers. According to the 1781 legislation, all medical officers appointed by Congress who remained in the service for the entire war would receive half pay for life, but the Director was paid as if his rank were that of a lieutenant colonel. Medical officers also received at this time compensation for the effects of depreciation, a measure they had been supporting since 1780.[69]

The ability of the department to function was further diminished by stories of great abuses within the Hospital Department, spurred by Rush's almost continuous criticisms, which again began to carry considerable weight in 1779, when demands for further reform reappeared. A request for $1 million for the Hospital Department was halved after violent debate on the waste believed to characterize its operations, especially as far as food and wine were concerned. Benjamin Rush, who had resigned his commission in the Hospital Department as a result of his quarrels with Shippen and was by now considered to be the Director General's bitter enemy, accused Shippen of trading in the very hospital stores with which Congress was most concerned, especially wine and sugar. In June 1779, his own name cleared, Morgan joined Rush in clamoring that Shippen be court-martialed. Since Washington insisted that nothing be done until the campaign of that season was complete, however, Morgan's demands that Shippen be at least suspended from office until he could be brought to trial were in vain.[70]

By December 1779, preparations for the court-martial of the Director General were under way, but the Hospital Department was facing further hardships. The winter of 1779–80 was unusually bitter, food was scarce, and the deep snow hindered the delivery of provisions. When a thaw set in, the resulting mud made roads impassable. By March 1780, when the case against Shippen was ready for trial, hospital stores, according to Cochran, were exhausted.[71]

Most of the accusations which were formally placed against Shippen originated in the period of Rush's service in 1776 and early 1777 when, as Shippen pointed out, Morgan had voluntarily remained in enemy-occupied Philadelphia.[72] Morgan was, therefore, forced to rely heavily upon Rush in his attempts to disgrace his old enemy. Rush was a man of obvious charm but questionable integrity. A contemporary, Dr. Thomas Bond, who was described by Whitfield Bell as "one of the sanest of the Philadelphia physicians" and at one time praised by Rush himself,[73] commented bluntly that Rush was "capable of LYING in the WORST SENSE of that approbrious [sic] word" and called him "an unprincipled man."[74]

In the spring of 1780, Morgan and Rush were ready to present five formal charges against their enemy. Shippen was accused of fraud in selling hospital stores as his own and moving them at government expense in government-owned wagons, of speculation in hospital stores and adulterating hospital wines at Bethlehem, of keeping no regular set of accounts for the Hospital Department, of neglect of his hospital duties to the point where soldiers died as a result, and of behavior unbecoming an officer and a gentleman in his alleged attacks upon Morgan. Unfortunately, the official records of the prolonged trial have not survived so that only the correspondence of that period and the newspaper evidence of the struggle in the form of "letters to the editor" can shed light upon the nature of the testimony offered by both sides during the trial and during the hearings of the Continental Congress which followed it.[75]

The reputations of Shippen and Morgan are still controversial. The documents of the time, however, indicate that the major difficulties of the Hospital Department were not only frustrating but also inevitable and not to be blamed upon any single man or group of men. It seems likely, furthermore, that neither Shippen nor anyone else could have emerged unscathed from an attack by Morgan and Rush once their ire had been sufficiently aroused. Shippen appears to have been the kind of man the ambitious Morgan (and perhaps Rush also) wished to be and to have won without great effort the acclaim Morgan was struggling so fiercely to gain for himself. On the other hand, Shippen does not seem to have been, for all his charm and talent, capable of great self-sacrifice. The basic conflict here appears to have been not so much of principle as of personality and ambition.

On 27 June 1780, the court-martial acquitted Shippen of all the charges against him, noting in the instance of the speculation charge, however, that Shippen had indeed speculated in stores of the kind used in hospitals and that this was "highly improper and justly reprehensible." The final charge, that of conduct unbecoming an officer, was dismissed as "groundless and malicious." [76]

The results of the trial established that, despite their claims, Morgan and Rush could not find witnesses to prove the first charge of selling stores belonging to the hospital for his personal profit. Dr. Bond's testimony that the third charge, of not keeping proper accounts, was false was apparently convincing. The charge of neglect made public much conflicting testimony, possibly including letters dated 1777 from Rush himself in which he praised Shippen's conduct of the department. The trial also raised questions as to the propriety of the ways in which Morgan and Rush had gathered their testimony on this charge.[77]

Since the court-martial had taken place at the request of Congress, Washington wished its verdict to have congressional approval, but he urged that it hurry its decision because of the disordered state of the Hospital Department. After some delay in coming to a decision, on 18 August 1780, a month after it received the court's verdict, the Continental Congress resolved that "The court martial having acquitted the said Dr. W. Shippen, *Ordered*, that he be discharged from arrest." [78]

This was by no means the end of the matter, however. Morgan, despite his earlier firm assurances that he would abide by the court's decision no matter what it might be, joined Rush in criticizing the verdict, the court's methods of handling the trial, the officers conducting it, and Shippen's witnesses, using as their vehicle a newspaper, the *Pennsylvania Packet*.[79]

Although Shippen remained as Director General of the Hospital Department, Congress still believed that reform was desirable. The Medical Committee brought in a report in July, and a reform resolve was finally adopted on 30 September, to be followed on 6–7 October by the election of officers for the newly reorganized department.[80]

The new legislation increased the role of Congress in choosing department personnel, who were reduced in number through a reorganization which no longer called for a separate staff for each geographical division. (*See Appendix F.*) The posts of Deputy and Assistant Deputy Directors General were among those eliminated. The office of Purveyor was officially created; the Purveyor was required to render his accounts to the Board of the Treasury rather than to the Director General. Three chief hospital physicians were responsible for the general hospital system and a chief physician for each army supervised the regimental medical staff. The fifteen senior hospital physicians, in addition to the highest ranking members of the department, were all to be elected by Congress. Any participation in trade by employees or members of the department was forbidden, and all medical officers from surgeon's mates upward were to receive allotments of land upon retirement just as had been voted line officers earlier, the Director ranking for this particular purpose as brigadier general and the surgeon's mates as captains. The Army hospitals from North Carolina to Georgia, however, were to continue under the old organization.[81]

When elections were held for the newly reorganized department, Shippen, rather than being quietly dropped, as might have been expected had serious credence been given to the charges so recently placed against him, was reelected as Director General. John Cochran and James Craik, both recommended by Washington, in addition to Malachi Treat and Charles McKnight, received other top posts. The next day the rest of the medical staff was selected; [82] it was apparently determined at this time that only one Chief Physician and Surgeon General for the Army was needed and the position was given to Cochran.

Officers of the Army Hospital Department as of 7 October 1780 were:

Director General, William Shippen, Jr.

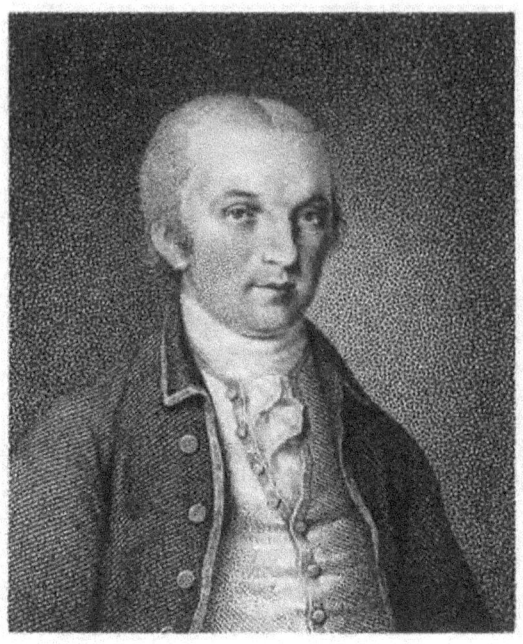

JOHN COCHRAN. *(Courtesy of National Library of Medicine.)*

Chief Physician and Surgeon General of the Army, John Cochran
Chief Hospital Physicians and Surgeons, James Craik, Malachi Treat, Charles McKnight
Purveyor, Thomas Bond, Jr.
Assistant Purveyor, Isaac Ledyard
Apothecary, Andrew Craigie
Assistant Apothecary, William Johonot
Hospital Physicians and Surgeons, James Tilton, Samuel Adams, David Townshend, Henry Latimer, Francis Hagan, Philip Turner, William Burnet, John Warren, Moses Scott, David Jackson, Bodo Otto, Moses Bloomfield, William Eustis, George Draper, Barnabas Binney.

SOURCE: Ford, *Journals of the Continental Congress,* 18:908-10.

Despite repeated reorganizations, the old problem of supply remained. In December, the Medical Committee admitted to the Continental Congress "That on account of the failures in obtaining money, the sick are in a suffering condition; The Physicians unable to proceed to their respective charges, and the business of the Department greatly impeeded [*sic*] in every part." Bond, as Purveyor, was unable to obtain even such funds as had been voted to him. As the winter deepened, transportation difficulties once more complicated the desperate supply situation and the lack of funds further hindered attempts to obtain horses and wagons. With conditions becoming ever more grave, on 3 January 1781, Shippen resigned, claiming that he did so because Congress had decided that the duties of a professor of anatomy and those of the Director General of the Hospital were not compatible.[83]

THE HOSPITAL DEPARTMENT UNDER COCHRAN

On 11 January, John Cochran and two others were nominated for the post of Director General, and on the 13th, John Morgan was added to the list of candidates. On the 17th, Cochran was elected. The new Director was known to his contemporaries as "an able and experienced practitioner." He also apparently possessed considerable administrative ability, badly needed at this time.[84] He had achieved an enviable professional reputation without the benefit of graduation from any formal medical school, having been entirely apprentice trained, but had gained military experience as a surgeon's mate in the French and Indian War. Not as personally ambitious as his predecessors, he once wrote that his "appointment was unsolicited, and a rank to which I never aspired, being perfectly happy where I was." He openly maintained that he preferred James Craik for the post. He had considerable experience in the Continental Army, having been appointed Assistant Director of the flying camp hospital in 1776, Surgeon General of the Middle Department in 1777, and Chief Physician and Surgeon of the Army in 1780.[85]

On the same day that Cochran was appointed Director General, several changes were made in the rules governing the Hospital Department. The power of the Chief Physician and Surgeon of the Army to remove regimental surgeons and mates for neglect of duty was modified so that these officers could only be suspended until they could be court-martialed, hospital physicians were empowered to appoint matrons, nurses, and other lesser figures necessary to the smooth functioning of Army hospitals, and the half-pay provision was passed.[86]

Various other changes in the organization of the Hospital Department followed one upon the other throughout the last three years of the war. In March 1781, the Southern Department was at last brought directly under the Director General, although in his absence from that area, its administration was placed under its own Deputy Director, Dr. David Oliphant. The entire staff in the South included, in addition to the Deputy Director, a Deputy Apothecary, a Deputy Purveyor, a Chief Physician of the Hospital who was required also to have the skills of a surgeon, two hospital physicians also to be qualified as surgeons, four surgeon's mates, one assistant each to the Deputy Purveyor and Deputy Apothecary, and lesser figures as necessary. Named to these positions were men who had served under Oliphant in the South before this change, including Dr. Peter Fayssoux as Chief Physician of the Hospital.[87]

In May 1781, the Medical Committee which had for so long supervised the affairs of the Hospital Department was discontinued and the department was required to submit its returns to the Board of War. The board was itself superseded later in the year by the War Office under Secretary of War Benjamin Lincoln. The following July, a hospital board was established, consisting of the Director General, the Chief Physician of the Army or one of the Chief Hospital Physicians, and two hospital physicians, with a general officer presiding who could exercise a tie-breaking vote as necessary. This board was assigned the task of determining the fitness of applicants for positions applied for in the Hospital Department.[88]

Still not satisfied with the operations of the Hospital Department, the Continental Congress began in the fall of 1781 to consider complex proposals for yet another reform. Among the ideas examined was a suggestion that a complete turnabout be made and the use of regimental hospitals strongly encouraged. By early January 1782, however, the committee studying the matter had determined that, since the war was apparently near an end, such a complete change was not appropriate and that lesser modifications would be satisfactory. The offices of the Chief Hospital Physician and of the Chief Physician of the Army were abolished and a three-man hospital board was set up to examine all candidates for promotion and to give advice.[89]

Under the new legislation, the Purveyor, under whom the stewards were to serve, was to report to the Superintendent of Finance, Robert Morris, appointed in 1781 to bring order to the chaotic finances of the Revolution. Further steps were also taken to tighten accounting methods. A committee investigating this matter recommended in July 1782 that an invariable standard of prices be established in the apothecary's office to systemize accounting. Accounting procedures were carefully outlined in detail so that this aspect of the department could function in as orderly a manner as possible. The committee also requested an immediate inventory of all the public property held by any medical officer. By October 1782, Morris was ready to appoint commissioners to settle the Hospital Department's accounts.[90]

The winter of 1780–81 was a tragic one for the Continental Army and particularly for the Hospital Department. Shortages were extremely severe, to the point where some hospital physicians were unable to make out their returns because of the shortage of paper. Cochran wrote repeatedly to the President of Congress, emphasizing his belief that "unless some speedy and effectual means are taken to relieve the sick, a number of valuable soldiers in the American Army will perish through want of necessaries." In February, Cochran was ordered to take over all publicly owned stores being held in private hands and, in at least one instance, Washington stated that, if necessary, force should be used to acquire this property. Specifically mentioned at this time were the medicines of Dr. Isaac Foster, former Deputy Director General in the Eastern Department and former acting Director after Church's disgrace, who, maintaining that he had not been reimbursed for drug purchases, refused to turn over his supply.[91]

The appointment of Morris as Superintendent of Finance on 29 February 1781 led to a gradual improvement in the young nation's finances, which in time favorably affected the supply problems of the Hospital Department; in January 1781, the Army was experiencing mutinies, and by March, the staffs of some hospitals were reduced to sending ambulatory patients into the surrounding communities to beg for food. Even in the summer of 1781, Army patients were "suffering extreme distress for stores of every kind," physicians were being asked to furnish their own instruments, and Bond, as Purveyor, was being urged to turn once again to the ladies of surrounding communities to obtain old linens for dressings.

Although the decisive battle of Yorktown culminated in the British surrender in October 1781, the Continental Army was still experiencing supply shortages well into the summer of 1782.[92] Many suppliers had not been paid and, as a result, were reluctant to continue to deal with the Continental government. By early 1782, Bond was being accused of using the money sent him "to different Purposes from those which were intended," and of delaying the sending in of his reports. Morris sharply informed the Purveyor in February 1782 that "Until I am possessed of these Things, I will not advance one Shilling for the Purpose." Bond's deficiencies as far as reports were concerned so distressed Morris that, in June 1783, he wrote the unfortunate physician that he would very much regret it if he were forced by Bond's delinquency to request these documents "in Terms which might excite your Painful emotions."[93]

By the fall of 1782, however, supplies and gold were beginning to arrive from France,[94] by which time, of course, the need for supplies was dwindling as the pace of the war slowed.

When Cochran became Director General of the Hospital Department in 1781, however, the personal financial situation of the officers of the department still was neither clear nor strong. The most immediate problem at this time was the tardy arrival of pay, which in some instances was two years overdue. This situation led even to resignation on the part of physicians unable to support themselves and their families under such circumstances. Cochran himself was at times unable to pay his way to Philadelphia to bring the department's problems before Congress. When Congress did issue warrants for pay, inflation seriously undercut their worth. "For God's sake," Cochran wrote Robert Morris on 26 July 1781, "help us as soon as you can. Most of our officers have not received one shilling of pay in upwards of two years." Furthermore, Cochran noted that the French paid their military doctors over half again as much as the American doctors were supposed to be receiving and that even the British medical officer was better paid than his colonial counterpart.[95] Although legislation calling, on paper, for compensation for depreciation had been granted to medical officers, when attempts were made to execute this law, difficulties were encountered. The warrants for this purpose were to be drawn on the states, but New York refused to go along,⁹⁶ and none of the states was in a position to pay a lump sum all at once. Pennsylvania, for example, decided to issue "Certificates of Indebtedness" as compensation.

The problem of half pay was only partly settled, although the original resolution on this subject was dated January 1781. In March 1783, a new modification was proposed, permitting the officers of the Hospital Department, as well as line officers, to receive five years of full pay in money or securities at 6 percent rather than half pay for life, if they so voted as a group.⁹⁷

Resignations, often prompted by financial problems, left openings within the Hospital Department and raised the question of standards for promotion. Men such as Dr. James Tilton favored a general promotion by seniority, but Cochran noted the possibility of the promotion of unqualified men and pointed out that the British did not promote in this manner. "It affords me but Melancholy Prospect," he wrote, "when Gentlemen, who are capable and willing to do their Duty, . . . take their departure from us. . . . God knows, with what kind of Cattle their Places will be supplied." ⁹⁸ Less than three weeks later, Cochran pointed out in a letter to the President of Congress that he had several vacancies and suggested that the most senior mates could move up. By July, there were seven vacancies among the fifteen positions of hospital physician. Congress ordered that vacancies in the state lines be filled as would any other vacancy within the regiment and that the Director appoint men to fill any positions vacant in the regiments not of state lines. By August, Washington was urging that an overall solution be developed for the problem, and Cochran was wondering if Congress had forgotten the wounded and sick. By September, there was also an urgent need for physicians within the Southern Department, but Cochran believed that these vacancies should be filled by southern physicians who could report for duty at once rather than by men promoted to these positions from the north.⁹⁹

On 20 September 1781, the matter finally reached a vote and Tilton's recommendations for promotion by seniority were adopted. Senior hospital physicians from hospitals recently closed were to receive first consideration for vacancies at that level. Hospital mates of the greatest seniority and regimental surgeons held the next priority, the two classifications to be equally ranked and examinations necessary for both. Appointments to the highest positions were still to be made by Congress, in theory on the basis of merit alone.¹⁰⁰

On 21 September, however, once again a motion was put before Congress to completely rescind a resolution just passed the previous day. This attempt to rescind Tilton's proposal failed of passage, but on the 22d, a motion to suspend the promotion of mates to physicians passed. On 3 January 1782, Congress ordered that hospital physicians be appointed from amongst hospital mates and regimental surgeons. The latter, to qualify ahead of the former, would have to take an examination to prove their competence. The obvious reluctance of Congress to promote physicians apparently stemmed from the conviction that the department already had enough officers in each rank.¹⁰¹

During the summer of 1782, Washington was in correspondence with the British general, Sir Guy Carleton, over the matter of granting immunity from prisoner-of-war status to hospital officers as first proposed by Carleton. By September 1782, Washington was able to notify his generals Heath and Knox that Congress had, on 9 September, resolved that captured surgeons, hospital officers, and chaplains were no longer to be classified as prisoners of war.¹⁰²

Even before the British surrender at Yorktown in October 1781, however, Cochran received totally unexpected orders from the Board of War to start closing hospitals, beginning with those at Yellow Springs, Pennsylvania, Albany, and Boston. He found these orders most confusing, since the cost of closing the Boston and Albany hospitals and transferring the patients elsewhere would be great both in money and in the danger to the patients. Some who were interested in the problem were now raising once again the old matter of the death rate in general hospitals, as Cochran noted in a letter to Craik, and were saying that general hospitals should be eliminated entirely in favor of regimental hospitals. Cochran likened this attitude to the notion that one should never go to bed because so many people died there; he told the President of Congress that he feared that Congress was not so familiar with the medical establishment as it might be and was being unduly swayed by the advice of those who were seeking their own advantage. "I fear we have some evil Counselors who are endeavoring to lead us astray, for astray we are going, as fast as the devil can drive us," he wrote to Dr. Barnabas Binney.[103]

Cochran apparently resigned himself to the closing of the Boston unit in the face of the argument that it held few Continental patients and that the state should assume the responsibility for returning prisoners and Massachusetts recruits. He believed, nevertheless, that the breakup of the Boston and Albany hospitals would be very expensive. Money would be necessary to procure accommodations for the patients who were put out of these facilities when the nearest hospital still open was 200 miles away. To save a relatively small sum, the Board of War, in Cochran's opinion, was spending a large sum.[104]

Although Cochran wrote to Dr. John Warren in Boston in October 1781 that the Boston hospital must be closed, he hoped to delay the closing of the Albany hospital, especially since he had just ordered 200 more men to be sent there. Cochran seems to have had his way as far as the Albany hospital was concerned, for it was still in operation in November of 1782.[105]

It was almost two years after the Yorktown victory that, on 3 September 1783, the Peace of Paris was finally signed. On 18 October, Congress resolved to disband the Army as of 3 November, and on 23 October, the wartime Hospital Department was replaced by an institution to aid those "invalids of the army and navy"[106] still in need of care.

During the most active years of the Revolution, the Continental Army's Hospital Department had been crippled by confused legislation. Its staff, often unpaid, frequently without needed medicines and supplies, torn by feuds, its reputation tarnished by the ambitions and greed of a few, struggled against hopeless odds in the often vain attempt to provide adequate care for the sick and wounded. Death rates in Continental hospitals in this period were high and conditions in them, particularly at those times when the Army was suffering its greatest reverses, were often horrible. The most vocal critics of these institutions, however, were physicians whose comments were their weapons in their bitter feuds. It should be noted, furthermore, that even the civilian facilities of Europe, which in some instances were housed in magnificent buildings designed specifically to serve as hospitals, might shock those who visited them; the Paris Hôtel Dieu, for example, with its four to six patients in a bed, its stench-filled rooms, and its appalling death rate, which at times reached a reported 33 percent, was notorious.[107] In the eighteenth century, hospitals established on an emergency basis in hastily procured buildings and filled to overflowing with patients from a lice-infested, starving, wretched, and retreating army could not be expected to exhibit conditions which were other than frightful.

Only in the closing years of the Revolution did the picture brighten, when the chain of command was clarified, the most contentious physicians were no longer with the department, and money and supplies began to come in from France just as the lack of major engagements began to reduce the patient load. It was at this point in the war that the officers of the American Army's first Medical Department began to receive recognition of their devotion to duty when the Congress granted them the same pensions, allowances, and other considerations which had already been awarded to officers of the line.

3

From Siege to Retreat, 1775 to May 1777

The months between 27 July 1775, when the Hospital Department was established, and the late spring of 1777, when General Washington's army left its winter camp at Morristown, New Jersey, to begin another campaign, saw the scope of Continental Army operations broaden from a largely inactive siege of Boston to action on two fronts, along the Canadian border and in the general vicinity of New York City and northern New Jersey. It was a time of limited successes for the new army and of increasing strain upon the Hospital Department.

THE BOSTON AREA, 1775 TO 1776

The 17,000-man New England army, composed for the most part of Massachusetts units, which was positioned outside of British-occupied Boston in July 1775, was both disorganized and undisciplined. Enlisted men generally ignored both camp and personal hygiene and regarded attempts to discipline them as tyranny, but when General Washington assumed command, only 9.5 to 12.5 percent of them were

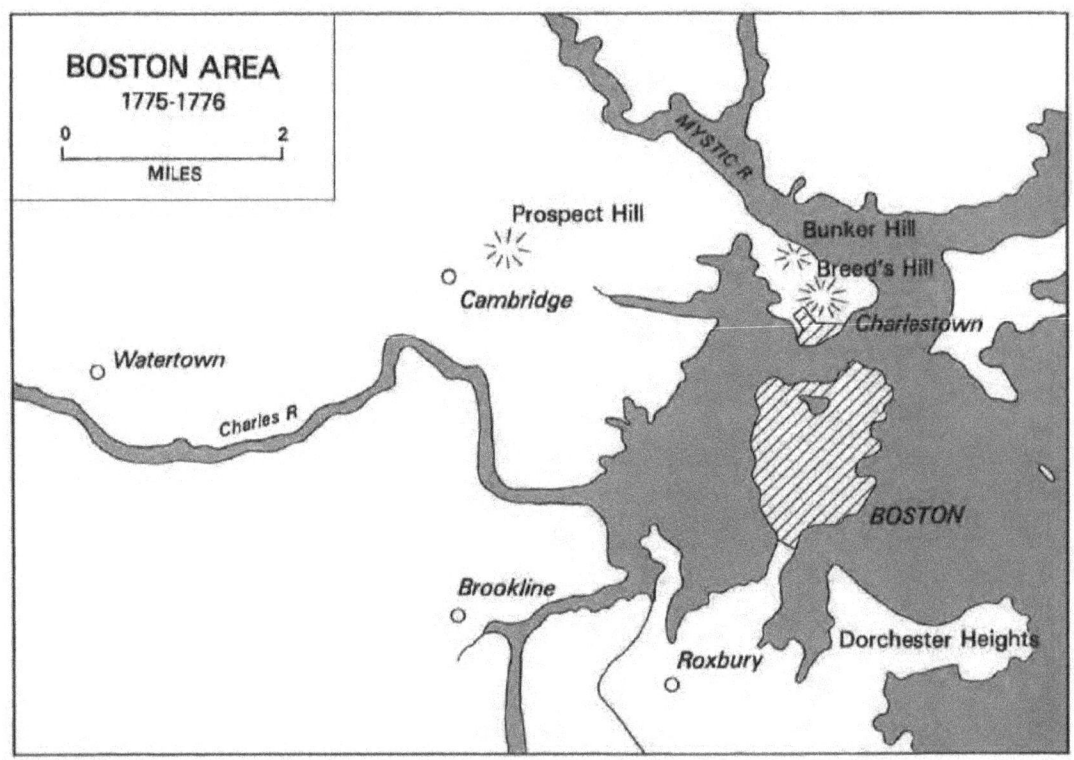

MAP 1

unfit for duty. Except for makeshift regimental facilities, the only hospitals available were those managed by Massachusetts at Cambridge, Roxbury, and Watertown. (*Map 1*) These hospitals seem to have made no attempt to segregate those with contagious diseases from the wounded, visitors were allowed unlimited access to patients, and the most elementary rules of hospital discipline were ignored.[1]

During his short time as Director General, however, Benjamin Church managed to instill some order into the medical service of Washington's army. By the late summer he had divided the Hospital Department's patients among six buildings, 200 in houses named after Generals Washington, Lee, and Putnam and served by surgeons Isaac Foster, John Warren, Samuel Adams, Jr., and Charles McKnight in Cambridge, and 170 in three others serving the Roxbury

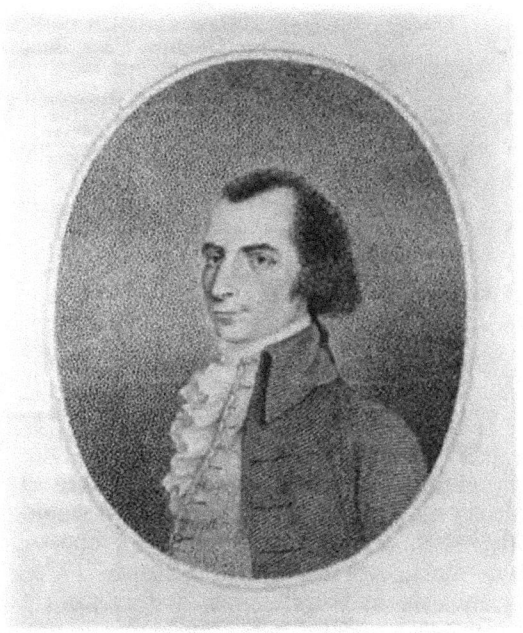

CHARLES MCKNIGHT. (*Courtesy of National Library of Medicine.*)

camp but actually located, according to Church, in Brookline. The care of Roxbury patients was supervised by William Aspinwall, Lemuel Hayward, and Elisha Perkins, all three in the pay of individual colonies rather than that of the Hospital Department. Church, however, urged that three more surgeons be appointed to serve with the department.[2] In December, John Morgan referred to Aspinwall and Hayward as "additional surgeons," so apparently they were by then members of the department staff. However, no records exist giving exact information on this point. Church also planned in August to acquire more beds so that he could expand the Cambridge hospital to a 240-bed capacity.[3]

Church had noted that his patients were returning to duty before fully regaining their strength and that, as a result, as many as four of five relapsed and had to return to the hospital. He urged the creation of a unit specifically for convalescents where,

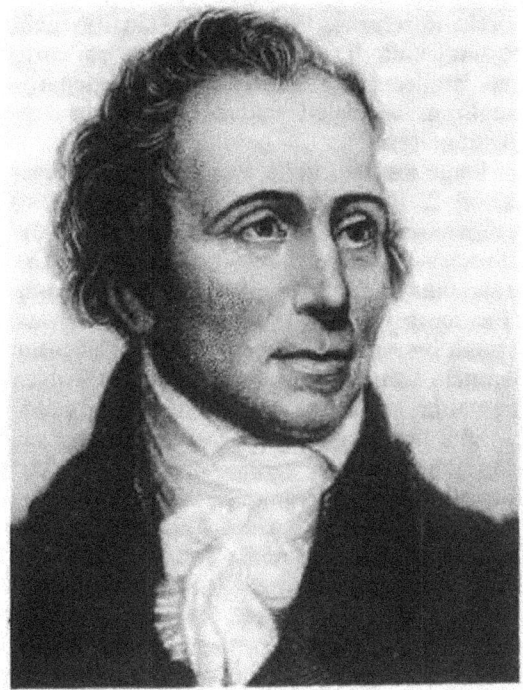

JOHN WARREN. (*Courtesy of National Library of Medicine.*)

TABLE 2—HOSPITAL DEPARTMENT UNITS IN THE BOSTON AREA WITH THE STATUS OF PATIENTS DURING WEEK PRECEDING 2 DECEMBER 1775

Hospital	Admitted Since Last Return	Dismissed Fit for Service	Discharged From the Army	To Convalescent Hospital	Absent With Permission	Absent Without Permission	Dead	Remaining
Total	128	95	5	51	1	6	13	ᵃ 377
At Cambridge:								
Washington House	25	8	0	15	0	1	2	69
Lee House	13	10	0	0	0	1	2	65
Putnam House	12	5	0	12	0	0	2	47
Convalescent House	26	30	2	0	0	4	0	80
At Roxbury:								
Ward House	18	0	1	19	0	0	5	39
Thomas House	14	17	0	5	0	0	2	50
Spencer House (convalescents)	20	25	2	0	1	0	0	37

SOURCE: John Morgan, Return of the Sick & Wounded in the General Hospital at Cambridge & Roxbury, 25 Nov 1775–2 Dec 1775, RG 93, M246 roll 135, folder 3–1, item 15.
ᵃ Morgan's addition.

if a Hospital Department physician were to check on them each day, such patients would otherwise need merely the care of one or two mates. By the end of October 1775, a convalescent hospital was in operation in Cambridge, and by late November, it was apparently caring for as many as seventy to eighty patients at a time.[4]

On Church's recommendation, General Washington took action designed to improve hospital discipline. On 21 August, he assigned a guard consisting of a sergeant, a corporal, and nine men to one of the hospital buildings. The following day, commenting that Church had informed him that patients were suffering as a result of "having improper things carried to them to eat" and that many of the illnesses afflicting them might have been brought in by visitors, the general ordered that no enlisted man or noncommissioned officer be allowed to enter a hospital without written permission from either his commanding officer or a surgeon. A week later, the general decided to organize the separate guards being set up at individual hospitals into one guard, to consist of "one Sub three Sergeants one fife Three Corporals & Thirty men," taking their orders from Church.[5]

Despite Church's efforts, when John Morgan became Director General, much was yet to be accomplished if the Hospital Department were to care for the sick and wounded of General Washington's army efficiently. Since his first inspection revealed that no one could tell him the number of patients for whom the department was responsible, Morgan ordered that weekly reports, or returns, be made to him by each hospital unit. It is from these that we learn the details of the structure of the department as it existed under Morgan in the Boston area.

Four hospital units were in Cambridge as of 2 December 1775, when the first return was made, the three named during Church's administration after the three generals plus the newer Convalescent House. The return from Washington House was signed by surgeon John Warren. Doctors Samuel Adams, Jr., and James McHenry, the latter apparently a regimental surgeon at this time, signed the return from Lee House, where five wards were named after patriots Henry, Franklin, Gadsden, Rodney, and Gates. Charles McKnight signed the report from Putnam House, where six wards were named after famous physicians, Pringle, Monro, Black, Shippen, Cullen, and Hunter. Surgeon's mate Daniel Scott signed the return from the Convalescent House. Cambridge patients ranged in age from 16 to 60 and the most frequent diagnosis was "fever." There were also three

TABLE 3—HOSPITAL DEPARTMENT UNITS IN THE BOSTON AREA WITH THE STATUS OF PATIENTS DURING WEEK PRECEDING 16 DECEMBER 1775

Hospital	Admitted Since Last Return	Dismissed Fit for Service	Discharged From the Army	To Convalescent Hospital	Absent With Permission	Absent Without Permission	Dead	Remaining
Total	a 155	117	5	29	1	4	11	341
At Cambridge:								
Washington House	23	11	1	7	0	0	0	73
Lee House	22	0	0	10	0	0	3	62
Putnam House	21	8	2	6	0	2	3	52
Convalescent House	29	25	2	0	1	2	0	67
At Roxbury:								
Ward House	11	29	0	2	0	0	2	15
Thomas House	16	19	0	4	0	0	3	49
Spencer House (convalescents)	23	25	0	0	0	0	0	23

SOURCE: John Morgan, Return of the Sick & Wounded in the General Hospital at Cambridge & Roxbury, 9–16 Dec 1775, RG 93, M246, roll 135, folder 3–1, item 16.
a Morgan's addition.

units at Roxbury, Thomas and Ward Houses and the convalescent hospital, Spencer House. Since the Roxbury returns were not signed, the surgeons or mates in charge there remain anonymous.[6]

The Director General's report to General Washington of this same date was typical in its form and its casual arithmetic of the many which Morgan was to submit from the Boston area in the following months. (*Table 2*) His patients during these first weeks did not total the 676 he claimed, although this figure has been uncritically repeated by subsequent historians.[7] In reaching his overall total in this instance, Morgan apparently added together the totals from all of the individual columns, thus counting both convalescents and newly admitted patients twice. A more accurate figure would appear to be 497. In his report of 16 December 1775, as an example of his arithmetic, Morgan not only incorrectly totaled the number of admissions to Hospital Department units (ten too many) but also concluded that the department cared for 512 patients, a figure at which it is difficult to arrive using Morgan's figures. (*Table 3*) It is interesting to note that, while these early returns were entirely handwritten, beginning with that of 2 March 1776, Morgan used preprinted forms into which the appropriate entries were made.[8]

The health of the army besieging Boston when Morgan became Director General was considered by contemporaries to have been unusually good, although the number of men unfit for duty after General Washington took command apparently ran from less than 14 percent to approximately 17 percent per month, if one can trust monthly strength reports. The number of patients actually in Hospital Department units varied from 320 to 550 in the period 16 December 1776 to 30 March 1777 and the death rate from 1.4 percent of these patients to 4 percent.[9] (*Table 4*) The most greatly feared threat to the health of the army came from within the city of Boston, where for months smallpox raged.

TABLE 4—MORTALITY, 16 DECEMBER 1775–30 MARCH 1776

Date	Total Patients	Dead
16–24 Dec 1775	439	8
23–30 Dec	465	9
30 Dec–6 Jan 1776	442	18
13–20 Jan	419	7
26 Jan–3 Feb	504	12
3–10 Feb	497	13
17–24 Feb	520	16
24 Feb–2 Mar	550	11
2–9 Mar	485	7
11–17 Mar	404	6
23–30 Mar	320	6

SOURCE: Returns of the Sick & Wounded in the General Hospital at Cambridge & Roxbury, 16 Dec 1775–30 Mar 1776, RG 93, M246, roll 135, folder 3–1, items 17–27.

RETURN SIGNED BY CHARLES MCKNIGHT. (*Courtesy of National Archives.*)

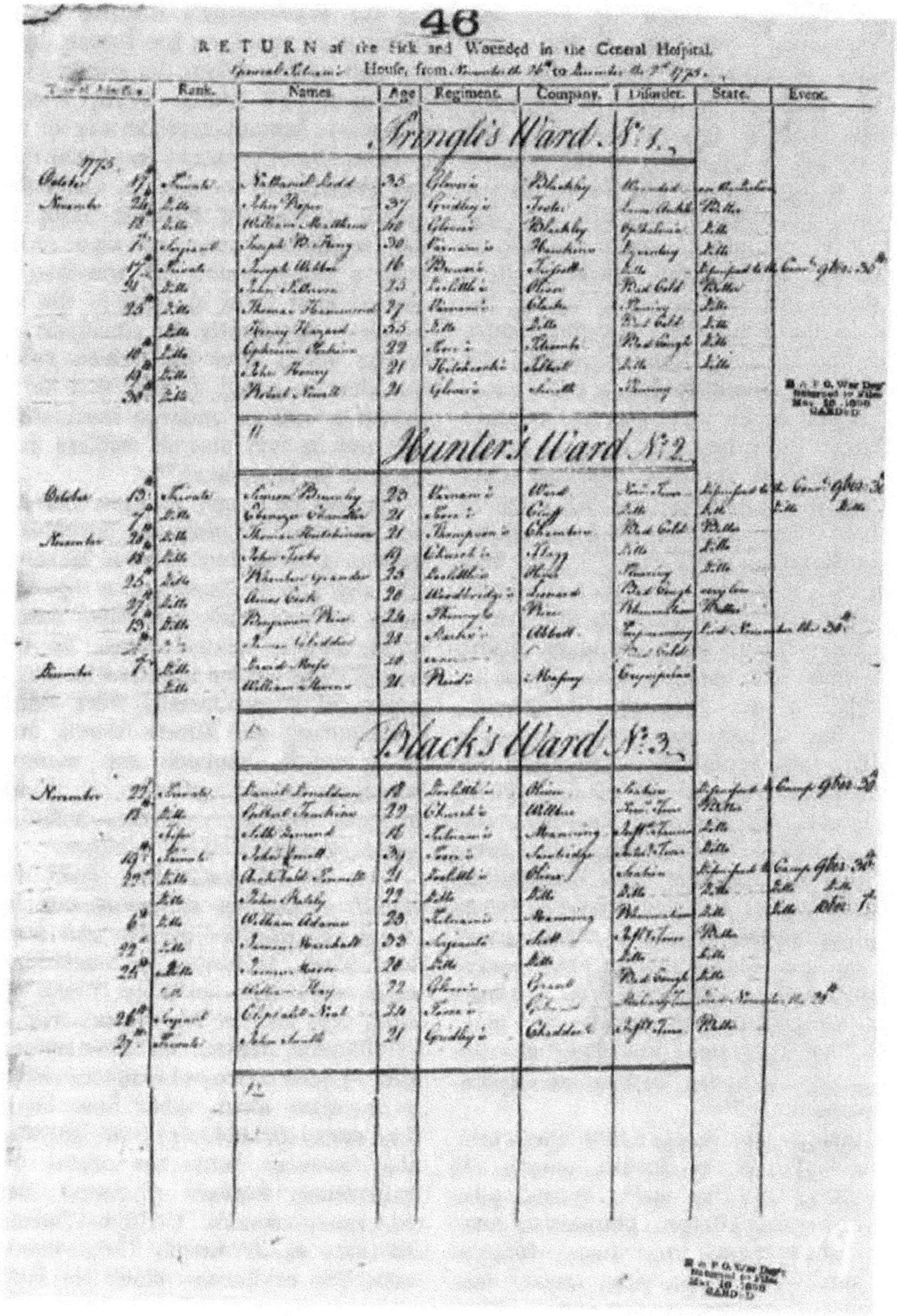
46
RETURN of the Sick and Wounded in the General Hospital.
House, from
Rank.
Names.
Age
Regiment.
Company.
Disorder.
State.
Event.
Pringle's Ward. No. 1.
Hunter's Ward No. 2
Black's Ward No. 3.

In the fall and winter of 1775–76, rumors abounded that the British were deliberately attempting to infect their enemies by sending diseased or recently inoculated civilians out of the city. The records on the hospitalizing of the Army's smallpox victims during this entire period are incomplete, but a smallpox hospital had been in operation, under the supervision of Dr. Isaac Rand, since 27 June 1775. Rand was among those caring for patients in the Cambridge hospital under Church, but at some time thereafter the threat posed by smallpox waned and General Washington decided to close the hospital. In December 1775, however, Morgan noting that smallpox had appeared "several times in the army," requested that the care of its victims once again be assigned exclusively to Rand and his mate.[10] The first mention of a smallpox hospital as reestablished under Morgan appears in the Director General's report of 20 January 1776. At this time, five patients were listed as "remaining" in the Cambridge institution, implying that it had gone into operation before that date. From the returns that followed through the end of March 1776, it would seem not only that smallpox was a minor problem for Washington's army at this time but also that mass inoculation of soldiers was not being undertaken, since the greatest number listed as "remaining" at any one time was twelve and the weekly admission never exceeded six. James Thacher, a regimental surgeon at this time, recorded that the most prevalent diseases were actually autumnal fevers and dysenterylike conditions.[11]

Nevertheless, the threat of smallpox continued to hang over the Boston area in the early months of 1776, and a Boston publisher even reissued Baron Dimsdale's pamphlet on inoculation, for which Morgan wrote a preface. It has been argued that the presence of smallpox in the city of Boston was actually to some degree responsible for Washington's reliance upon siege rather than attack on the British during the fall and winter. When the enemy evacuated Boston on 17 March 1776, Washington, still wary, initially forbade any of his men to enter the city except for 1,000 men who had already had the disease, under the command of General Putnam. Both hospital and regimental surgeons were ordered to keep a sharp watch for smallpox victims and to send them at once to the isolation hospital. Apparently the contagion was still feared weeks after the British evacuation, for Thacher noted in May that he had believed it wise to undergo inoculation himself and in July that all soldiers in Boston were to be inoculated.[12]

During the siege, Morgan met the supply shortage affecting the hospitals in the Boston area by buying what he could himself and also by launching a vigorous campaign to have both individual citizens and states donate needed items. In Morgan's behalf, Washington appealed to the governments of Massachusetts, New Hampshire, Connecticut, and Rhode Island, and within a month blankets and materials for bandages were arriving at Cambridge. Morgan then set everyone, including surgeons, to work making bandages.

One of Morgan's first tasks after the British evacuation of Boston was to locate drugs and supplies for the new hospital in New York. In Boston he found that medicines were often held by Tories who hid what they had or by owners who, in fear of inflation, insisted on cash payments. In time, a good source of medicines also proved to be prize ships, taken from the British. The drugs left behind by the British in Boston, however, were the source of much controversy because of reports that they had been poisoned. Dr. John Warren testified that on 29 March 1776, when he entered the workhouse which the British had used as a hospital, he found the medicines in great disorder with small amounts of yellow and white arsenic mixed in with them. After learning that another physician had already removed twelve to fourteen pounds of this poison from among the drugs, Warren recommended that no attempt be made to use them. On Washington's orders and after offering to pay for what he took, Morgan did confiscate the drug supplies of two Tory physicians in Boston, one of whom was reputed to have the largest pharmaceutical business in the city.[13]

By June, having taken over a large quantity of abandoned British property and using every other means available to him, Morgan had acquired a large collection of bedding, medicines, furniture, and other supplies which, with the exception of the materials needed for medicine chests for five regiments left to defend Boston, he then had moved to Connecticut, as ordered by Washington. He was quite optimistic about the adequacy of his stock for the coming year, believing that he could easily obtain the little he still needed in Philadelphia. His optimism, however, was not entirely justified, since as early as April one of his principal suppliers was running low in items needed for regimental chests and by May was out of bark, ipecac, and cream of tartar, among other popular items.[14]

In anticipation of the active campaign against Boston, which the formation of new army units in March had made possible, Morgan also prepared a barracks at Prospect Hill which could care for at least 100 wounded. The fortification of Dorchester Heights by the Americans made the British position untenable, however, and they evacuated Boston. American losses in action, therefore, were slight, and Morgan's planning remained essentially untested.[15]

Almost immediately after the British left Boston, the Continental Army moved south to the defense of New York City, leaving Morgan with the dual problems of caring for the approximately three hundred patients left behind in the Boston area and of preparing to establish a new hospital system. Maj. Gen. Charles Lee, sent in January 1776 to prepare the defense of New York, had written Washington as early as 9 February to request the establishment of a hospital there, but it was not until 3 April that Morgan received official orders to do so. He was at that time told to leave behind in Boston only those surgeons and attendants necessary for the care of soldiers too ill to move with the army. Morgan placed Isaac Foster in charge of these patients, who did so well that the death rate among them was very low and by 22 April only eighty remained in department hands. Within six weeks of receiving orders to move the department's main operations from Boston, he discharged the last man and settled all his accounts for the Boston hospitals.[16]

THE NORTHERN
DEPARTMENT

In the Northern Department in the late summer and early fall of 1775, preparations were under way for an attack on Canada under the command of Maj. Gen. Philip Schuyler. (Map 2) These preparations left much to be desired. No department physicians were assigned to the expedition and some units even failed to bring regimental surgeons. Furthermore, General Schuyler still had no hospital supplies by the first week of August, when 100 of his 500 men were ill. On 6 August, he reported this situation to the Continental Congress, stating that he had already given up his own personal wine supply for the sick of his regiments and that he must have medical supplies even if he had to pay for them himself. He added that he had hired a surgeon from Albany on his own authority and that he would also meet this expense personally if Congress failed to act.[17]

Samuel Stringer, the physician appointed by General Schuyler, was requested to

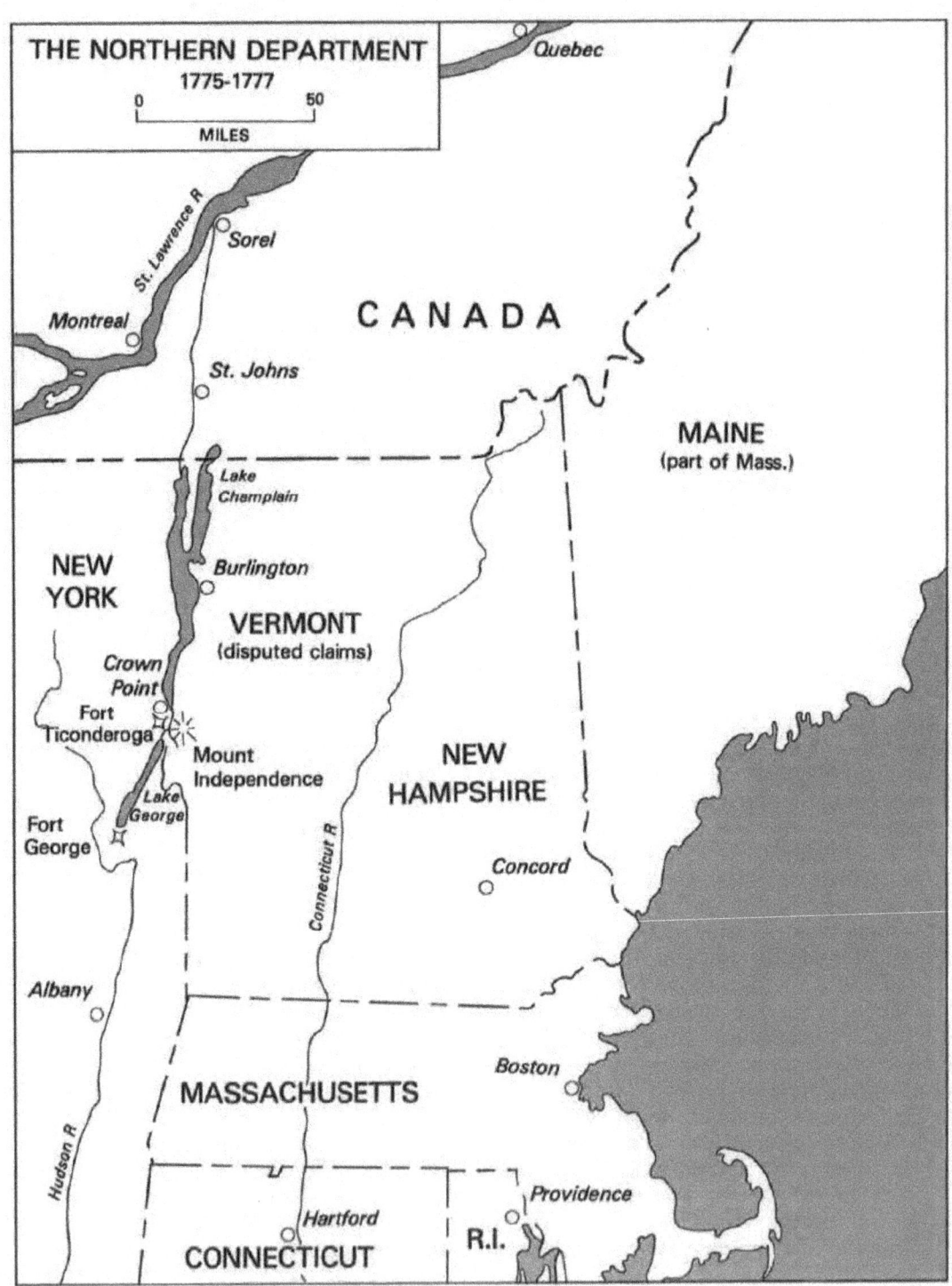

MAP 2

bring with him as many of the supplies he believed to be needed for Schuyler's army as time permitted him to gather. By 14 September, however, when Congress officially approved both Stringer's appointment and his reimbursement for the medicines he brought with him, General Schuyler had become too ill to continue in command and had been replaced by Brig. Gen. Richard Montgomery.[18]

Stringer's headquarters and that of Montgomery's 2,000-man army appear to have been at Fort George, at the southern end of Lake George. Stringer's only assistance here seems to have come from regimental surgeons and mates, but on 25 October, he requested the assignment of Hospital Department surgeons to serve under him. Stringer apparently accompanied the army only to Fort George, but General Montgomery continued to Montreal, taking the city on 12 November. By this date, however, disease, desertions, and expiring enlistments had reduced his army to 500 men. When he marched from Montreal to Quebec in December, 300 of the Montreal army went with him and they carried with them the seeds of a devastating epidemic of smallpox.

While General Montgomery's army moved on Montreal, Col. Benedict Arnold led approximately eleven hundred men on a second operation against Canada, aimed at the city of Quebec. The only medical attendants to accompany him on the grueling march through thick New England forests and swamps were the 22-year-old regimental surgeon Isaac Senter and his assistants. Senter organized the hospital used for the Continental troops before Quebec, but although this institution was called the "General Hospital," it received its name from the fact that the building housing it already bore that designation. While most of the Northern Army was at Quebec, the smallpox epidemic first struck. It continued through the spring and summer of 1776 and eventually involved not only the regimental surgeons and mates but also Stringer and the Hospital Department.[19]

By the spring of 1776, Brig. Gen. David Wooster was in overall command of the troops in Canada, General Montgomery having been killed in action in January, and almost half of the approximately 1,900 men before Quebec were sick. An abortive attempt was made to start an official inoculation program, since many officers and men were secretly inoculating themselves and were thus intensifying the epidemic. When British reinforcements arrived at Quebec and the colonial army fell back on Sorel, many smallpox victims left their beds to join the flight. The epidemic worsened at Sorel and the men in the Montreal area were in no better condition, 1,200 of the approximately 3,200 there in early May being unfit for duty, according to General Arnold, most of them sick with smallpox.[20]

The Hospital Department was by no means prepared to deal with the rapidly growing epidemic. Stringer wrote from St. Johns, where the army from Quebec retreated when it left Sorel, that he had neither medicines nor instruments and no way of obtaining either. It was in late May, however, that he finally received permission to hire a larger staff.[21]

A committee of the Continental Congress urged in early May, when new units were arriving and the total number of men in Canada was approaching 8,000, that Dr. Jonathan Potts be hired by the Hospital Department for assignment to either Canada or Fort George. By the end of May 1776, the situation of patients in the Northern Department was "almost Sufficient to excite the pity of Brutes, Large barns [being] filled with men at the very heighth [sic] of smallpox and not the least things, to make them comfortable"[22] "and medicines being needed at both Fort George and Ticonderoga."[23]

By 6 June, as estimated by the recently created Brigadier General Arnold, who was now in command at Montreal, only 5,000 of the men in Canada were fit for duty. Smallpox threatened the destruction of the entire army. On 15 June, General Arnold evacuated Montreal and by the time he arrived at St. Johns, two days later, half of his army was sick and the condition of all his men so poor that to remain at St. Johns seemed unwise. Maj. Gen. John Thomas, who took command of the army at Quebec on 1 May, himself died of smallpox on 2 June. "The smallpox," mourned John Adams, "is ten times more terrible than Britons, Canadians and Indians, together." [24]

The misery of the men who had so recently set off to conquer Canada was total. One hospital was described, for example, as a "dirty, stinking place" in a camp which "echoed with execrations upon the musketoes." "Language cannot describe nor imagination paint, the scenes of misery and distress the Soldiery endure," and the patients crowded into the barn which served as the hospital were in such condition that many "could not See, Speak, or walk. In one day two had large maggots, an inch long, Crawl out of their ears." [25]

It was only in June, however, that the Continental Congress, while leaving Potts's exact status unclear, officially ordered him to go as Physician and Surgeon to the North. Washington was at first undecided as to whether to send Potts or Stringer to aid Arnold's men who were then still in Canada, but by 26 June, when Potts and a supply of medicines from the Hospital Department headed north with Brig. Gen. Horatio Gates, who was to assume command of the Northern Army in the field from Brig. Gen. John Sullivan, General Thomas's successor, General Arnold had left Canada. When Potts arrived at Fort George, he found approximately one thousand patients suffering from smallpox, dysentery, and fevers, cared for by four surgeons and four mates. The number of patients there was still growing when the bulk of the Northern Army, which had been first reunited at Crown Point, fell back further in early July to Ticonderoga. Their seriously ill were rowed in small boats to the Hospital Department's Fort George facilities. [26]

By mid-July, an estimated three thousand of the men of the Northern Army were sick, for the most part with smallpox, three thousand well, and five thousand unaccounted for. Stringer, now also at the Fort George hospital, was close to desperation. More units were being sent to join the Northern Army, yet except for those which Potts brought with him, there were no drugs and the hospital was "in the utmost distress for both assistants and medicines." [27] Stringer had even been reduced to suggesting to Potts that "hemlock tops" be used for bedding. His request to Washington of 10 May 1776 for help had not been granted, the number of patients for whom he was responsible was still rising, and men were dying for lack of aid. On 26 July, the hospital at Fort George, reporting for a two-week period, noted 1,497 admissions, 439 discharges, and 51 deaths,[28] with the deaths in a five-week period estimated by one regimental surgeon at 300 or more. "In the name of God," Stringer asked Gates, "What shall we do with them all, my dear General?" [29]

Morgan, meanwhile, noted in a letter to Samuel Adams that he was lacking instructions as to how he should help Potts. He had, nevertheless, appointed Dr. James McHenry to serve under Potts, instructing him to go first to Philadelphia to obtain medicines with which to resupply the hospitals of the Northern Department. He had also assigned Potts the assistance of an apothecary, Dr. Andrew Craigie. Morgan ordered Potts to supply medicines both to the department's unit and to regimental surgeons and to require an accounting from regimental surgeons for whatever they used.

Returns of the Sick of the General Hospital at Fort George from the 12th to the 26th July 1776 inclusive

Regiments					
Col. Patersons	70	26	8		89
Burrels	164	69	8	2	85
Bonds	116	31	3		82
Artillery	16	24			32
Col. De Haas	118	22	1		95
Beedles	21	1			20
Reeds	127	40	3		84
Maxwells	172	83	5		84
Porters	59	9	3		47
Greatons	43	15			28
Winds	129	35	5		89
Starks	105	6	3		96
Battean Men	2				2
Artificers	12				12
Col. Vanschaicks	113	55	5		53
Wynkoops	14	3			11
Waynes	6	4			2
VanDykes	4	1			3
St. Clairs	83	13	6		64
Ivenes	31	2	1	1	27
Doors	49				49
	1497	439	51	3	1004
Men for Nurses					106
Total					1110

Return of the Sick of the Gen'l. Hospital at Fort George from July 12 to 26, 1776.

Numerical only
Not signed

RETURN OF THE SICK OF THE HOSPITAL AT FORT GEORGE. (*Courtesy of National Archives.*)

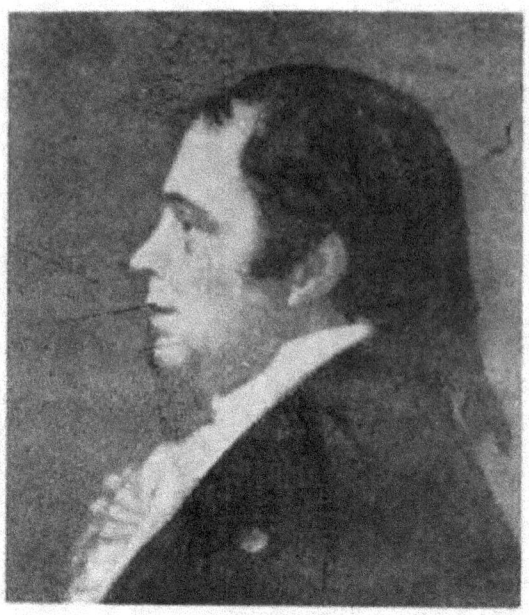

JAMES McHENRY. *(Courtesy of National Library of Medicine.)*

He was to report to Morgan monthly on the hospitals under him and their expenses.[30]

McHenry had not arrived by the end of July and the drug shortage was so severe that Stringer received permission from General Gates to go to New York himself to obtain medicines. Unable to fill his requirements in New York, however, Stringer hurried to intercept McHenry, who was preparing to travel north with the few drugs he had been able to collect. Although he obviously and desperately needed a larger staff, Stringer attempted to show his own independence by dismissing McHenry as soon as he encountered him, in so doing apparently failing to take over the drugs McHenry had with him. In August, however, Potts was still in ignorance of this development and anxiously awaiting the arrival of his new assistant with his supply of medicines. His own dismissal of McHenry did not keep Stringer from eventually blaming Morgan for the shortage of supplies in the Northern Department, because the Director General had failed to forward the medicines which McHenry had obtained. "A tissue of misunderstanding and mistakes seem to be the fate of your district," McHenry commented to Potts.[31]

By the second week in August, although he still believed he should have been independent of Stringer, Potts had resigned himself to working as Stringer's subordinate and acted as Director while Stringer was absent from his post, still ostensibly seeking drugs. There had been no enlargement of the staff caring for the patients at Fort George and the situation at the hospital had not otherwise improved since his arrival a month earlier. Patients were "without clothing, without bedding, or a shelter sufficient to screen them from the weather." There were no jalap, bark, salts, or opium available and the number of sick was, according to Stringer, still increasing.[32]

Although the urgent need to improve the care given patients in the Northern Department was recognized by the Continental Congress by the late summer of 1776, there were occasional optimistic reports in mid-August and the smallpox threat was diminishing. Samuel Adams believed that the number of patients was no longer increasing at Fort George, Stringer maintained that he had located a supply of medicines and sent a portion of them to Potts, and, on 28 August, General Gates was able to write Washington that "the Smallpox is now perfectly removed from the Army." For the disappearance of this disease, Potts should receive some credit, since he apparently did go forward with the inoculation not long after his arrival, as ordered by Stringer, although exact figures are not available.[33]

Nevertheless, despite these hopeful comments, the shortage of medicines was by no means relieved, self-inoculation by newly arriving militia was threatening a renewed epidemic, and Stringer was still absent from his post. When he had not returned by 22 August, General Gates became angry that the Director of his department's hospitals would go "preferment hunting . . . while the troops here are suffering inexpressible distress for want of Medicine." Begging that medicines be sent to Potts at Fort George, Gates added a request that General Washington be informed of Stringer's behavior. He followed this letter by comments in his General Orders of 31 August which emphasized that, although Stringer had been ordered to obtain the needed drugs and return at once, he had now been absent from duty 33 days.[34]

Smallpox did not reappear in Gates's army, but other diseases also afflicted his men, among them dysentery at a time when the accepted remedies for this condition were scarce, bilious, remittent, and intermittent fevers, and scurvy; even worms apparently added to the miseries of the Northern Army. In September, one regimental surgeon at Ticonderoga reported that half of his regiment was unfit for duty because of dysentery, jaundice, and various fevers. Returns of late September suggest that in the Northern Army at this time, as many as 50 percent of all the enlisted men assigned to the camp may have been sick. Two to four times the number sick away from camp remained under the care of the regimental surgeons in their tents or, quite possibly, within regimental hospitals, a situation which may have resulted from the fact that the general hospital staff had not grown as rapidly as the size of the army in the North.[35]

A committee of surgeons had drawn up a list of the minimum drug supplies required by a battalion, which included twenty pounds of bark, four pounds each of gum camphor and powdered jalap, three pounds of powdered ipecac and tartar emetic, two pounds of powdered rhubarb, and fifteen pounds of Epsom salts, along with quantities of more than a dozen other medicines. Several of these drugs might be used to treat any one collection of symptoms, tartar emetic, followed by a combination of nitre, camphor, and tartar emetic, for example, being one treatment for the "ague and chills; a violent pain in the head, back, and in every bone . . . with loss of appetite, Nausea, and considerable degree of weakness . . . succeeded with an inflammatory fever" which was seen in the fall of 1776 in the North.[36]

Recognizing that the department's inability to provide adequate care for its patients threatened future recruitment, Gov. Jonathan Trumbull of Connecticut wrote General Schuyler that, rather than waiting for a specific order from Congress, he would send on clothing and medicines whenever informed of the need.[37]

The Continental Congress reacted to reports of the situation in the Northern Department by ordering that the necessary medicines be sent to the northern hospitals and by sending an investigating committee to Ticonderoga. In view of reported shortages of all kinds of food except bread and meat, the Congress also ordered that not only sheep but also cornmeal, rice, oatmeal, and molasses be sent at once to the Army's patients in the Lake George and Ticonderoga area.[38]

Early in October, apothecary Craigie commented that, although he had received a wagonload of herbs, half of it consisted of varieties he could not use, but Stringer, now in Albany, wrote General Gates only a few days later that he had been most successful in obtaining medicines. He wrote Potts, as he had on another occasion, that he was sending along a portion of his supply, this time enough to fill two barrels and a box, and added that he had more on hand should it be needed later. The picture brightened further in November when a member of Congress noted with satisfaction that "Medicines are sent in sufficient Quantities for the Army at Ticonderoga," and Potts was able to begin distributing generous quantities of medicines to his regimental surgeons.[39]

The alleviation of the drug shortage did not mean that the problems of the Northern Department were over. Items valued for the hospital diet were still in short supply, especially sugar, vegetables, and "spirits," money to pay the medical staff was almost nonexistent, and the Fort George hospital was badly overcrowded. Alarmed by the possibility of an enemy attack which could further burden this facility, Stringer attempted to reduce its population by urging that no more patients be sent to Fort George, by discharging some from the Army, and by sending still others to the Albany unit, recently set up in a building originally constructed as a military hospital during the French and Indian War. In November, when the anticipated attack seemed imminent, despite Arnold's successful delaying action against British naval forces seeking to gain control of Lake Champlain, he sent 130 patients to Albany; housing for as many as 500 patients and an adequate supply of food were available there, but medical attention was inadequate. Because of his need for medical attendants, Stringer was unable to have a senior surgeon escort these men.[40]

Complaints about the number of patients Stringer's department was discharging from the Army, however, apparently began to appear in the summer of 1776, and in September, Potts was ordered to discontinue the practice. Stringer protested this order to General Gates, maintaining that the number for which he was required to care was growing daily and that he had but three surgeons and two mates at Fort George to handle them. He added that he believed that such discharges as had already been granted would have met with the general's approval.[41]

The committee sent by Congress to investigate Northern Department hospitals reported in November that the Fort George General Hospital contained 400 patients who lacked only an adequate supply of vegetables, "good female nurses and comfortable bedding." Concluding that the Fort George unit was too far from Ticonderoga to serve the troops there, it also recommended that a building designed to serve as a general hospital be constructed on Mount Independence, a hill across a narrow stretch of Lake Champlain from Ticonderoga, where Potts was apparently already prepared to care for the wounded if any enemy attack should occur.[42]

When no British attack had materialized by December 1776, the Fort George hospital was closed and all of its patients apparently were moved to Albany, while Potts was preparing to go home to Pennsylvania on leave late in 1776. Having now dismissed Stringer, the Continental Congress ordered Potts to return north at once in February 1777, however, and by the end of March he was again on duty in the Northern Department,[43] this time as its acting Director.

By the time Potts arrived in the Northern Department, conditions were sufficiently stabilized for improvements to be scheduled and carried out in a coherent manner. General Schuyler suggested that Potts leave the Albany hospital to the care of others and concentrate on preparing the Fort George facility to house patients with contagious diseases, as suggested by the congressional committee the preceding November. It was planned to house newly inoculated patients there, but one wing of that hospital had never been finished. A general hospital was now being prepared on Mount Independence, and General Schuyler wished patients from the Fort George garrison, presumably those not afflicted with diseases considered contagious, to share this hospital with those from Ticonderoga. Since the Congress wished in addition to have a vegetable garden planted on Mount Independence, Potts had the additional problem of obtaining an adequate supply of seeds.[44]

The staff assumed by Potts when he succeeded Stringer in the Northern Department apparently consisted of three surgeons, an apothecary, nine mates, and a clerk. The new Director had the same difficulties as his predecessor in meeting the payroll and also began to receive complaints about the pay scale. Early in April, however, he wrote General Gates that he believed he had succeeded in persuading all but one of his subordinates to stay on even though the promised pay increase had not yet materialized.[45]

The new appointments for the Hospital Department made in April (see Chapter 2) designated Potts Deputy Director for the Northern Department and assigned him as assistants, among others, Dr. Malachi Treat, reputed to be "clever," and another physician,[46] whose surgery the new Director General, William Shippen, Jr., described as "elegant." His new and enlarged staff at this time apparently consisted of an Assistant Director, a Physician General, a Surgeon General, a Physician and Surgeon General of the Army, an Apothecary General, six senior surgeons, seven mates, a Commissary General and his assistant, two clerks, and one steward.[47]

By the end of May 1777, conditions in the Northern Department with its three general hospitals at Mount Independence, Fort George, and Albany were much improved. The general hospital at Mount Independence, for example, on 21 May reported no great incidence of any one disease among its patients but rather a variety, from asthma and measles to inflammation of the liver and "cough and hectic." Although Potts had appointed a private physician, one Dirk Van Ingen, to care for army patients near Schenectady, there is no evidence that this was done because of crowding in the nearby Albany hospital. Smallpox was under control, supplies were adequate, patients were, for the most part, housed in buildings specifically designed for their care, the staff was large in proportion to the number of patients, fresh vegetables were available from local gardens, and evidence even indicates that sheep and cattle were now being delivered on the hoof. By May 1777, therefore, the Hospital Department in the North was well prepared to handle the casualties of another hard campaign.[48]

NEW YORK AND NEW JERSEY, 1776 TO 1777

For the estimated forty regiments defending New York City, hospitals were initially established not only within the city but also on Long Island, where one of the five divisions forming Washington's army of about twenty thousand was stationed.[49] (Table 5)

On the island of Manhattan, hospital units were located in the City Hospital, newly rebuilt after a disastrous fire, in the City Barracks, and even in rows of private houses appropriated for the purpose by the New York Convention, in some instances outside the most populous areas, but the principal unit was at King's College. Morgan later maintained that he had experienced considerable difficulty in using private homes. The state militia actually turned patients out of houses on the Bowery and one belonging to the Stuyvesants, where they had been placed by the state legislature. There were also instances where regimental surgeons took over buildings

TABLE 5—PATIENTS IN HOSPITAL DEPARTMENT UNITS, NEW YORK CITY AREA, APRIL-JUNE 1776

Hospital	Admitted Since Last Return	Dismissed Fit for Service	Dead	Remaining
New York City				
24 Apr–4 May [a]	70	7	3	57
4–11 May	60	15	1	101
11–18 May	85	28	2	156
18–25 May [b]	37	22	1	165
9–16 Jun [c]	20	31	4	136
Long Island				
4–11 May	7	2	0	5
11–18 May	19	6	0	18
18–25 May	27	18	2	25
Smallpox Hospital, Montresor's Island [d]				
4–11 May	4	0	0	5
18–25 May	8	0	3	25
9–16 Jun	0	1	0	6

SOURCE: Return 24 Apr–25 May, 9–16 Jun 1776, signed by Isaac Foster, RG 93, M246, roll 135, folder 3–1, items 4–8.
[a] Three absent without permission.
[b] Three removed to the smallpox hospital, two absent without permission.
[c] Two discharged from the Army.
[d] No return submitted for 11–18 May.

assigned to the general hospital. Asked to collect herbs, however, the local populace also helped to supply other needs of army patients in the area, giving the hospitals 2,000 sheets, hundreds of shirts, and similar supplies.[50]

To Maj. Gen. Nathanael Greene's division fell the assignment of holding Long Island, and it was at General Greene's request that a branch of the general hospital was established to serve his troops. Morgan assigned this Long Island unit to Dr. John Warren when it began operations in the summer of 1776 and ordered him to take three hospital mates with him. Any further assistance Warren might need could come from among the surgeon's mates of General Greene's brigade. On the question of what medicines to bring with him, Morgan told Warren to consult with physicians Foster, Adams, and McKnight.[51]

Morgan gave Warren detailed instructions on how the Long Island hospital was to be managed. Careful records must be kept of its patients, the time of their entering and leaving the hospital, and their diseases. In this instance, they could also be allowed to remain under the care of their own regimental surgeons in whatever quarters General Greene might see fit to set aside for this purpose. These surgeons were even to be permitted to draw upon the Hospital Department's stores, but when so doing, they were to consider themselves a part of the Long Island hospital and under Morgan's authority. No supplies were to be issued to patients not reported to and considered as a part of the general hospital. Nurses must be hired and each nurse paid 50 cents a week. The regulations for the unit's personnel and patients should be agreed upon by the surgeons, read to the occupants of each ward, and then posted, along with the rules for diet. Both sets of rules must be most strictly enforced.[52]

The regimental surgeons were to be required to keep careful records of their patients and to submit weekly returns to Warren of those of their patients being cared for through the Long Island unit. Once each month a roll was to be made out for ration money and signed by the general. The rations for these men to their regiment were to be stopped while they were in the care of the Hospital Department. Morgan assigned a storekeeper to Warren's staff and he was to apply, as appropriate, to either the Commissary General or the Quartermaster General for what he needed, keeping strict accounts of such transactions. Warren was instructed to obtain 100 blankets and 100 beds to take to Long Island, applying to the Quartermaster for straw, and he was to be sure to have the nurses and washerwomen clean these beds "from time to time." An "orderly Mate" was to be placed in charge of hospital furniture and bedding and to keep careful records, which were to include notations on what equipment and clothing each patient brought with him to the hospital.[53]

Warren's hospital was not long established, however, before the British attack in late August 1776 drove the Long Island division, now under Maj. Gen. John Sullivan because of General Greene's illness, from the island. American losses ran high, 970 officers and men killed or wounded. The patients from Warren's hospital had to be moved in considerable haste to New York City and placed in the barracks there. A heavy rain was falling as the patients were landed at various wharves and many inevitably suffered as a result, but Morgan personally took part in caring for them and later maintained that he had not only attended all the operations of which he was aware but also dressed all the patients himself.[54]

When operations in the New York City area were just in the planning stage, it had been assumed that the city itself could not be successfully retained unless, by holding Long Island, the Continental Army could make the city also untenable for the British. It was, therefore, obvious that if the British were to take Long Island, New York City was doomed, patients in the New York hospitals would have to be evacuated, and hospital supplies and medicines would have to be quickly moved to a safer place for storage. (Map 3)

On General Washington's order, Morgan went to Newark several days before the evacuation from New York was scheduled to take place to set up a hospital for the approximately one thousand patients from Long Island. Here he established Foster and Dr. William Burnet plus seven or eight mates to assist them. Morgan had sent Dr. Barnabas Binney to Philadelphia in July to round up additional hospital stores and in August had located some himself. Although Binney could find no instruments, the supplies arrived at Newark just before the patients themselves were expected and were deposited at the new hospital under the care of Assistant Apothecary John B. Cutting.[55]

Despite Morgan's efforts, however, the move of patients from New York City to Newark led to a "dreadful scene of confusion and disorder." Some mates had been taken prisoner and many nurses and other attendants had fled. The militia had impressed a considerable number of wagons in the course of their flight, complicating the moving of seriously ill and wounded patients to boats. The boats themselves were late in arriving. Furthermore, the neighbors of the new hospital were not pleased to have an institution assumed to be a source of fatal infections established near them. It was also becoming difficult to obtain nurses to care for the growing numbers of sick because, Washington believed, they were not being paid enough. Men from the regiments, therefore, were used even though their services were of questionable value to the sick.[56] On 18 September, Washington was forced to authorize regimental surgeons to care for their own patients "until the General Hospital can be established on a proper footing." [57]

The situation at Newark was made more difficult by the Morgan-Shippen feud over control of department hospitals in the New Jersey area. Shortly after Morgan's departure from Newark, he received a visit from Foster, whom he had left in charge of the hospital there. Foster reported that Shippen had attempted, albeit unsuccessfully, to assume control over both the hospital and the stores left in Newark. Washington, in response to Morgan's complaint about this situation, wrote Shippen that he wished Foster to remain in charge at Newark.[58]

In addition to the Newark hospital, Morgan also set up other hospitals in New

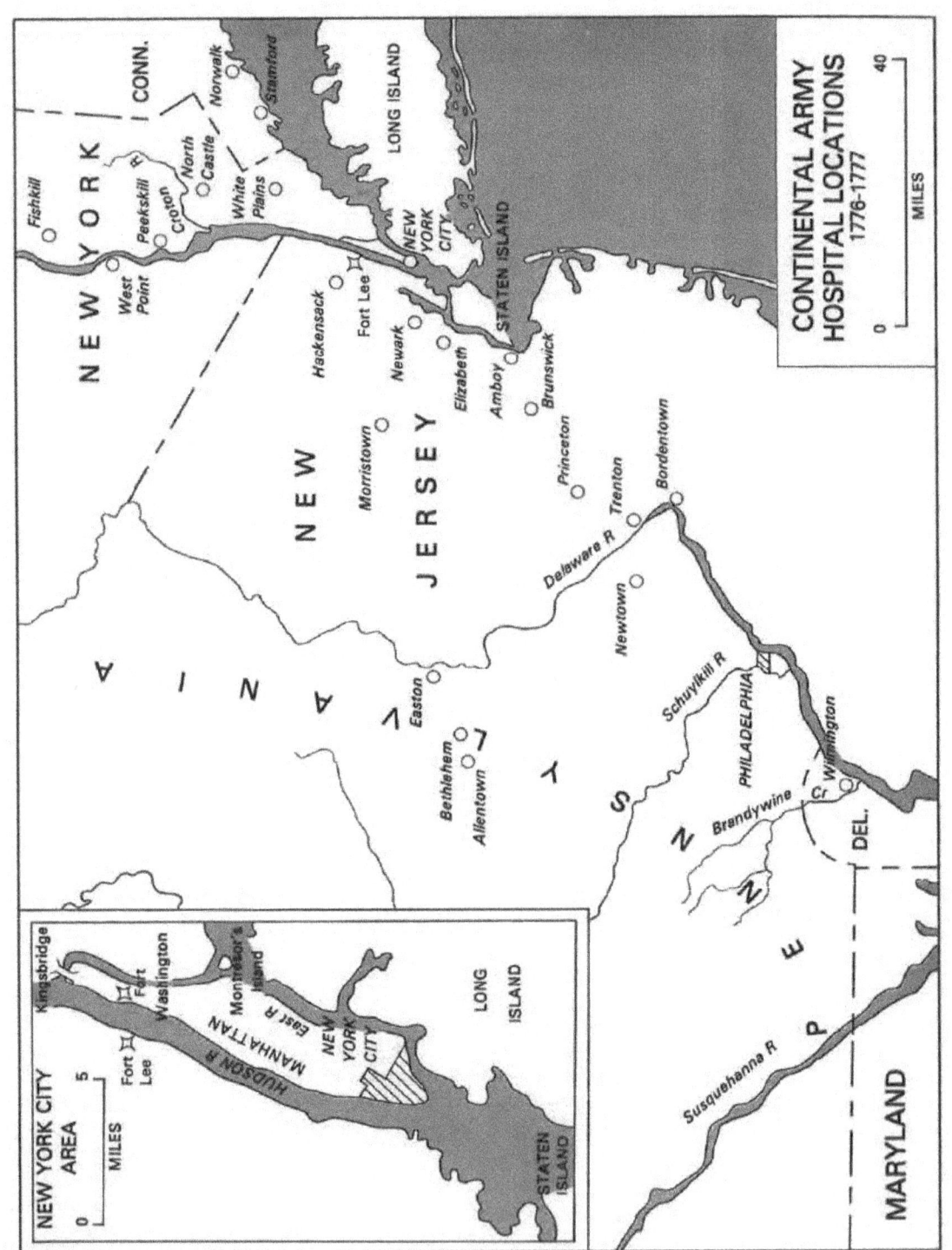

Jersey for the sick and wounded of General Washington's army. He supervised the establishment of a 300-bed facility at Hackensack, New Jersey, where hospital supplies had also been stored, a few days after he opened the Newark hospital. By 18 October, Morgan was able to move "several hundreds" of patients to Hackensack despite the fact that he had only three mates and a surgeon to help him, that he had been forbidden the use of army workmen, that several days' more work was needed, and that he had no guards to help him because the fifty assigned managed within a short period of time and on various pretexts to disappear. Morgan was particularly anxious to have his hospital in Hackensack running smoothly so that he could leave it in Warren's hands and join General Washington at White Plains, New York, where action was momentarily expected.[59]

While Morgan attempted to care for the men of Washington's army, Shippen was with the men of the militia's flying camp at Amboy. Chosen chief physician for the camp on 15 July 1776, at a time when fewer than 3,700 men had come in, he was quite confident of success in spite of his lack of military experience and the greenness of the new recruits which predisposed them to illness. He at once placed appeals in local papers asking the citizens of Philadelphia and nearby areas of Pennsylvania as well as those of New Jersey to send old sheets and linens to him for his hospitals and he also began to collect a staff.[60]

By mid-September, however, Shippen found himself hard pressed and in great need of surgeons, especially, he stated, in view of the fact that seven or eight battalions in the flying camp had neither regimental surgeons nor mates of their own. He was forced to act personally as both director and surgeon at the Amboy unit as well as apothecary for nine battalions. By the end of September, however, he had added to his staff at least two former regimental surgeons, Bodo Otto, a native German who had served with Pennsylvania troops in the Battle of Long Island, and William Brown, who had been recommended by both General Washington and the flying camp's Brig. Gen. Hugh Mercer. It is interesting to note that even before the 9 October resolve which placed him in command of all army hospitals in New Jersey, the Continental Congress apparently considered Shippen chief physician for the entire New Jersey area. Thus, in appointing Brown as Shippen's assistant, the Congress named him assistant for the "flying camp and troops in New Jersey." [61]

As General Washington's army retreated south through New Jersey before the British in the fall of 1776, the sick and wounded, often numbering one-fourth to one-third of the total, were sent ahead and placed in temporary hospitals at Amboy, Elizabeth, Brunswick, Trenton, Fort Lee, Newark, and Morristown. On 1 November, Shippen submitted an optimistic report to Congress on the hospitals in five of these towns, saying that his two units at Amboy contained 90 sick and 7 wounded, that at Brunswick 10 sick, and that at Trenton 56 sick. At Elizabeth he recorded 54 sick, 3 wounded, and 25 "sick from Canada" and at Fort Lee, 75 sick, 9 wounded, and 19 "distressed New-England Troops." It should be noted that even at a time of action, the sick outnumbered the wounded sixteen to one. Shippen predicted that four-fifths of his patients would recover but noted that 2,000 more patients who were not yet under his control were scattered in barns around the countryside. By late November, in spite of Shippen's optimism, patients from the flying camp, unattended by physicians, were pouring into Philadelphia, arriving in wagons and threatening to spread putrid or camp fever among the citizens of the city. Although he must have been aware of the sickliness of green troops, Benjamin Rush later tried to claim that Shippen was to blame for the flying camp's high death rate at this time. In November 1776, however, he wrote Shippen that everyone was praising the work he was doing. Washington personally ordered the sick from Trenton moved to Philadelphia so that his troops might use the barracks which had formerly sheltered Shippen's patients and gave Shippen permission to use supplies in New Jersey which Morgan had been moving about without using.[62]

Hospital units in Philadelphia were under Morgan's direct control, but such a great number of the Army's sick was coming into the city that the Council of Safety asked the vacationing Jonathan Potts early in December to take charge of them, apparently under Morgan. Bodo Otto took over the city's Bettering House, and several stores and private houses were also pressed into service as hospitals. Philadelphians were asked to help to obtain the supplies the Hospital Department needed and many citizens served as volunteer nurses. Morgan, with a possible British occupation of Philadelphia in mind, asked faculty members of his own medical school to stand by to care for patients too ill to be moved. Soon, however, so many disabled soldiers were quartered on local citizens that Morgan ordered Potts to send flying camp patients belonging to Maryland units back to Maryland, adding that Potts was to be sure that these men received the best care, including warm housing and blankets. A hospital was, therefore, established in Baltimore under Dr. Samuel MacKenzie and a mate. Morgan urged that others be accommodated in towns outside Philadelphia. Despite the care and attention devoted to the patients remaining in the city, however, the death rate was very high. On 16 February 1777, a total of 4,745 of the 17,449-man army was reported to be ill or unfit and some claimed that as many as 2,000 military patients were buried in the Philadelphia potter's field.[63]

Washington was concerned with the threat of contagion posed by the large numbers of the Army's patients housed in Philadelphia and wished from the beginning to see hospitals established at a safe distance from that city. Shippen moved his family to join him at Bethlehem in early December and, with the cooperation of the Council of Safety of Pennsylvania, established hospitals at Bethlehem, Allentown, and Easton, Pennsylvania. In a letter urging that he be sent the funds he was totally lacking for the care of his patients, he reported to his brother-in-law, Richard Henry Lee, that as of 17 December his patients were much reduced in number and doing well.[64]

The main hospital in Shippen's system occupied the former Single Brethren's House of the Moravian Order in Bethlehem. This 83- by 50-foot building dated from 1748 and contained eight rooms on the first floor of the main section. There were also refectories, a chapel, and superintendent's rooms on the second floor and dormitories plus several smaller rooms on the third. More recently built east and west wings housed further accommodations, including workshops. Completing the complex was a 40-foot belvedere or summerhouse open to the outside air. Shippen filled the cellars of the former church storehouse with hospital supplies and medicines and assigned officer patients the upper rooms. The hospital guard, surgeons, and convalescents were housed in shops and other buildings on the western side of town. A Moravian minister, the Reverend John Ettwein, visited all the patients at Bethlehem, the single brethren aided patients, the women made lint bandages, and Moravian carpenters made the coffins and dug the graves for 110 patients before the survivors were transferred to Philadelphia late in March 1777.[65]

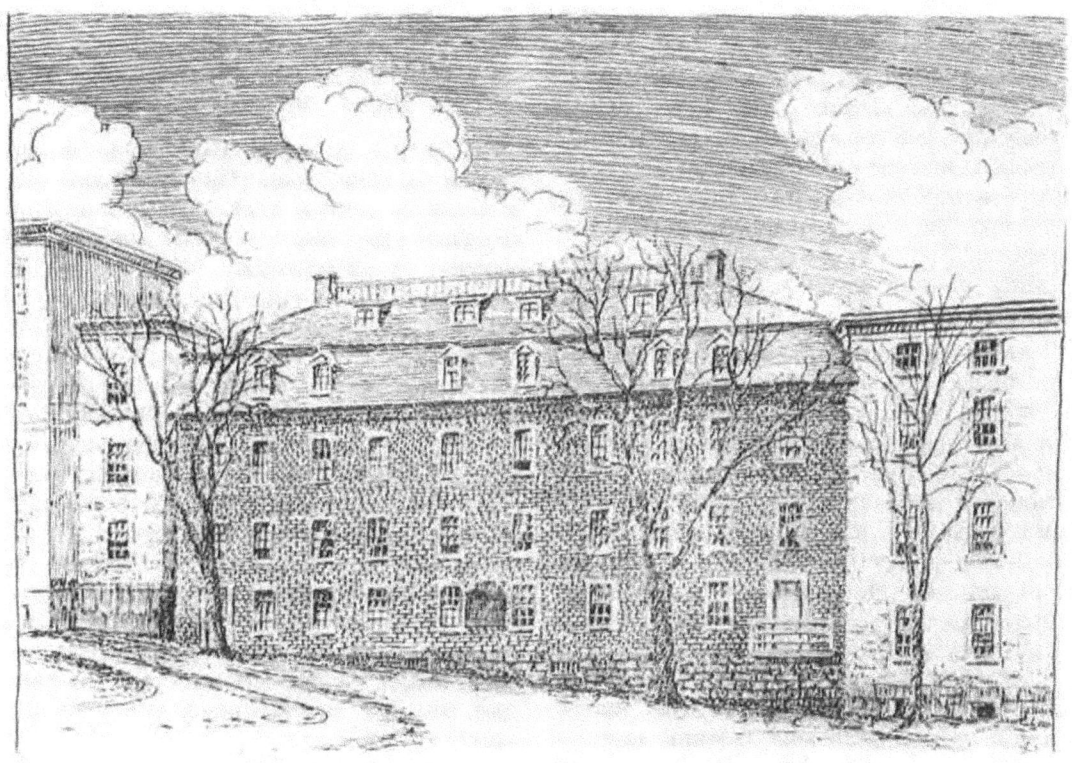

BRETHREN'S HOUSE AT BETHLEHEM. *(From Duncan, Medical Men.)*

Patients began arriving in Bethlehem early in December 1776 in all sorts of transport and were initially so short of food that the Moravians fed them for three days until the Army's supplies arrived. Shippen was touched by the cooperation of the townspeople and decided to house as many of the former Morristown patients as possible at Easton and Allentown. These units also were closed in March 1777 and patients too sick to be discharged as convalescents were sent to Philadelphia. The men who had been serving as nurses or orderlies returned to their regiments, while the department began efforts to find women to replace them.[66]

The last action before the Army went into winter camp at Morristown involved Washington's surprise Christmas attack upon Hessian units at Trenton and his early January success against the British at Princeton. The wounded from these operations and the sick from the camp at Morristown required the opening of new hospitals and the reopening of some old ones in New Jersey.

Christmas celebrations at Bethlehem were interrupted by General Washington's call to Shippen and his principal surgeons to join him as he moved against Trenton. It would appear, however, that Shippen did not reach the general in time to take immediate charge of the wounded, as on 29 December the general ordered that the wounded from the initial Trenton engagement be taken to Newtown, Pennsylvania, just across the Delaware River from Trenton, until Shippen and John Cochran could have them moved farther.[67] Fortunately, few Americans were injured in this engagement, but seventy-eight wounded Germans surrendered. Since the Americans wished to encourage such mercenaries to desert the British cause, they paroled these men and provided them with hospital facilities and the care of their own surgeons. An attempt was even made to give the German surgeons instruments, but it was reported that at least some of the amputating instruments so supplied were unusable.

Benjamin Rush had offered his services to General Washington's army after the Continental Congress adjourned on 12 December, and he and Cochran assumed responsibility for the Continental Army's wounded at Trenton just before the general began his withdrawal toward Princeton. It would appear that General Washington not only took no physicians with him on this march but also failed to inform Rush and Cochran that he was leaving. Cochran discovered the Army's departure on 3 January 1777 only when he rode out in search of it. Rush and Cochran were at the time caring for about twenty American wounded who were in danger of being captured by the British. The surgeons hastily obtained wagons and horses and removed their patients to Bordentown, southeast of Trenton, apparently assuming that this would be Washington's destination. Three days later they moved their unit to Princeton, where on 7 January 1777 Rush wrote Richard Henry Lee of the serious (and soon to prove fatal) wounds of General Mercer. Since many other Americans were also wounded in the Princeton engagement, a hospital was set up in the College's Nassau Hall. Here Rush and the other surgeons, possibly including Potts, with the aid of a surgeon and five privates left behind for the purpose by the British, cared for both American and enemy wounded until the end of the month when Rush, considering his patients to be out of danger, left to rejoin the Continental Congress.[68]

HOSPITALS IN NEW YORK STATE AND NEW ENGLAND AFTER THE EVACUATION OF NEW YORK CITY

Some of the wounded from action in the vicinity of New York City were cared for in hospitals in New York State and in New England. (*See Map 3.*) After opening the hospital at Hackensack, New Jersey, in October 1776, Morgan had hurried toward White Plains, New York, where action was momentarily expected. When he arrived at his destination, he found that the department's surgeons had already decided upon a church at North Castle as the site for a general hospital. The supply situation, however, had not been solved, since, despite orders to the contrary, the regimental surgeons of Maryland units had arrived at White Plains expecting Morgan to let them have what they needed. Many regimental surgeons were not even present, despite both orders to the contrary and the fact that the sick and wounded were numerous.[69]

As soon as action was joined, on 28 October, Morgan and his surgeons set out for White Plains from North Castle, while mates followed them with wagons carrying instruments and dressings. They established themselves near the front lines in houses along the road to North Castle and remained there, according to Morgan, about a week, until the enemy withdrew and Washington left to cross the river in an attempt to defend Fort Washington, on the northern end of Manhattan Island. During this engagement, Morgan was able to return to North Castle only briefly and at least one surgeon and three or four mates were also on duty at White Plains, awaiting possible further action. Morgan kept surgeons Samuel Adams, Jr., and Charles McKnight at North Castle, and sent some one thousand patients to Stamford and Norwalk, Connecticut, under the care of physicians Philip Turner and William Eustis.[70]

While Morgan was at White Plains, the British took Fort Washington and also Fort Lee, opposite Fort Washington on the west bank of the Hudson River, and then began to drive General Washington south through northern New Jersey. After leaving instructions with his surgeons, therefore, Morgan moved to join General Washington, catching up with him not long after the army crossed the Delaware River.[71]

Among the hospitals Morgan left behind him was that at Stamford, in charge of Turner, whose unit cared for 1,200 to 1,300 patients from early November to February 1777, by which time only 25 remained. Eustis was in charge of the hospital at Norwalk, where approximately 700 patients were sheltered in the course of the late fall of 1776 to March 1777, when only 8 to 10 patients remained.[72]

For help in supplying these two hospitals, Morgan was forced to turn to Gov. Jonathan Trumbull of Connecticut, who sent Turner a significant supply of necessary items. It was ironic that Morgan's need in Connecticut was so great, for about eighteen tons of supplies from New York City had been moved by boat to Stamford just before the evacuation of that city and stored in a private home there. Not long after these supplies arrived in Stamford, they were moved, without either Morgan's knowledge or General Washington's approval, but their new location was only fifty miles from Stamford and Morgan could easily have reached them. Unfortunately, however, while Morgan's most urgent need at this time was for medicines, the bulk of these supplies consisted of blankets, bedding, sheets, and new shirts.[73]

Among the hospitals set up by the Hospital Department in New York State were units at Kingsbridge, on the east side of the Hudson opposite the northernmost tip of Manhattan Island, and at Fishkill, on the Hudson River not far from West Point, both of which served the men of Maj. Gen.

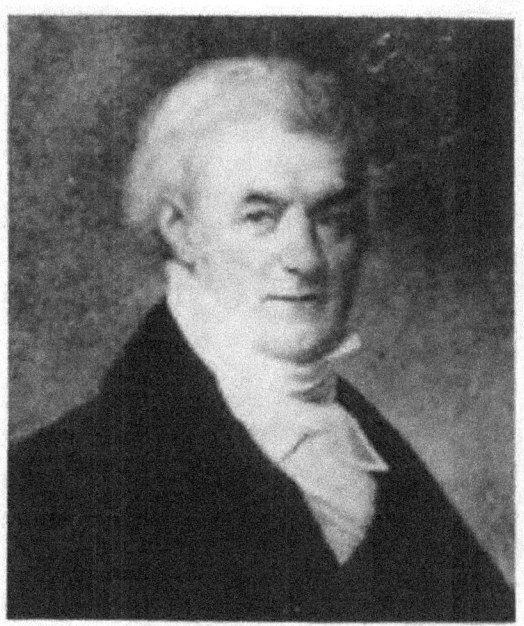

WILLIAM EUSTIS. *(Courtesy of National Library of Medicine.)*

William Heath's army. The hospital at Kingsbridge cared for the sick and wounded of a still raw and undisciplined army in a filthy camp entirely devoid of sanitation. A form of diarrhea termed "putrid" resulted from the unhealthy conditions, and one surgeon commented that "Many died, melting as it were and running off by the bowels." Aid from the Quartermaster's Department was almost impossible to obtain for this hospital, according to Morgan, and medicines were so short that the capture of a chest of medicine from the enemy was deemed a noteworthy event.[74]

After the loss of the White Plains engagement, General Washington sent General Heath's division north to Peekskill and West Point and stationed General Lee on the Croton River south of Peekskill. Both divisions thus remained on the east side of the Hudson River, where Morgan still directed the department's hospitals. Before leaving to join General Washington near Trenton, New Jersey, Morgan set up a hospital for General Heath's division at Peekskill, in response to the complaint that the sick and wounded of this 5,000-man division were receiving inadequate care. Morgan initially suggested that General Heath find appropriate quarters to shelter 300 sick and that the Hospital Department, now free to expand its staff to match the Army's growth, then staff the unit. The Director General added, however, that he believed Peekskill to be an unhealthy location for a hospital. Morgan put Adams and McKnight in charge of the new hospital, but they were unable to find a satisfactory site near the town and finally took over accommodations at Fishkill, twenty miles to the north, for their hospital. General Washington, however, ordered that convalescents be sent to Peekskill. On Morgan's dismissal in January 1777, General Washington requested that Dr. Isaac Foster, as the "eldest surgeon," take over the temporary supervision of these hospitals on the east side of the Hudson River.[75]

Until mid-1776, official policy called for the prevention of smallpox epidemics through isolation only and rejected planned inoculation. When General Washington's army moved south from Boston, a smallpox isolation hospital was established on Montresor's Island (now Randalls Island) in the East River and a twenty-three-man guard of men who had already had the disease was assigned to it. Although there had been some inoculations at the Montresor's Island hospital in the spring, in May, General Washington ordered that there were to be no more. All those already inoculated or exposed to the disease were to be sent there. (See Table 5.) The general warned that "any disobedience to this order will be most severely punished." The Continental Congress supported Washington's stand and when a private physician in the State of New York was discovered to have been inoculating soldiers, he was jailed.[76]

Despite these precautions, the fear of smallpox grew among the men of the Continental Army. Recruiting was threatened, and by late June, official attitudes toward inoculation began to show signs of change. The Maryland Council of Safety, noting the presence of smallpox among some of the Maryland troops, suggested that inoculation be tried and even offered to pay for such a step, but the Council of Massachusetts, learning that Maj. Gen. Artemas Ward was permitting the inoculation of some of the troops outside Boston, where this procedure was illegal, asked that the practice be stopped.[77]

General Washington found that, despite all precautions, most units contained a few infected men who posed a threat to the entire regiment in which they served. And by August official attitudes were apparently changing in favor of inoculation in segregated camps. Orders again were issued specifically forbidding private and secret inoculation, but the prohibition brought protests, since it was believed that such a rule would hinder recruiting, especially for the Northern Army.[78]

Since General Washington and the Hospital Department still feared the possibility of triggering an epidemic, careful precautions were planned to ensure the isolation of soldiers undergoing inoculation. The general suggested moving them out of Philadelphia and into nearby segregated hospitals. And when he sent John Cochran to Newtown, Pennsylvania, to oversee inoculation there, he suggested that houses in the remote countryside be used to shelter newly infected soldiers. General Washington urged that those already inoculated not be moved until entirely recovered and that when they left the hospital they be equipped with either new or "well washed, air'd and smoaked" clothing. By mid-February, he was also suggesting that the individual states immunize their recruits before sending them to join the Army. Rush, as chairman of the Medical Committee of the Congress, wrote Washington that troops coming in from the South were terrified of contracting smallpox naturally and, since the disease was raging in Philadelphia, should be inoculated somewhere outside of that city.[79]

It was in February 1777, while the bulk of Washington's army was in winter camp at Morristown, that the official order to proceed with the inoculation of the entire army was given. The Continental Congress, then meeting in Baltimore, ordered specifically that the troops there be immunized and requested the Maryland Assembly to give MacKenzie the necessary medicines. On 5 February, the general, convinced that only inoculation would prevent the destruction of his army, decided that all soldiers, including recruits, at Morristown and in the Philadelphia area should undergo the procedure.[80]

The Hospital Department, although now without a Director General and in a state of disorganization after the dismissal of Morgan, nevertheless immediately moved to carry out the wishes of Congress. Shippen ordered Dr. Bodo Otto to leave Philadelphia for Trenton, where he was to set up an inoculation hospital in an old barracks originally constructed for British troops in the French and Indian War. General Washington personally told Dr. Nathaniel Bond to prepare to inoculate troops in the Morristown area, emphasizing that he wanted the procedure administered secretly and as quickly as possible. Bond was to immunize not only the troops already in Pennsylvania and New Jersey but also all those coming into the area, upon arrival.

A few minor complications arose as the process of immunizing General Washington's army began. The general was unhappy that so many troops were being marched all the way to Morristown before being inoculated, since the facilities were not as good there as elsewhere. Some confusion existed in the area supervised by Foster, and that doctor claimed that he had been told that the order to inoculate the troops in the Fishkill area had been countermanded. General Washington told Foster that he had never intended to cause any delay in the inoculation of these troops, since waiting so long to begin the procedure had already had harmful effects.[81]

Distressed that Virginia still did not permit inoculation, General Washington wrote Gov. Patrick Henry to support the repeal of such restrictions, adding that smallpox "is more destructive to an Army in the Natural way, than the Enemy's Sword." [82] These regulations were apparently changed shortly after General Washington's request, since on 23 April, the Continental Congress ordered Dr. James Tilton to Dumfries, Virginia, "to take the charge of all continental soldiers that are or shall be inoculated" there and on 30 April decreed that troops from Carolina stop at Dumfries, Colchester, and Alexandria, all in Virginia, to undergo the procedure.[83]

In having his entire army inoculated during the winter and early spring of 1777, General Washington took a great risk. The procedure would in a short time greatly strengthen his army, but it temporarily weakened his forces in the face of the enemy. Only four of every 500 of his men died as a result of inoculation, however, and the gamble was so successful that he repeated it in the Valley Forge winter of 1778.[84]

By March, General Washington had sent a large proportion of his troops north to the Hudson River, and only 3,000 remained at Morristown, two-thirds of them militia whose terms of enlistment were about to run out. French arms and supplies were now arriving, however, and in a short time new units also began to come in. By May there were 8,000 men at Morristown, but

2,000 of them were soon sick. Furthermore, an epidemic of fever was raging in one of the Army's facilities in Philadelphia, where Benjamin Rush reported that most of the staff had been ill at one time or another and several surgeons and mates had died.[85] Thus, despite his precautions, it was with an army weakened by sickness that General Washington opened the spring campaign in May 1777.

4

Year of Despair and Hope, June 1777 to June 1778

During the 1777–78 campaign season, the crucial victory over the British at Saratoga in October 1777 brought action in the North to an end for the season and, for all practical purposes, for the war. In the Middle Department, however, repeated military setbacks as Washington unsuccessfully attempted to defend Philadelphia and the grim winter at Valley Forge which followed placed demands upon the Hospital Department in the New Jersey-Pennsylvania area which it could not meet.

THE MIDDLE DEPARTMENT

As Washington retreated before the British in Pennsylvania, the Hospital Department was forced to move seriously wounded and ill patients from place to place in all kinds of weather in open and springless wagons. Villagers who lived along the evacuation routes long remembered hearing "the wounded cry as they passed over the stones."[1] The shortage of both housing and clothing led to the overcrowding of poorly clad patients in inadequate facilities and the rapid spread of what was then called putrid fever, making a shambles of whatever hopes may have arisen as a result of the reorganization of April 1777 under the leadership of the new Director General, William Shippen, Jr.

Troops in the New Jersey-Pennsylvania area saw no major action until September of the new season since during the early summer the maneuvers of the British general, William Howe, in an attempt to force the Continental Army to give battle in the vicinity of Brunswick and Amboy, New Jersey, were in vain. In July he embarked 15,000 men, about two-thirds of his army, in the waiting ships of the British Navy and disappeared over the horizon. During the following six weeks, several sightings of the enemy fleet led to varying predictions of General Howe's ultimate intentions, and General Washington, trying to anticipate the enemy's next move, led his forces north to the Hudson River and then south again to New Jersey and Pennsylvania.[2]

General Washington's troops were far from healthy during this time. Of an army of roughly 18,000, more than 3,500 were sick, according to a Medical Committee report of 5 August 1777.[3] The general blamed the high rate of sickness upon the excessive use of "animal food, untempered by Vegitables, or Vinegar, or by any kind of Drink, but Water and eating indifferent Bread" and continued his efforts to improve not only the diet and camp sanitation affecting his troops but also the conduct of his regimental surgeons and the management of the hospitals caring for his men. He ordered that a list of the sick in each regiment be made every day and turned in to the regimental surgeon. He required that these doctors neither go on leave nor hospitalize a patient without permission from Dr. John Cochran, Physician and Surgeon General of the Army, or his deputy.[4]

By July, however, the situation had not improved and Cochran's problems were multiplying. Although his letters do not reveal

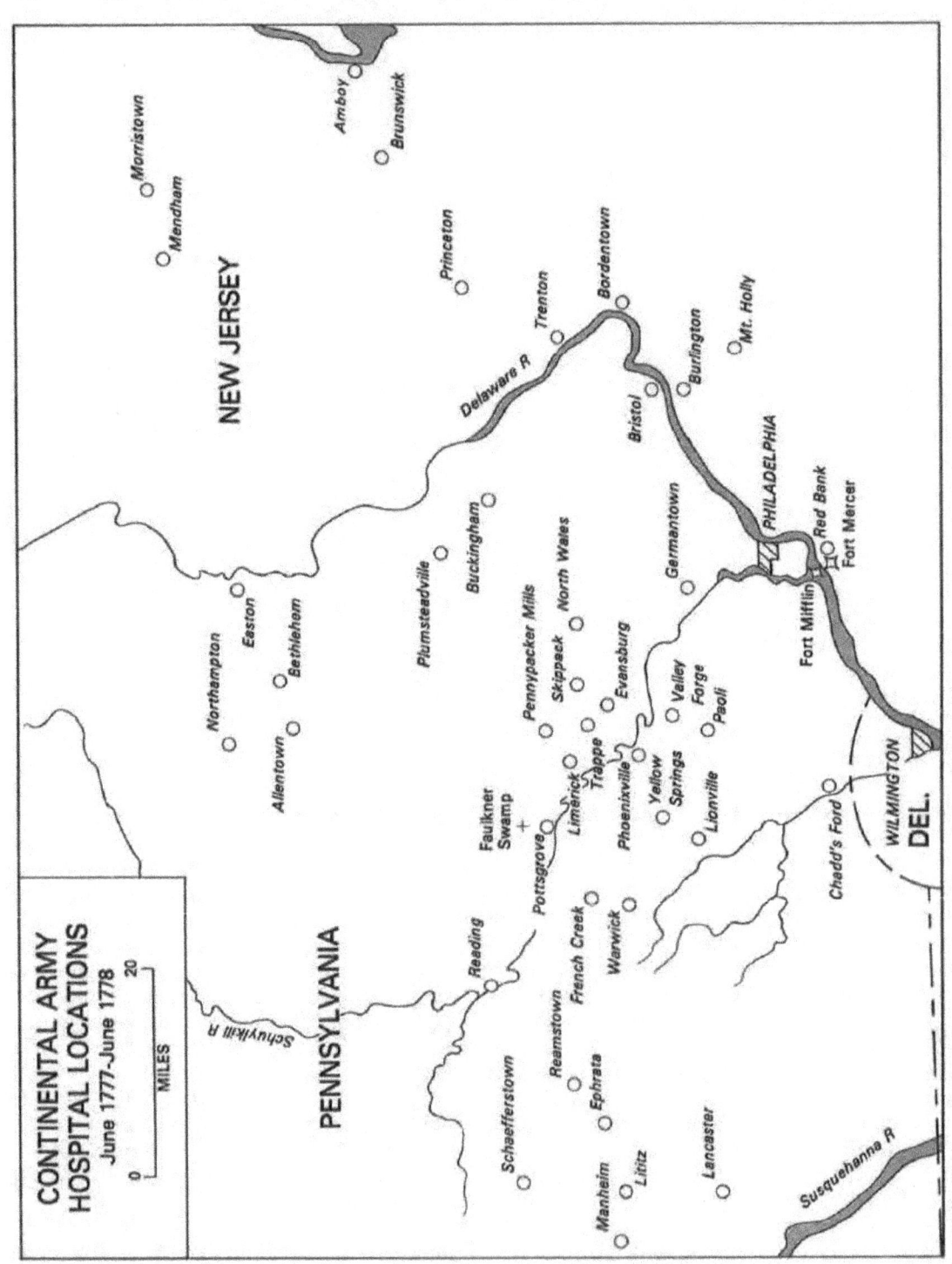

precisely what it was that Cochran had done to offend, Cochran was under fire from Maj. Gen. John Sullivan, who regarded this physician's attitude as insulting. Furthermore, General Washington's very recently issued orders that regimental surgeons report twice weekly to Cochran on the patients in their care were apparently all too frequently ignored. On 9 July, he announced that surgeons continuing to disobey him in this matter were to be arrested.[5]

When the general turned his attention to the facilities caring for his men, he discovered that interference from his officers was undermining the authority of hospital physicians. Commenting that doctors should be in complete control of these units, he ordered that no officer visit such a facility except to check on the treatment of its patients or to help maintain order and discipline. In September, he also ordered that officers not remove patients from hospitals without the written permission of the physician in charge.[6]

The situation as far as hospitals were concerned seems to have been satisfactory in August 1777, however, Dr. Benjamin Rush claiming at that time that "great order, cleanliness, and the most perfect contentment prevail in our hospitals." By the end of that month, his army's march slowed by the presence of unfit soldiers still under the care of regimental surgeons, General Washington had decided to turn all the sick over to the hospitals rather than attempt to take them with him on further moves about the countryside.[7]

In September, the British landed at the head of the Chesapeake Bay and Continental units saw their first real action of the season when General Washington attempted to stop the enemy at Chadd's Ford on the Brandywine Creek in Pennsylvania on 11 September 1777. (*Map 4*) Contemporary estimates of the losses suffered here by General Washington's army vary widely, but a modern authority estimates 200 killed and 500 wounded. Failing to stop the British at the Brandywine, the Continental Army moved northeast to the Schuylkill River and then retreated northwest along that river. After using a surprise bayonet attack to defeat Brig. Gen. Anthony Wayne at Paoli on 21 September, on the 26th the enemy occupied Philadelphia unopposed. The Continental Army lost an estimated 100 wounded at Paoli and another 500 in wounded on 4 October through the defeat of General Washington's army at Germantown. By 24 November 1777, wounds and disease had crowded Middle Department hospitals with approximately three thousand men, a figure which did not include those under the care of regimental surgeons.[8] (*Table 6*)

The walking wounded from the Brandywine defeat appear to have been directed toward the Hospital Department's facilities in Philadelphia, and the more seriously injured were taken in open wagons, escorted by physicians, to such New Jersey hospitals as those at Trenton and Princeton. Dr. John Augustus Otto, one of the sons of the Dr. Bodo Otto who was director of the barracks hospital at Trenton, accompanied one group of wounded to his father's unit. Here he stayed until the fall of Philadelphia necessitated the abandonment of that hospital. Another group of the wounded, escorted by Dr. James Tilton, went in slow stages to Princeton, stopping on the way in Philadelphia and Bristol, Pennsylvania, and Trenton. Tilton later claimed that the quarters these men were assigned at Otto's hospital had not been cleaned and that his patients contracted putrid fever there. The commissary of the Trenton hospital, Otto, and a second son, Frederick, who also worked with his father, however, maintained that the rooms had been cleaned before Tilton's arrival and that there had been no putrid fever in their hospital for three weeks before that date. It was true, at any rate, that Tilton and many of the Brandywine

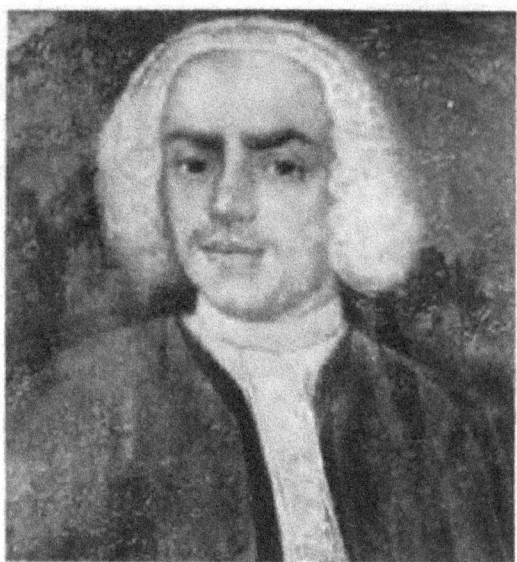

BODO OTTO. *(From James E. Gibson, Dr. Bodo Otto and the Medical Background of the American Revolution, 1937. Courtesy of Charles C Thomas, Publisher, Springfield, Ill.)*

symptoms appeared, and "the pulse began to sink, a dry tongue, delirium" developed. Tilton noted that "If I ever saw the *petechiae*, so much dwelt upon by Pringle and Monroe, I have forgotten all about them. This I am sure of, they were not regarded as essential to the disease."[9]

The most seriously injured from Brandywine received emergency care in buildings near the battlefield and were then collected by the victorious British and removed to the Wilmington area. General Howe told General Washington shortly after the battle that Continental physicians would be permitted to visit and treat wounded Americans held by the British. The Continental general responded by sending Rush, whose subsequent experience with the British system left a lastingly favorable impression, four other doctors, a hospital mate, and several other attendants through the lines.[10]

The fall of Philadelphia forced the evacuation of facilities within the city and rendered nearby hospitals vulnerable to surprise raids by the British. It also made necessary the establishment of new units at more distant locations. After the Brandywine defeat, Shippen had written a Moravian leader at Bethlehem, Pennsylvania, to ask the aid of his order in locating permanent

wounded with him did develop "languor and listlessness of the whole body, and a peculiar sensation of the head, as if it were tightened or compressed" shortly after their arrival in Princeton. After some days, other

TABLE 6—MIDDLE DEPARTMENT HOSPITAL PATIENTS, 24 NOVEMBER 1777

Location	Sick	Wounded	Convalescent	Total
New Jersey				
Burlington	80	10	11	101
Trenton	112	0	102	214
Princeton	139	130	10	279
Pennsylvania				
Buckingham	239	10	10	259
North Wales	100	0	59	159
Skippack (Shippack)	90	0	20	110
Easton	253	40	107	400
Bethlehem	161	80	142	383
Allentown	81	9	100	190
Reading	....	....	....	290
Lancaster	....	....	....	300
Manheim ^a	17	5	40	62
Maryland				
Baltimore	....	....	....	37

NOTE: Excluding regimental and brigade hospitals; as reported by William Shippen.
^a Mistakenly listed as Mendham in Duncan, *Medical Men*, p. 239.

accommodations in that area for an estimated two thousand patients; and in late November and December, many of the patients from New Jersey facilities at Mount Holly, Bordentown, Burlington, and Trenton were moved to Princeton. General Washington feared for the safety of the Princeton unit and urged unsuccessfully that it, too, be moved. Other patients, including those from such Pennsylvania hospitals as the units at Bristol, Pottsgrove, and Buckingham, were evacuated to the west and northwest deeper into Pennsylvania, where new hospitals were established at Lancaster, Lititz, Ephrata, Reading, Easton, Allentown, Warwick, Reamstown (Rheimstown), and Northampton. The closing of so many hospitals, however, and the distance to the new facilities made it necessary to open temporary hospitals at Evansburg, Trappe, Pennypacker Mills, Faulkner Swamp, and Skippack, Pennsylvania. These units handled the 421 wounded from Germantown before they were moved even farther west within the state.[11]

Those patients in General Washington's army who had accumulated under the care of regimental surgeons since the army had first seen action in the fall of 1777 were removed to units of the general hospital when the army went into winter camp at Valley Forge. Reports to the Adjutant General concerning the number and location of patients still with the army were required in anticipation of this move. Dr. Charles McKnight and a colonel were told to provide wagons, but only for those patients unable to walk even when relieved of their packs. Three days' provisions were to be sent with these men and one officer from each brigade was to accompany them to ensure their receiving proper care. Dr. Jonathan Potts, again on leave from the Northern Department, had volunteered his help in this massive evacuation, and Shippen wrote him to point out that patients being taken to hospitals on the west side of the Schuylkill River would eventually pass through Potts's hometown of Reading. Shippen asked his colleague to supervise these men during their stay in Reading and to do what he could to obtain for them comfortable transportation to their final destinations.[12]

The evacuation of so many hospitals, the overall increase in the patient load, and outbreaks of disease added to the burden of the Hospital Department even in hospitals which were not relocated. Nevertheless, in early December, although Tilton maintained that the Princeton facility's patients at this time were vermin-infested and filthy, Rush did not seem unduly alarmed. When he wrote Shippen from Princeton, he limited himself to explaining his need for cooking utensils, straw for bedding, and similar items and mentioning plans to take over the local Quaker meetinghouse and the home of a Tory to expand to 1,000 the capacity of his unit, which was already using the college's Nassau Hall and a church. Rush's letter of the same day to Maj. Gen. Nathanael Greene also gave no indication that the doctor was particularly upset by conditions at Princeton, although he did note that since many of the patients in his hospitals were only slightly ill and tended to spend their time stirring up trouble, he needed two or three officers to enforce discipline. In mid-December, however, Rush pronounced the situation at Princeton frightful. One building, which was large enough for only 150 men, now held 400, he said, and in one three-day period, twelve soldiers had died of putrid fever. Since the past spring, he added, six surgeons had died of fevers contracted at the Princeton hospital and there were still no guards present to enforce discipline.[13]

The necessity for reopening the hospital at Bethlehem had apparently distressed Shippen, who wrote the Reverend John Ettwein of his regret that he was "obliged by Order of Congress to send my sick and wounded to your peaceable village . . . I am truly concerned for your Society and wish sincerely this stroke could be averted." By the end of September, both civilians and soldiers were pouring into the village. Less than three weeks after the defeat at Germantown, there were reportedly more than 400 men in the Single Brethren's House, where physicians considered 360 to be an absolute maximum. The wounded coming in after the Germantown engagement were frequently sent on to Easton, but those too seriously injured to be moved farther were placed in tents at Bethlehem. Despite the crowded condition of the Bethlehem hospital, in October, Rush, as Physician General, ordered that 100 more be taken in.[14]

Because of such severe overcrowding in the Single Brethren's House, steps had to be taken to add to the available accommodations. Early in November, seventy patients were sent to a nearby farm. Rooms not previously used for patients, such as the kitchen, also were taken over. A separate hospital was set up nearby at the Fulling Mill, where woolen cloth was made. The suggestion that one or more of the women's buildings be used, however, caused so much dismay among the Moravians that the idea was abandoned. Sixteen members of the Continental Congress, including Richard Henry Lee, John Hancock, and both Samuel and John Adams, signed a message at this time recognizing the Moravians' "humane and diligent attention to the sick and wounded" and calling for the protection of their "persons or property."[15]

The situation in the middle states as General Washington's army prepared to take up winter quarters at Valley Forge did not inspire optimism. Shortages of all kinds, especially of housing, made it impossible to provide care compatible with the standards of the time. Severe overcrowding alone was considered by one physician to have been responsible for at least half of the large number of deaths which occurred in the early winter, although precise recordkeeping was often impossible where the turnover was so great.[16]

A large number of the higher officers of the Hospital Department came into Pennsylvania during the winter at Valley Forge. Among them were, in addition to the Director General, the leading members of the staff for the Middle Department, including the new Deputy Director and Purveyor, Dr. Jonathan Potts; the Surgeon General (soon to succeed Rush as Physician General), Dr. William Brown; and Cochran, the Physician and Surgeon General of the Army. Also serving in this area were two Assistant Directors, Dr. Thomas Bond, Jr., and Dr. James Craik; and two Apothecaries General, Dr. Andrew Craigie, who left the Northern Department at about the same time as Potts, and Dr. John Brown Cutting, who had apparently been asked in the summer of 1777 to take charge of the buying of drugs of the entire Hospital Department. Also present at Valley Forge was Baron von Steuben, whose *Regulations for the Order and Discipline of the Troops of the United States,* enacted into law by Congress in March 1779, formalized those doctrines on hygiene long preached by British and Continental military physicians.[17]

Food, clothing, bedding, drugs, instruments, bandaging, even wagons for moving supplies were all very difficult to obtain at this time. The spring of 1778, furthermore, brought an increase in the number of men sent to hospitals because of disease, enhancing the effects of these shortages and leading Craik to warn, "if I am not supplied with what I write for, it will be impossible for me to give satisfaction here."[18]

The scarcity of clothing affected not only patients being treated in hospitals but also those ready to return to duty. Those who entered more or less fully clothed often could not leave when recovered because the clothes they had turned over when they were admitted could not be found. Those in the hospital, moreover, had so little to wear while in bed that an adequate supply of blankets assumed a crucial importance. General Washington ordered that the items of clothing a patient wore on entry into the hospital be carefully recorded before storage. Those belonging to patients who died in the hospital were to be saved for men returning to duty. The Continental Congress appealed to the clergy in the Middle Department for donations of linen and woolens for the sick and wounded, and in February, General Washington ordered the Clothier General to supply both sick and convalescent patients.[19]

General Washington also was distressed by the inadequacy of supplies of food and bedding for hospitals. In January 1778, he ordered the Quartermaster General to draw upon his supplies of straw to meet the requests of army doctors and to see that the huts used for the sick at Valley Forge be kept well supplied. In February, he also ordered the Commissary General, Ephraim Blaine, to keep the army's sick supplied with rice, or, if it could not be found, at least with the ubiquitous cornmeal. Blaine and Potts, however, were in conflict for the purchase of many items and Blaine attributed some of the higher prices to the competition from Potts, so that wholehearted cooperation between the two men was unlikely. Furthermore, since Blaine was not always able to meet his regular commitments, it was not easy for him to aid Potts significantly. A more direct approach to the problem of buying food for the sick involved sending several men from each regiment out to scour the neighborhood for such food as could be obtained from local farmers and transferring supplies from the Northern Department where, after the victory at Saratoga, the demand had begun to drop. Because of these steps, combined with the efforts of the new Quartermaster General, Nathanael Greene, and the milder weather which facilitated transportation, by April, adequate amounts of flour, beef, and bread were available in the Middle Department. In May, however, when the army was preparing for the new campaign, many other items were still in short supply, among them sugar, tea, coffee, chocolate, salt, wine, and vinegar as well as bedding, paper, and pots. By June, difficulties obtaining food for the sick led General Washington to direct the Commissary General of the Army to be prepared at all times to supply the sick with fresh foods.[20]

Medicines were difficult to obtain throughout the entire winter of 1777–78. General Washington's January order that the Director General furnish medicines for regimental chests was not carried out until April because of the shortage of the required drugs. Department members traveled to neighboring colonies in their search for medicines and considerable ingenuity was shown in acquiring what was needed; the Department turned to the Commissary of Military Stores for sulfur and oil and to the Northern Department for other medicines.[21]

The shortage of instruments experienced in the early weeks of Dr. John Morgan's administration also continued during the winter of 1777–78, when many regimental surgeons were still unable to obtain so much as a lancet. Lint and bandages were also hard to find in Pennsylvania. To alleviate this problem the department encouraged Moravian women at Bethlehem and Lititz to make lint and drew once more on the generous supplies of the Northern Department. Apothecary General Craigie also suggested that the shortage of bottles be relieved by reopening the glassworks at Manheim, Pennsylvania.[22]

The shortages of medicines, bottles, instruments, and other items usually contained in the regimental surgeon's medicine chest led inevitably to delays in the distribution of these chests. Cutting sugested that when the new, smaller, and standardized chests were ready, the larger ones be called in for replacement. Concern over the need for these medicine chests was expressed by General Washington himself, who ordered that regiments without chests be reported to Cutting as Apothecary General of the Middle Department. In May, however, Cutting "went away before the regimental chests were finished" and there was "a great clamor about them," since sufficient medicines to keep all regiments supplied were still lacking.[23]

Such drugs as were available to the Hospital Department in Pennsylvania were apparently stored initially at Manheim, but in March 1778, Shippen ordered them moved to Yellow Springs. Craigie, however, under the assumption that there would be some consolidation of hospitals in the area in the future, wanted to locate the main depot at Carlisle, Pennsylvania, and to have medicines and chests prepared there. He noted, however, that he had not been able to induce the masons at Carlisle to complete the required construction for such a depot and commented in a letter to Potts that "The department is at present in chaos—no regularity—no system," even though needs were "great and many." [24]

In addition to the shortage of supplies and medicines, many serious conditions afflicted the men at Valley Forge. Those most frequently experienced included a typhus-typhoid type of fever and smallpox, the latter for the most part apparently through inoculation. While neither of these conditions posed a serious problem in the camp until spring, frostbite injuries during the winter were at times so severe as to necessitate amputations. There was, moreover, at least one minor ailment which, without threatening life, tormented the men at Valley Forge. This was "the Itch," or scabies. Baron de Kalb wrote back to France that Continental soldiers were severely affected even before they camped at Valley Forge, and General Washington ordered regimental surgeons to obtain the necessary sulfur from Cochran and to see that men with this condition were "annointed for it," as quickly as possible.[25]

Large orders for lime juice suggest that scurvy was present in General Washington's army in the spring of 1778. Dysenterylike conditions were also being encountered, but the greatest burden on the entire hospital system in the Middle Department during the period spent at Valley Forge seems to have resulted from the repetition of the previous winter's smallpox immunization campaign. It was believed that not only the ever-present possibility of action but also the heat itself made the procedure inadvisable in the summer, so despite the fact that spring inoculation slowed the preparation of the army for a new season of campaigning, the step was again undertaken in the winter and early spring of 1778. Attempts to determine how many men would require immunization began late in 1777, and by January, the effort to inoculate all susceptible soldiers in General Washington's army was under way. The progress was slowed, however, both by the tendency for some surgeons to slip away from camp and by the lack of straw to serve as bedding. By March, inoculation had progressed to the point where, along with the lack of proper clothing, it was rated as one of the principal factors which "certainly emaciate the effective column in our returns," [26] and the rate of sickness for General Washington's army exceeded 48 percent.

Recruits for General Washington's army who had to come through Virginia were for a time inoculated at Alexandria, Virginia, under the supervision of Dr. William Rickman, Director of the Continental hospitals in Virginia. In the fall of 1777, however, rumors began to circulate that the procedure was being mishandled there and that patients were dying with putrid fever. Rickman was temporarily recalled, but the committee

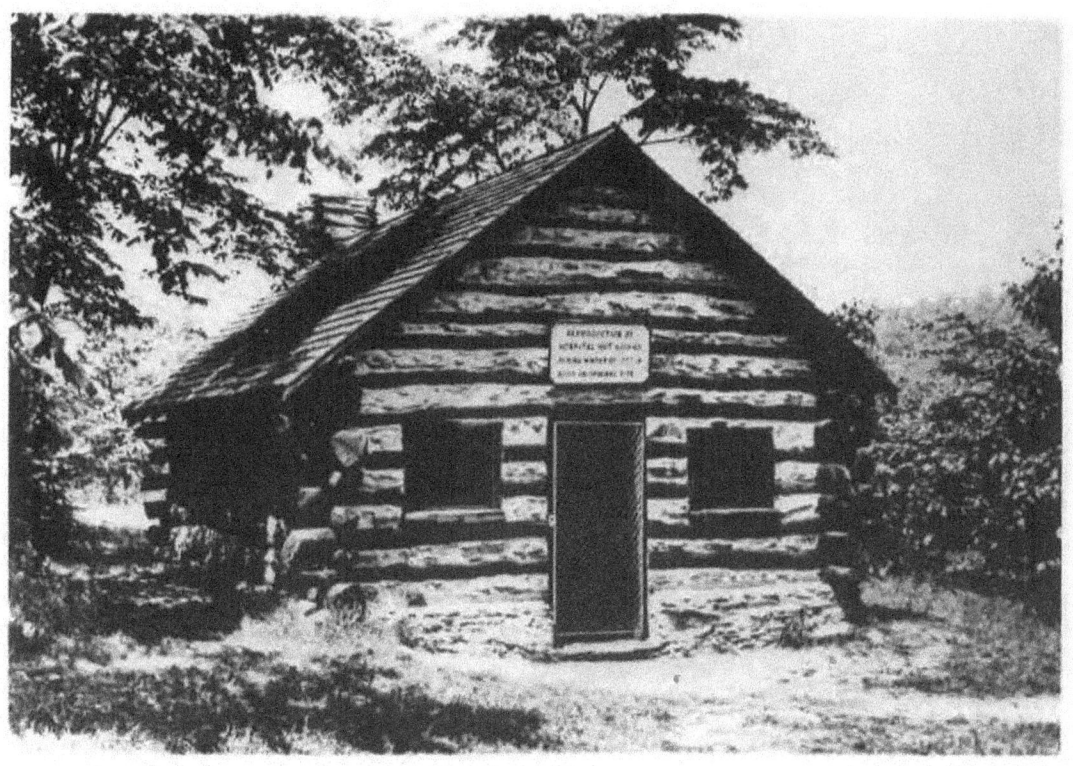

VALLEY FORGE HOSPITAL HUT. *(Courtesy of Historical Society of Pennsylvania.)*

investigating his conduct determined that the high death rate was attributable to the poorly clothed and exhausted condition in which the men arrived at his hospital and that the doctor had done as well as could have been expected under the circumstances.[27]

In March, it was decided that in the future troops coming in from the south should not be inoculated until they reached the Valley Forge area. Orders were issued to the effect that as they moved north, these troops should avoid all towns where smallpox might be present. In anticipation of the inoculation of these men and apparently believing it a necessary ingredient of the diet of the smallpox patient, Cochran urged that Potts send him "Molasses in abundance." By the end of April, approximately one thousand men were in various stages of inoculation at Valley Forge and 50 to 100 more were undergoing the procedure in a hospital near Wilmington, Delaware.[28]

It is in the documents dating from the winter at Valley Forge that one first encounters with any frequency the use of the term "flying hospital" in connection with the Continental Army. Like so many other designations in this army, however, the phrase was casually and imprecisely employed. In this instance, the flying hospital was managed not in the British manner as part of the general hospital (see Chapter 1) but rather as a large and more formal version of the regimental hospital. The flying hospital at Valley Forge consisted of a series of brigade hospital huts whose man

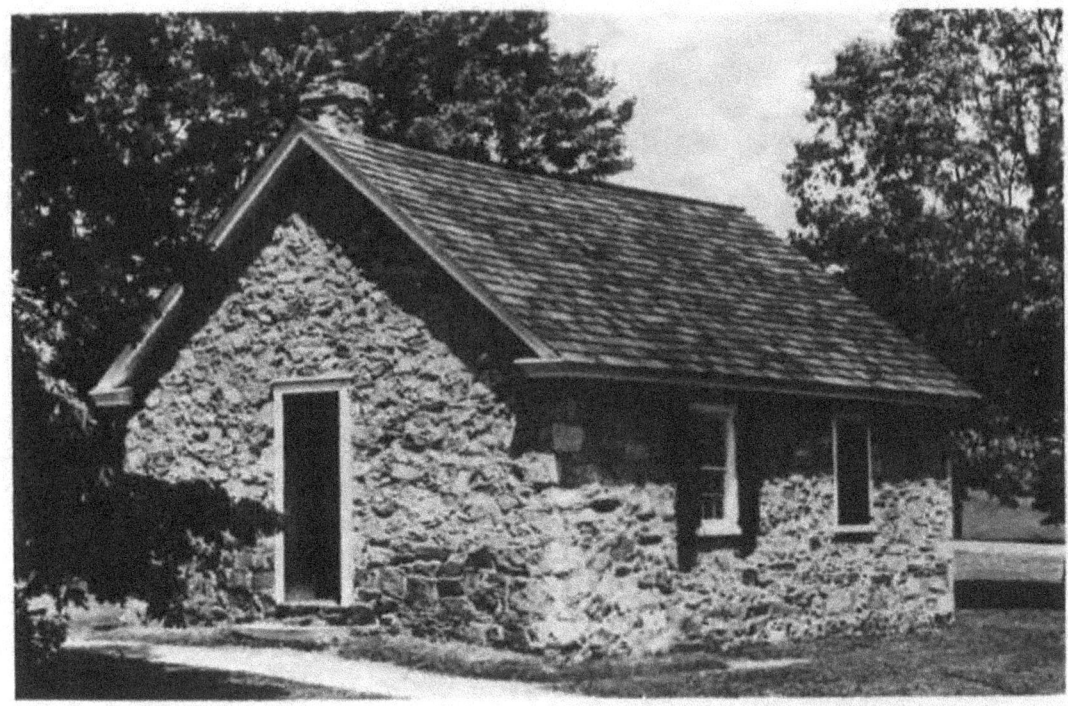

SCHOOLHOUSE USED AS HOSPITAL AT VALLEY FORGE. *(Courtesy of Historical Society of Pennsylvania.)*

agement was the responsibility of Physician and Surgeon General of the Army Cochran. In these units were kept, as was the custom also with regimental hospitals, only those who would be ready in a short time to return to duty and those who would be moved to a general hospital as soon as their conditions permitted.[29]

General Washington issued the order which led to the establishment of the Valley Forge flying hospital early in January. He required his generals to have two huts built for each brigade at appropriate locations 100 to 300 yards to the rear as soon as men could be spared for the work from constructing shelters for the rest of the army. These hospital huts were to be 15 feet wide, 25 feet long, and at least 9 feet high. They were to be covered with board or shingles, the cracks were to be left unfilled in the interests of ventilation, and there were to be a chimney at one end and a window on each side.[30]

General Washington wanted patients to be kept as close as possible to camp, which necessitated the opening of new units near Valley Forge, for which the Hospital Department at that time had "neither utensils nor necessities required to open new ones." Nearby buildings, therefore, including churches, barns, and even a schoolhouse, were pressed into service to house Valley Forge patients who could not be accommodated in brigade huts. The assignment of the individual patient to a hospital was always to be made by Cochran. General Washington pointed out that sending men to overcrowded hospitals or to units not prepared to receive them could have already caused some deaths.[31]

A lack of discipline among army doctors continued to plague the hospital system at Valley Forge. Although there were more than sixty surgeons and thirty-three mates serving with General Washington's army shortly before it entered winter camp, it was difficult to estimate the exact number actually on duty at Valley Forge because so many were able to wangle furloughs to which they were not entitled. At one point, the general forbade all leave for doctors, and in April, he ruled that only passes signed by Cochran were to be honored. In an attempt to further ensure that the sick of his army receive as nearly adequate care as was possible under the circumstances, General Washington also ordered the commanding officer of each brigade to appoint a captain to make daily visits to the sick of his unit who were hospitalized in the vicinity of Valley Forge.[32]

The casual attitude of so many Valley Forge physicians toward their responsibilities even thwarted General Washington's attempts to estimate the strength of his army. The reports of hospital surgeons on the number of men being cared for in their facilities differed markedly from those of regimental surgeons who were, despite the general's efforts, still careless, both in meeting the deadlines which had been set for their reports and in clearing hospitalizations with Cochran.[33]

By spring it was necessary to prepare the flying hospital for the new campaign season. Although the army was "becoming more sickly," the flying hospital itself was reported by Craik to be "in fine order." General Washington's principal concern in this connection seems to have been the speed with which the staff of the flying hospital could move the wounded after a battle back to a general hospital, since he did not wish to be again encumbered with disabled soldiers while his army was on the march. He therefore ordered the physicians of that unit to investigate the most efficient ways to move the seriously ill or wounded to permanent facilities, and by the end of June, approximately 85 percent of those under the care of surgeons appear to have been transferred to general hospitals.[34]

During the winter of 1777–78, patients from the camp too ill to remain in the flying hospital were cared for in the general hospitals nearest Valley Forge, while facilities at a greater distance sheltered the sick and wounded hospitalized during the fall's campaigns. In the first group, the Yellow Springs facility was by far the largest and most important. It was built during the early winter on land owned by an army physician, Dr. Samuel Kennedy, in an area already well known for the healing properties of its mineral spring.[35]

Unlike so many of the army's hospitals during this period, the Yellow Springs unit was carefully planned from the outset. The main building, later called Washington Hall, was specifically designed for the purpose and could comfortably shelter 125 patients. It was three stories and an attic high, 106 by 36 feet in dimension. The first floor held the kitchen, dining room, and service rooms, the second two large wards, and the third many small rooms. Nine-foot porches extended around three sides of the first two stories. Dr. Bodo Otto, formerly in charge of the Trenton hospital, was called to take over here, where he was joined by at least two of his sons and by Kennedy himself.[36]

Although Otto's patients began to arrive before the new building was ready for use and thus had to be sheltered in three nearby barns, the Yellow Springs unit quickly acquired a reputation for being "very neat, and the sick comfortably provided" for.[37] General Washington himself visited the hospital in May, speaking "to every person in their bunks, which exceedingly pleased the sick," and was apparently favorably impressed by the facility.[38]

Nevertheless, the Yellow Springs unit was not without its problems. Putrid fever raged

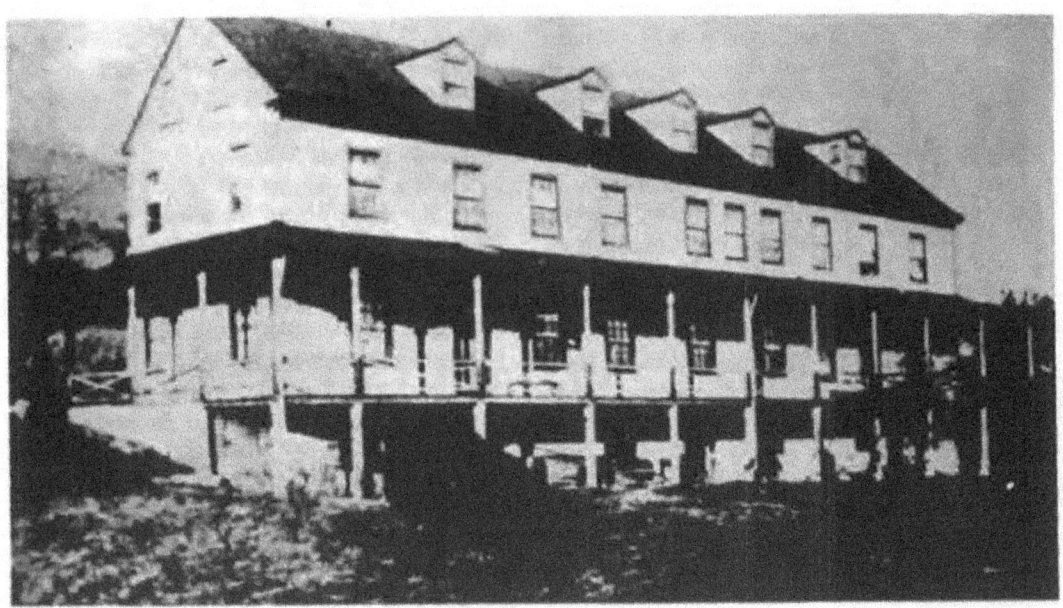

WASHINGTON HALL. *(From James E. Gibson, Dr. Bodo Otto and the Medical Background of the American Revolution, 1937. Courtesy of Charles C Thomas, Publisher, Springfield, Ill.)*

there as elsewhere, and Kennedy, among others, died from it. The staff found that a shortage of the wine so esteemed for its medicinal properties triggered problems with rowdy officers who "crowd in upon us and from the reputation of our hospitals, . . . call for wine and threaten excision if they do not get it." Furthermore, the number of patients was so great that other nearby buildings were pressed into service, the three barns were retained in use even after the main building was opened, and a convalescent unit was opened about two miles distant from Washington Hall.[39]

Among the units caring for battle casualties was the hospital reopened in Bethlehem, Pennsylvania, in September. At the end of November, Shippen recorded only 383 patients at this facility, but patients continued to arrive in the village throughout December. *(See Table 6.)* The total number of the sick and wounded in the Bethlehem Single Brethren's House alone by the end of December, after the arrival of fifty wagons laden with men from New Jersey on the 27th, was reported to be over 700. Many of these patients arrived after exhausting journeys through snow and rain clad "in rags swarming with vermin" and despite the Moravians' efforts to collect blankets, bandaging, and clothing on their behalf, continued even in the hospital to be poorly clothed and filthy. In this environment, of course, wounds quickly became infected and putrid fever appeared. It spread rapidly not only among patients but also among attendants, many of whom were Moravians,[40] and afflicted most heavily those on the upper floor, where "the stench and filth were bad indeed." The Reverend John Ettwein wrote in his account of the 1777–78 winter that among the Moravians, "several died (among them my best & dearest Son 20 Years old)."[41]

Preparation to close the Bethlehem hospital began in the spring of 1778, and in

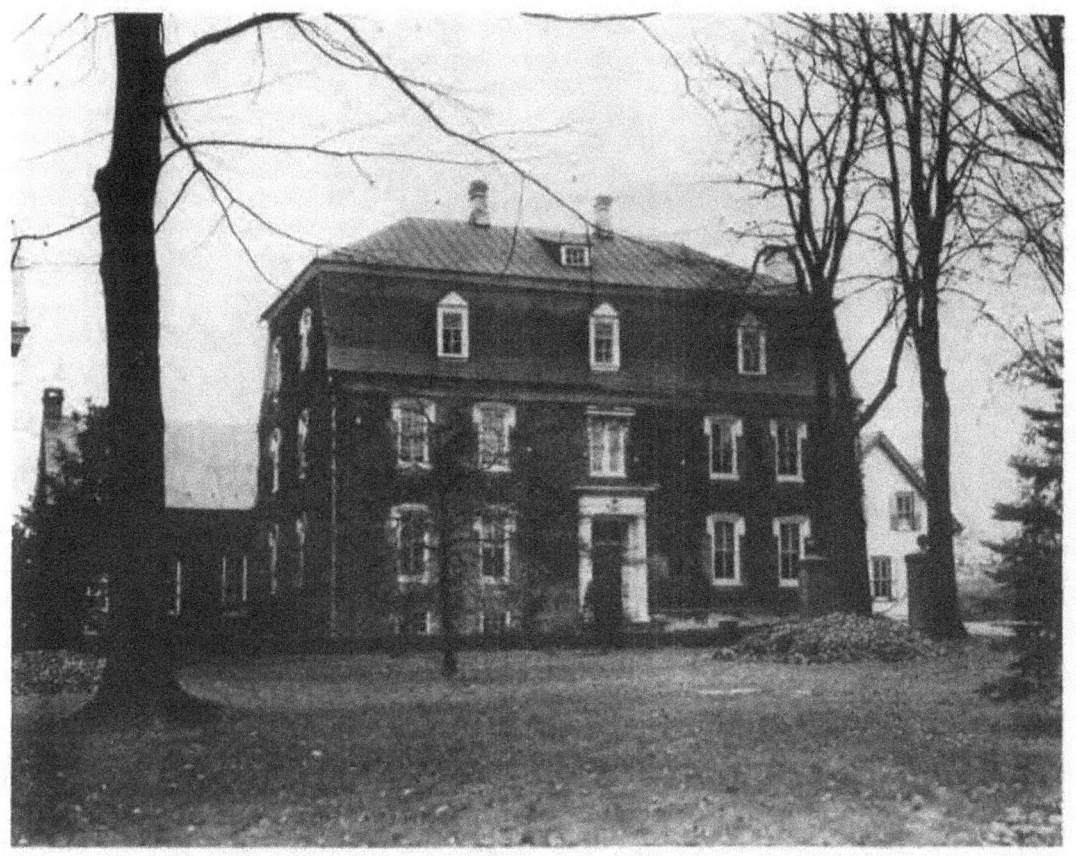

BRETHREN'S HOUSE AT LITITZ. *(Courtesy of Historical Society of Pennsylvania.)*

mid-April, a large number of the patients, about 100 of whom were classified as convalescents, were removed to the facilities at Lititz, Pennsylvania. A few still remained in Bethlehem in early May, however, and it was not until late June that the Moravian men were able to reoccupy their home. The staff of this hospital was moved to the Yellow Springs area to serve patients left behind at Valley Forge.[42]

The village of Lititz, to which so many Bethlehem patients were taken in April 1778, was a Moravian community about half the size of Bethlehem. Since here, too, the order possessed large buildings appropriate for hospital use, when hospitals near Philadelphia were being evacuated, a unit was established in the stone Brethren's House, which was three stories high, 60 feet long, and 37 feet wide. Dr. Samuel Kennedy was in charge of the Lititz unit from the time of the unit's opening until he moved to Yellow Springs, when he was succeeded by Dr. Henry Latimer. Dr. William Brown, best known as the probable author of the first American pharmacopoeia, made Lititz his headquarters after his selection as Physician General in February 1778.[43]

The hospital at Lititz, apparently overcrowded soon after its opening, was also swept by disease during the winter of

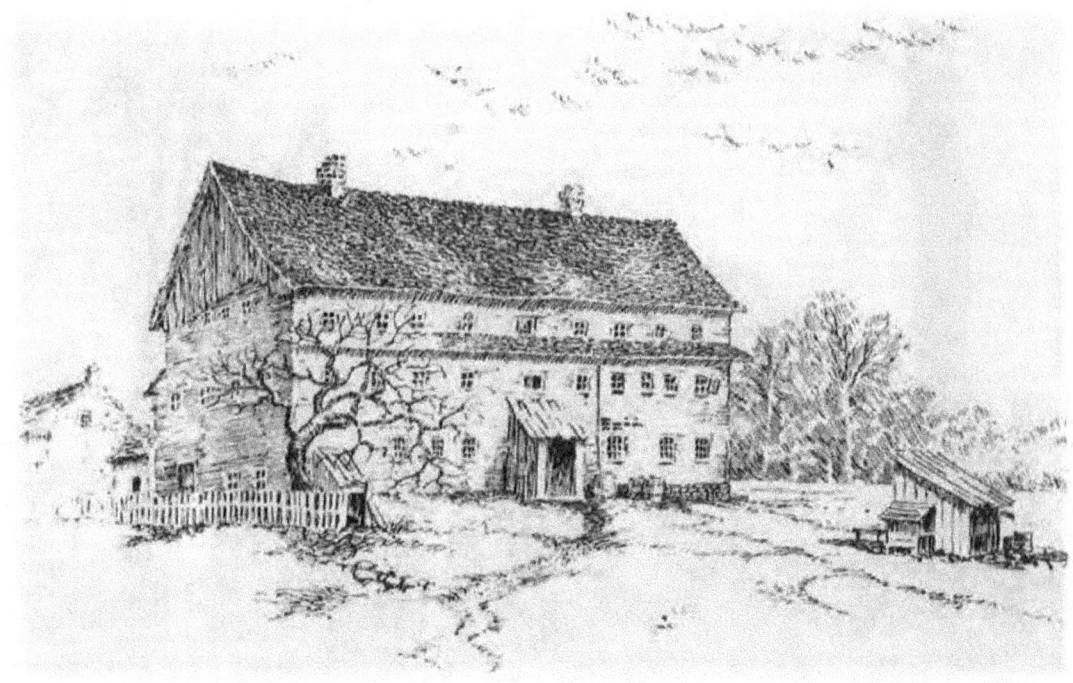

BROTHERS' HOUSE AT EPHRATA. *(From Duncan,* Medical Men.*)*

1777–78. Although the first eighty patients arrived in fifteen wagons on the evening of 19 December, only two days later the unit had become so crowded that its staff had to turn away 100 patients. Inevitably, in a very short time, putrid fever was raging. The hospital quickly ran out of medicine and members of the staff began to fall ill. In a ten-day period ending 1 January 1778, seven patients died. From 12 to 22 January 1778, there were 12 deaths and 25 cases of putrid fever among the 173 patients. In the course of the winter, both of the physicians serving the hospital contracted the disease at the same time, and civilian doctors had to be called in to care temporarily for military patients. Five Moravian nursing volunteers and the congregation's pastor died. The Sisters' House Diary of Lititz records in an entry at the end of December, "The misery of the lazaretto cannot be described; neither can it, without being seen, be imagined." [44]

The town of Ephrata, where a Hospital Department unit opened about the time of the Brandywine engagement, was another unusual religious community, not of Moravians, however, but of "Dunkards," after whom Ephrata was also called Dunkerstown. The Dunkards of Ephrata were actually a splinter from the original Dunkards, lived celibate and almost monastic lives, and observed the seventh day of the week as the Sabbath. At Ephrata, three surgeons and two mates apparently formed the staff which, during the course of the winter and spring, cared for about 500 patients. Although the buildings they used were relatively large, the Dunkards of Ephrata had made their rooms small and the doorways low, in an attempt to keep the occupants humble. [45]

The community kept the hospital well

supplied with veal and milk, and Shippen sent in all the required medicines, while the physicians in charge reportedly maintained a high level of discipline; but the death rate was still high. Putrid fever soon invaded this unit, too, and killed patients, staff, and Dunkards who had volunteered to serve as nurses. As many as 200 were rumored to have died and been buried on a hill in a plot belonging to the community, but Brig. Gen. Lachlan McIntosh reported that from 18 December 1777 to 26 April 1778, only 57 either died or deserted and 168 were discharged, with 34 remaining in the hospital as of that date.[46]

Ephrata was considered at the time to be "An inconvenient place for an Hospital," but an unknown number of the patients from the facility at Reamstown, Pennsylvania, were moved there, nevertheless, on 17 March 1778, when the Reamstown unit was closed. By June 1778, however, the Ephrata hospital, too, had been closed.[47]

Another important Pennsylvania hospital during this period was at Reading, often for patients whose ultimate destination lay further to the west. Beginning in September 1777, the courthouse, a potter's shop, several churches, a Quaker meetinghouse, and other buildings in Reading were used to shelter patients. Soldiers' wives were among the patients here and as many as eight of the nurses were women. These buildings quickly filled up and as early as mid-December men were being sent on to other hospitals, including that at Ephrata. On 30 March, 149 patients were reported to be at the Reading facilities, but by mid-April, only 32 remained. General McIntosh recorded a total of 132 as dead or deserted in the seven months of the hospital's operations to that date, 367 sent on to Lancaster County hospitals, 22 furloughed, and 513 more returned to camp.[48]

Other large general hospitals in Pennsylvania at this time included the units at Allentown and Easton. In November 1777, the Allentown facility held 190 men and that at Easton 400, but by March 1778, the two together held no more than 70 patients and were plagued by shortages, especially by a shortage of beef. Shippen, on visiting these hospitals in the spring, urged that both be closed and that any patients not ready to return to camp be sent to Bethlehem. The men at Easton were moved to Bethlehem on 27 March, but the unit at Allentown remained open through mid-April.[49]

The idea that the military hospitals in the Middle Department should be consolidated was put forward in the spring of 1778 by both Shippen and General McIntosh, who made an inspection trip among these hospitals at this time at General Washington's request. Both men envisioned a greater concentration of patients at the Lititz unit, to which General McIntosh recommended the removal of the Schaefferstown and Ephrata patients. He urged that all Pennsylvania hospitals except those in Lancaster County (which included the Lititz unit) be closed. Shippen, however, wished to go further and envisioned the expansion of the Lititz facility and the complete abandonment of the village by the Moravians. The Reverend Ettwein, however, wrote General Washington to emphasize that his people from Lititz would be rendered almost incapable of supporting themselves should this happen. Shippen finally abandoned his plan, but the Hospital Department continued to occupy the Brethren's House there for five more months and patients continued to come into Lititz not only from Bethlehem but also from Easton, Allentown, and Reading, as the hospitals in these towns were closed.[50]

In addition to the hospitals in Pennsylvania, at least two units east of Philadelphia remained open during the winter and early spring, one at Princeton and the other in Delaware. The latter facility averaged eighty patients, all from Brig. Gen. William Smallwood's brigade. Originally located at Newport, which General Washington considered to be too exposed, this hospital was moved to the Nottingham Meeting House near Wilmington some time shortly before 22 April 1778. The Princeton hospital, the only one outside of Lancaster County, Pennsylvania, which General McIntosh believed should remain open in the Middle Department, held only fifty-three patients as of 8 April. From 14 January to 8 April, 52 died or deserted from this hospital, while 135 were recorded as returned to duty.[51]

As spring approached, various proposals were put forth concerning the handling of the casualties which would be left behind when the army marched or would be sent to the general hospitals from the flying hospital with General Washington's army. Craik at one time envisioned continuing to use the huts at Valley Forge as units of the general hospital after the army itself had left. He assumed that 1,500 to 1,700 patients would be left behind and urged that Shippen send surgeons and mates to Valley Forge to care for them since, of course, the regimental surgeons would leave with their units.[52]

General Washington, however, was not happy with the use of these huts even for healthy men and had ordered some sickly regiments to vacate their huts as soon as tents could be obtained for them. The rate of illness continued to climb at this critical time, however, and there were not enough wagons available to move the ill to hospitals beyond Valley Forge. The general seemed to have at last resigned himself to the temporary use of huts for the sick, but he ordered that any mud used as plastering be removed and every effort be taken to improve ventilation.[53]

The general also ordered that officers be appointed to stay behind with the ill at the rate of one officer for every 250 men. He told his regimental surgeons to report to Cochran on the number of men who could not march with the army and required that medical attendants from each brigade remain to care for these men until hospital surgeons could remove them. An attempt was also to be made to find women to serve as nurses for the patients remaining at Valley Forge. On 1 June, General Washington appointed a colonel to supervise the care of the sick and to send them back to the army as they recovered. Finally it was decided to put Otto in charge of the patients left behind and to move them when possible either to Yellow Springs or to a new hospital to be established for them elsewhere.[54]

On 18 June, the British evacuated Philadelphia and General Washington led his army out of Valley Forge to reoccupy that city and then through Bucks County, Pennsylvania, across the Delaware River; on 28 June, the army was into the first action of the new season, at Monmouth, New Jersey.[55]

THE NORTHERN DEPARTMENT

Although the men under Maj. Gen. Philip Schuyler, like General Washington's men, continued to suffer from a lack of clothing, prospects for the new season of campaigning seemed reasonably bright as far as the army's health was concerned. The smallpox problem was under control, and newly planted gardens promised a reliable supply of fresh vegetables. The total number who were sick of the 4,533 men who were at Ticonderoga and Mount Independence on 25 June, however, is difficult to estimate. (*Map 5*) Samuel Adams reported 342 to be "Sick in camp, and in barricks" as of that date,[56] and since General Schuyler complained of the hospital under construction there that "not one single room . . . is yet finished, nor will it soon be in condition to receive a considerable number of sick,"[57] one might safely assume that there were few patients, if any, being cared for outside of "camp . . . and barricks," in this area. It is, therefore, surprising to note that

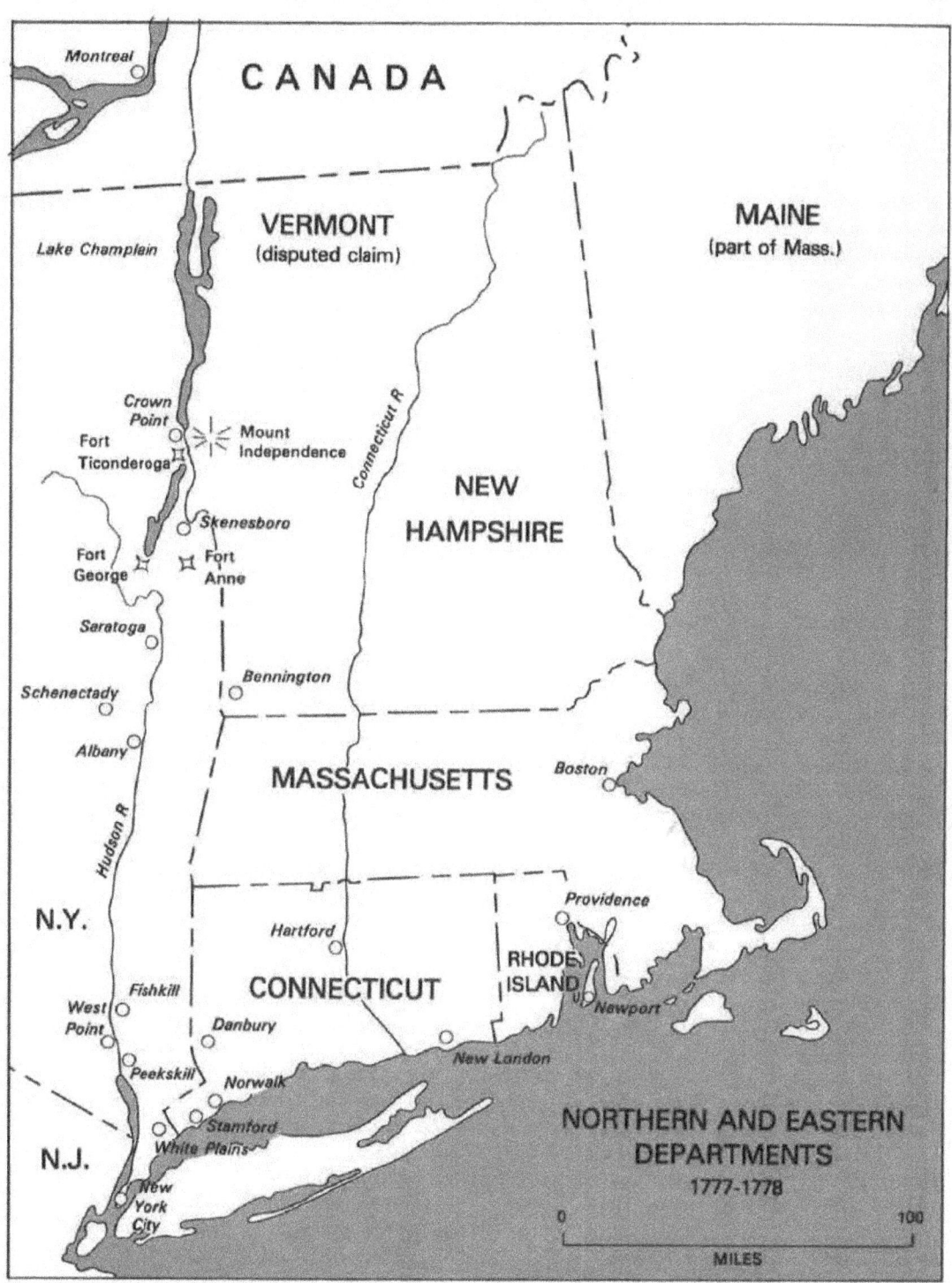

MAP 5

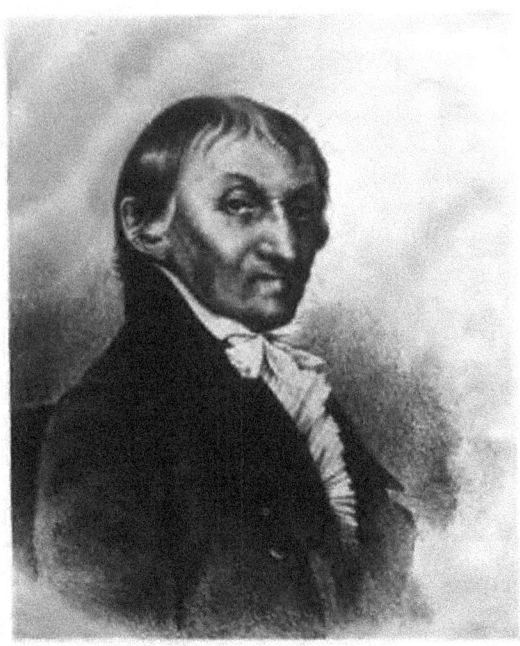

JAMES THACHER. *(Courtesy of National Library of Medicine.)*

in the entire Northern Department in July and August the overall sick rate, if monthly report figures are used, was just under 24 percent and that more than half of these were "sick absent." General Schuyler was distressed by the condition of the hospital accommodations on Lake Champlain and at the end of June had all the patients not likely to be ready to return to duty in a very short time moved in covered boats to the Fort George facilities where, he believed, there would also be a better supply of vegetables.[58]

The British, under Maj. Gen. John Burgoyne, had already begun their move south, and when, on 6 July, Continental forces abandoned Ticonderoga, the remaining patients, along with hospital and other supplies, were hastily loaded into 200 small boats. That night, escorted by five armed galleys and a guard of 600 men, these vessels slipped across thirty miles of water as still as glass to Skenesboro, at the southern tip of the lake. They were so closely pursued by the enemy, however, that they were unable to stop there and were forced to continue south along a small river to Fort Anne, in the process losing to the British several patients and most of their supplies. At Fort Anne, the sick were placed in tents where they remained until 25 July, when surgeon's mate James Thacher was ordered to take them by boat to Albany. Thacher and his forty patients arrived there safely, having covered approximately fifty-five miles in three days.[59] On 29 July, the British also took Fort George. If any of the patients who had been moved to Fort George from Ticonderoga were still there, presumably they also moved farther to the south before the British arrived.

Although the hospitals in the Lake Champlain-Lake George area were abandoned in the summer of 1777, a new unit was established at roughly the same time in the vicinity of Bennington, Vermont, to serve the militia units gathering there. American patients were cared for by regimental surgeons in whatever shelters could be found for them scattered about the countryside, but after the British were severely defeated in their raid on Bennington, Dr. Francis Hagan reported to Potts that a meetinghouse had been taken over for wounded prisoners and two German surgeons had been placed in charge of them. Stores were badly needed; this shortage was to continue throughout the summer and fall, causing unnecessary suffering for the unit's patients. Hagan could not find nurses for the wounded, and the local population was of no assistance to him, but his patients were in no condition to be moved. The situation here seems to have only deteriorated as the season progressed, for as late as 21 September, Hagan was writing Potts of his fear of the effects of cold weather upon his patients, of the poor condition of the prisoners, and of the additional problem posed by the fact that the British and Hessian patients were mutually antagonistic.[60]

Not all was gloomy at Bennington, however. Another physician there, Dr. Samuel MacKenzie, wrote Potts on 27 August 1777, "I want Doctr Treat here very much to prescribe leeks for the Doctrs as they seem very fond of bundling and the Tory girls seem to have no objection to that kind of amusement." [61]

The flying hospital for the Continental Army in the Northern Department, under the direction of Physician and Surgeon General of the Army John Bartlett, was also beset by many problems. Its location as the army prepared to meet General Burgoyne at Saratoga was considered unhealthy, and at times the sick entering and being discharged were too numerous to count, although on 18 August, Bartlett fixed the number of patients at 335, under the care of thirty-two nurses. Regimental surgeons contributed to the situation by complaining that Bartlett was refusing to supply them with medicines, lint, and bandages, a charge he vigorously denied. His staff was too small, he added, and he needed three more regimental surgeons and three more mates. By the end of the month, when he still had 192 patients in his hospital, such regimental surgeons as were available were refusing to help him, saying that Maj. Gen. Horatio Gates, who replaced General Schuyler on 19 August, had forbidden them to do so.[62]

Despite the good beginning, as the summer progressed, sickness increased in the Northern Army. The men were often in retreat, at times without shelter, and almost always short of every sort of supplies except food, and the quality of that food was open to criticism. Nevertheless, on 20 July 1777, of 6,023 officers and men, only 459 were reported to be in the general hospital, a figure which apparently represented about half of the total list of those sick and presented a marked contrast to the situation in the North the previous year. The staff of the department included fifteen surgeons and seven mates and the much feared putrid fever was not a great threat. Furthermore, during the period 1 March to 29 August 1777, only fifty-three of the men cared for by these doctors were reported to have died.[63]

General Gates's force grew rapidly in October 1777. He had approximately 8,000 officers and men on 4 October, 885 of whom were sick in the general hospital and another 4,000 men joined him in the course of the following three days. In contrast to the situation which developed in the North in the spring of 1776, however, the staff of the Hospital Department in the Saratoga area, responsible for both American patients and wounded prisoners, also grew rapidly until it was almost double its original size. From the end of August to mid-November 1777, however, another 150 men were reported to have died and the British complained that their wounded held by the Continental Army were not being well treated. In September, British Brig. Gen. Simon Fraser himself inquired with concern about sick and wounded prisoners in American hands after the British raid on Bennington and suggested that he could forward both medicines and surgeons to aid in their care, but General Gates appeared initially to have rejected this offer. The American informed his counterpart that his wounded prisoners were well supplied with "Surgeons, medicines, and attendance, with every comfort imaginable." After their Saratoga defeat in October, however, when the British were forced to abandon an entire hospital, including approximately 250 patients, five medical attendants remained with their patients in captivity.[64]

At some time in the fall, the British wounded were moved from the Saratoga area to the Albany facilities, where more than 300 American patients were being cared for, but their chief physician continued to complain of the treatment they received and of supply shortages. Among the enemy patients here who had the least cause for complaint, however, was one Maj. John Dyke Ackland (Acland), who was shot through both legs. His wife, who had accompanied him through the entire campaign, sailed down the Hudson River, accompanied only by a maid, a valet, and a chaplain, to join her husband at Albany and to nurse him back to health at the hospital. She apparently was treated with true gallantry by General Gates.[65]

Most of the American patients at the Albany hospital suffered from disease rather than from physical injuries; numbers of patients reported in mid-August were as follows:

Dysentery	81	Rupture	2
Intermittent fever	79	Scorbutic	4
Diarrhea	61	Pleurisy	3
Rheumatism	22	Hemorrhoid	1
Cough	25	Hemoptysis	2
Convalescent	17	Nephritis	3
Debility	17	Asthma	1
Lues venerea	14	Paralysis	2
Fever	13	Cholera	1
Whooping cough	10	Hypochondria	1
Head itch	9	Scrofula	3
Measles	8	Ophthalmia	1
Putrid fever	6		
Bilious fever	4	Total	396
Dropsy	4		
Jaundice	2	Surgical	53

SOURCE: A Return of the Present State of the General Hospital at Abany [sic] 20 Aug 1777, Potts Papers, 2: 283. This return, however, gives an incorrect total of 296.

In the fall of 1777 the patients with physical injuries included none other than Brig. Gen. Benedict Arnold (promoted to major general on 29 November 1777), who was again wounded, this time by a musket ball which had broken his leg. Of Arnold the patient, Thacher said, "He is very peevish and impatient under his misfortunes." Hospitalized for a time with Arnold was a young lieutenant colonel, James Wilkinson, who was to lead a colorful life after the Revolution and to serve with less than complete success as a major general in the War of 1812. While on duty in the North, Colonel Wilkinson became so ill that he had to be evacuated by wagon first to Albany and then, on 20 October, accompanied by a hospital surgeon, further south, taking with him the details of the Saratoga victory.[66]

By the end of October, the overflow from the main Albany unit had spilled over into private homes and a church. Enemy patients were being cared for by their own surgeons, but Thacher considered the Hessian doctors "uncouth and clumsy operators." The operations being performed consisted principally of amputations and trepanning, and some surgical patients for a time had to endure maggots which thrived in their wounds. Among the twenty patients Potts had assigned to Thacher was a particularly interesting one in the person of an American captain who had managed to survive a scalping at the hands of the Indians.[67]

The increase in the number of patients at the Albany unit strained the supply system in the Northern Department. For a time, no fresh straw was available, and with the harsh northern winter rapidly approaching, wood was also badly needed. In an attempt to relieve the pressure on the hospital, seventy to eighty men were returned to their barracks and steps taken to furlough an even greater number. By mid-November, however, 218 patients, 118 wounded and 100 sick, were still listed on the rolls at the Albany hospital, a figure which a month later had risen to a total of 297.[68]

The number of patients under the care of Dr. Dirk Van Ingen in Schenectady had also increased in this period to the point where by late summer Van Ingen had found it necessary to hire two men and two women to care for them in the two rooms which had been allotted them in a barracks. By mid-August, he needed bedding, medicines, and more attendants for his forty-three patients. In November the Schenectady unit was treating 72 patients and a month later 312, more than were reported for that period by the Albany unit. The subsequent decrease in the patient load by February 1778 led to the transfer of remaining Schenectady patients to Albany, where on 16 February 1778 there were only 304 patients, 24 of whom were children being wormed. (The records do not indicate whether these patients were military dependents.) [69]

Inoculation continued to be practiced in the Northern Department, although the evidence suggests that the procedure was undertaken earlier in the year in the North than it was in the Middle Department. Repeated references to the fact that inoculation was taking place can be found, but since the records remaining to us from this period rarely distinguish between smallpox deliberately and naturally acquired, we can only assume that most of the smallpox patients hospitalized in the Northern Department at this time had acquired the disease through deliberate immunization. Northern Department records list 68 smallpox patients at Albany and 260 at Schenectady in December 1777, but only 30 at Albany and 55 at Schenectady in January, and on 15 January, Dr. Robert Johnston noted that those patients who had been inoculated had done well and were almost ready to return to duty.[70]

The total number of patients in the Northern Department at the end of November was estimated by Director General Shippen at 1,000. Potts had been forced by ill health to return to Pennsylvania at the end of the campaign season and Johnston was asked by both General Gates and Potts to function as Deputy Director General in the Northern Department, although it appears that he was never actually named to the position. By the end of the year, since the patient load was diminishing and all of the twenty patients assigned specifically to Thacher's care had recovered, the young surgeon was permitted to go on a forty-day furlough.[71]

When Thacher returned in February 1778, although the hospital was in desperate need of money, the atmosphere was quite different from that prevailing in Middle Department hospitals at this time. "Several gentlemen belonging to the hospital being desirous of improving in the accomplishment of dancing," Thacher and his friends actually hired a teacher and every afternoon worked with him to prepare themselves to "figure in a ballroom." In the spring of 1778, with the patient load still steadily decreasing, the decision was made to move most of the Albany staff and supplies down the Hudson to the West Point area, since it was expected that in the future major Continental operations would not take place in the Northern Department. On 5 June, therefore, the staff, except for three doctors who stayed behind to care for the remaining patients, and the facility's stores were embarked on a sloop and taken down the Hudson. Two days after its departure, the unit stopped at Fishkill to replenish its food supply and on 10 June was ready to install itself on the east bank of the Hudson across from West Point. Large houses surrounded by extensive farms and gardens had been found for the hospital facilities to be established there; good pasture for horses and cows abounded, and a number of large orchards offered several kinds of fruit. The principal house used by the Hospital Department here was referred to as Robinson's House, after the wealthy Tory Col. Beverly Robinson, from whom it was confiscated following his flight to New York City.[72]

THE EASTERN DEPARTMENT

Despite several British raids in the area, there was no major action in the department east of the Hudson River in the period June 1777 to June 1778, and there were few patients for Eastern Department hospitals to treat, only 383 being reported there in late November 1777. Dr. Isaac Foster had been placed in charge of this department in April

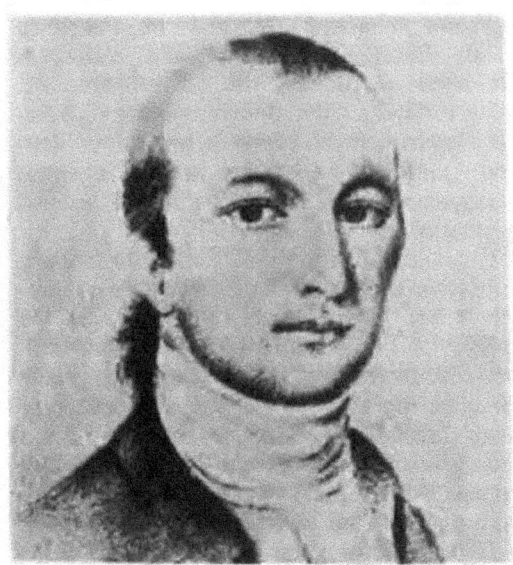

PHILIP TURNER. *(From Packard, History, I: 565; reproduced from Charles B. Graves, "Dr. Philip Turner of Norwich, Connecticut." Annals of Medical History 10 (1928). Courtesy of Harper & Row, Publishers, Inc.)*

1777 with physicians Ammi Ruhamah Cutter and Philip Turner as his Physician General and his Surgeon General, respectively, and Dr. William Burnet as his Physician and Surgeon General of the Army. Cutter apparently resigned his position in March 1778.[73]

The hospitals within this department included units at Danbury, to which the Stamford hospital had been moved, Hartford and New London, Connecticut, Providence and Newport, Rhode Island, Boston, Massachusetts, and Fishkill and Peekskill, New York. The assignment of patients to appropriate hospitals was the responsibility of Burnet, who also received reports from regimental surgeons reputed to be often careless with their reporting. Turner apparently made his headquarters at Danbury, where a five-room building housed the hospital, and traveled a 400-mile circuit to visit lesser units.[74]

The hospitals in his department, Foster maintained, were in excellent condition and "the sick soldiers are as anxious this year, to be admitted into them, as they were last, to avoid them." Rush believed Foster's division to be so superabundantly supplied with linen, bedding, and similar items that he suggested that the Director General send someone to New England to bring back a portion of their plenty to the Middle Department.[75]

The only real concern for the medical staff of the Eastern Department lay in the possibility of a smallpox epidemic among newly arrived troops during the active part of the campaign season, since, as noted in the section on health at Valley Forge, inoculation was not undertaken during the summer. As early as July 1777, therefore, Maj. Gen. Israel Putnam, commanding in the Peekskill, New York, area, ordered the immediate hospitalization and isolation of all who so much as seemed to be infected with the disease. Inoculation was undertaken in the late winter and early spring of 1778, however, and the existing records do not mention any type of epidemic in this department in the period June 1777 to June 1778. Foster was able to comment in March 1778 that "we do very little here."[76]

The 1777–78 season was characterized by inactivity in the Eastern Department and the end of large-scale operations in the North, but the Hospital Department had no reason to expect that their work would be easier in the 1778–79 season. The Continental doctors and their patients from General Washington's army had endured another year of agony, and the sickly condition of the men as they left Valley Forge gave little reason for optimism.

5

From Defeat to Victory, June 1778 to 1783

For three years after the battle of Monmouth in June 1778, the major operations of the Continental Army took place in the South, where the organization of the Hospital Department was either weak or nonexistent. The successful siege of British-held Yorktown, Virginia, by a combined French-Continental force in the early autumn of 1781, however, brought an end to all significant military activity in the American Revolution, while the signing of the Treaty of Paris in the early autumn of 1783 was followed by the disbanding of both the Continental Army and its Hospital Department.

NORTH OF THE POTOMAC: BEFORE THE VICTORY AT YORKTOWN

After evacuating Philadelphia in June 1778, the British forces withdrew to New York City, on their way defeating an attempt by the Americans to stop them at Monmouth, New Jersey. (Map 6) After the battle of Monmouth, General Washington also led his men north and established his headquarters at White Plains, New York. General Washington's army saw little action in the North from this point onward,[1] and the number of wounded was correspondingly small, but shortages of food, clothing, and supplies continued to have an unfavorable effect upon both the health of the army and the suffering of the patients in Continental hospitals.

The wounded from the battle at Monmouth were initially cared for in nearby buildings, including a courthouse and churches, where they lay upon straw on the floor. Many fell victim to the heat during the battle, and as the army continued northward, the number of those unable to keep up the pace without medical care increased, the temperatures being so high that a "vast number of our men fell down with the Heat . . . & Died." Early in July, General Washington, concerned lest the army's mobility be impeded by attempts to carry the sick and wounded with it, ordered that they be sent to a barracks in the town of Brunswick, New Jersey, and that the director of the flying hospital inform him at once how many of these men were left behind. Many who became ill after early July appear to have been carried along for a short time in wagons but at the end of the month were sent back to hospitals at Trenton and Princeton, New Jersey. It appears that somewhere in the course of the march to White Plains, men were also hospitalized at Springfield, New Jersey, in accommodations General Washington considered inadequate. Only one Hospital Department physician could be spared for this facility, but a regimental surgeon was assigned to assist him. The number of patients here rose to 200 before these men could be moved to the hospital opened at Morristown, New Jersey.[2]

In returning to New York State, General Washington's men crossed from the Middle into the Eastern Department, where Dr. Isaac Foster was the Deputy Director and Dr. William Burnet the Physician and Sur-

NORTHERN
DEPARTMENT
NEW YORK
Hudson R
New Hackensack
New
Windsor
Fishkill
Otterkill
West Point
Robinson House
Peekskill
Tarrytown
Susquehanna R
Delaware R
MIDDLE
DEPARTMENT
PENNSYLVANIA
Paramus
Jockey
Hollow
Morristown
Basking Ridge
Springfield
NEW
YORK
CITY
Sunbury
Pluckemin
Bound
Brook
Middlebrook
Brunswick
Princeton
Reading
Schaefferstown
Susquehanna R
French Creek
Trenton
Monmouth
Yellow Springs
Lititz
Downingtown
PHILADELPHIA
NEW JERSEY
MARYLAND
DELAWARE
BALTIMORE

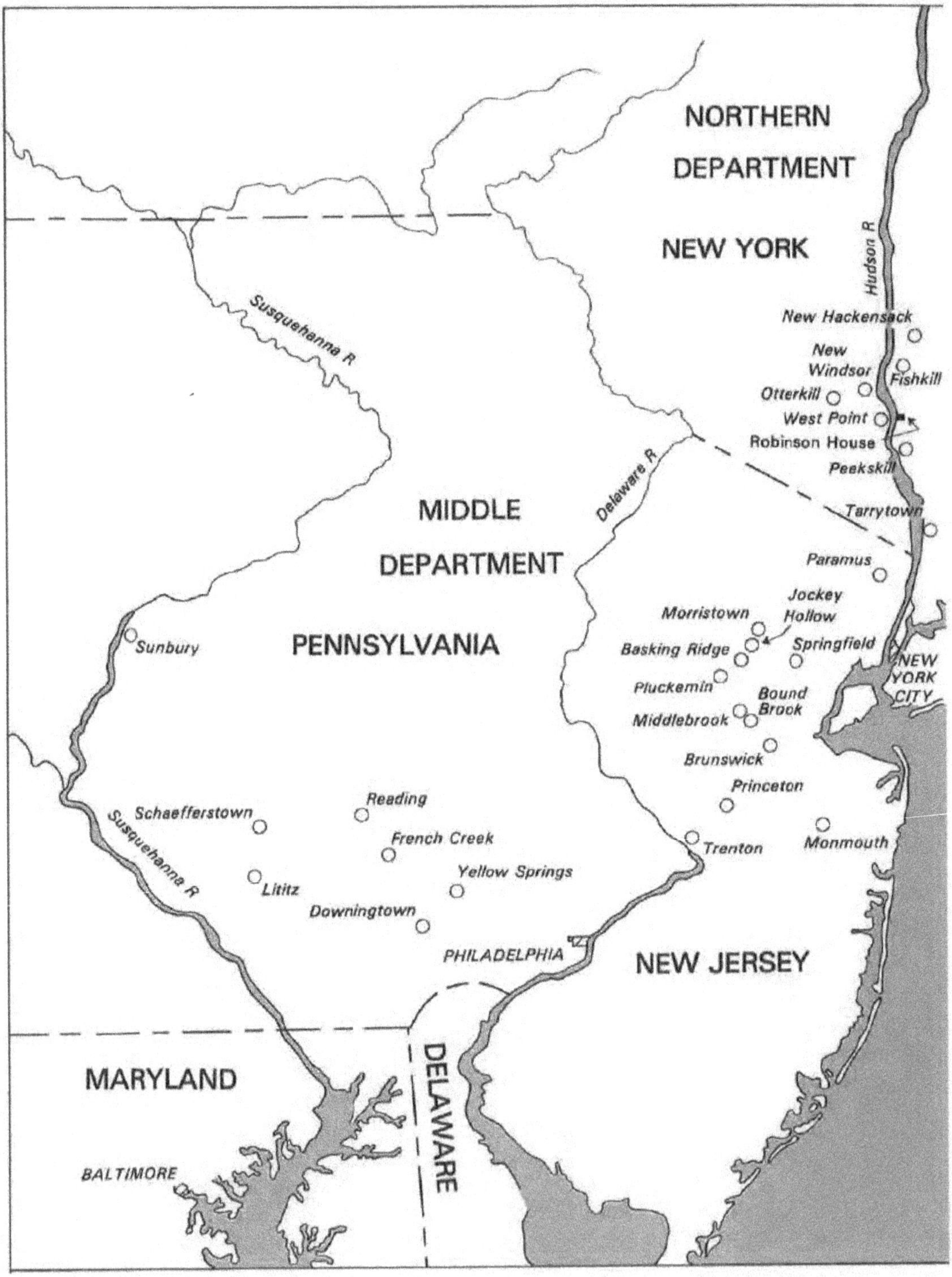

MAP 6

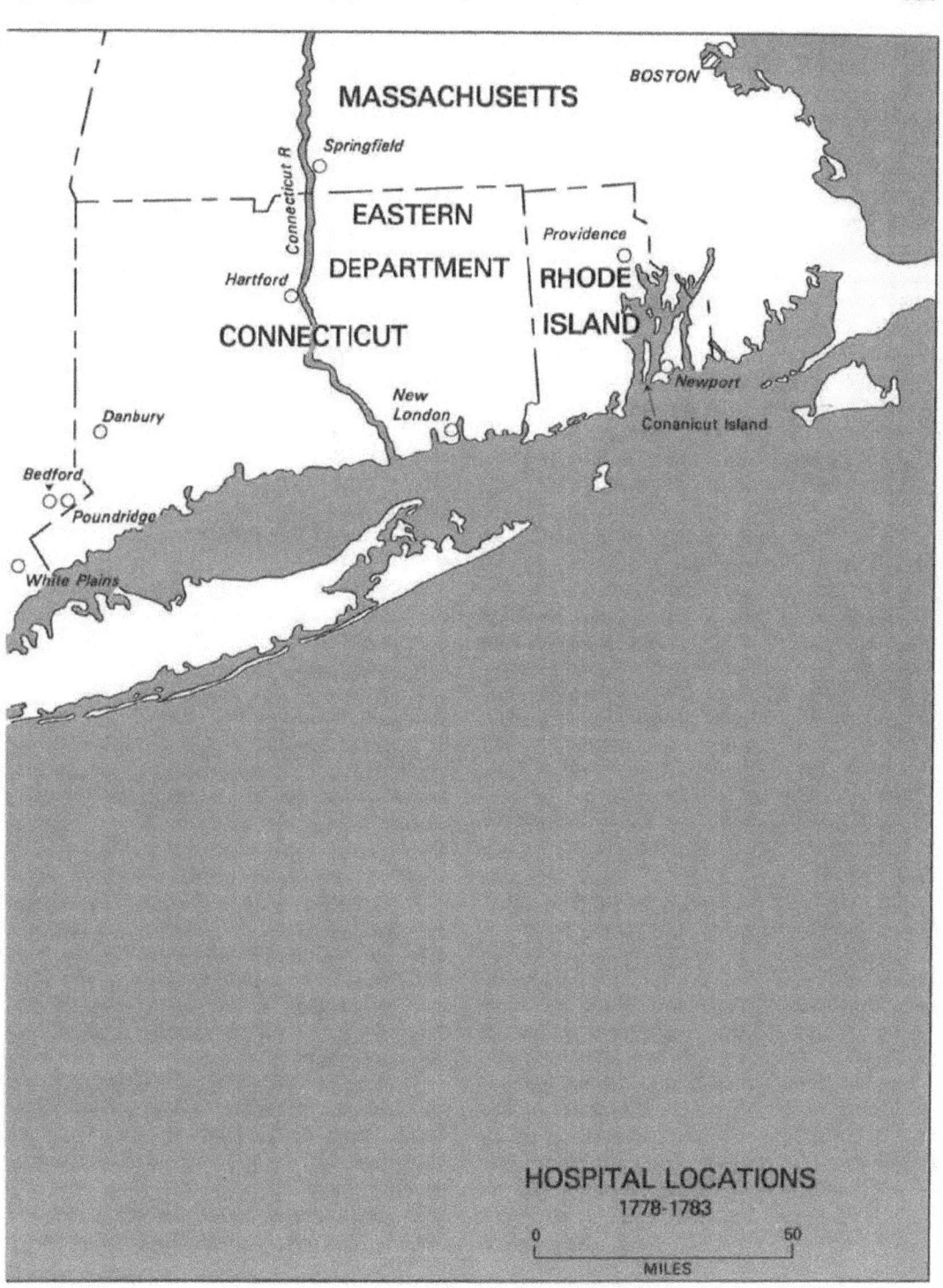

geon General of the Army. Dr. John Cochran, however, was still attached to General Washington's army as Physician and Surgeon General of the Army. The situation was further complicated by the fact that many surgeons from the Northern Department were still working in this area. Rather than grant either Cochran or Burnet supreme authority over flying and regimental hospitals there, General Washington ordered that they share the responsibility. Burnet apparently signed many, if not all, of the weekly returns submitted concerning these facilities,[3] but there does not seem to have been any friction between the two men.

Reports of the late summer of 1778 signed by Burnet as Physician and Surgeon General of General Washington's army suggest that the number of the sick within General Washington's army was running at 1,200 to 1,450 men per week, but not all of the sick soldiers were retained in the hospitals within the camp and the monthly strength report for the period indicates that the rate may have been 17 to 20 percent. On 12 September, a group of patients was moved to the general hospital at Fishkill. Water transportation was frequently resorted to for such moves, many of the patients on this occasion going by land to Tarrytown and thence by water to Fishkill. Those able to walk went on foot to Peekskill, where they boarded boats for the same destination, while their packs were sent separately by the Tarrytown route.[4]

Little detail is available on the management of medical support for the unsuccessful attempt by the Continental Army on Newport, Rhode Island, conducted from 29 July to 31 August 1778, but we know that the care of the 137 American wounded was assigned to Dr. Thomas Tillotson of the staff of the Northern Department and to an assistant, also drawn from the Northern Department staff. Tillotson reported to Foster, from whom he was ordered to obtain his medicine, instruments, and "such things as may be thought necessary in the formation of a military and flying hospital." [5]

When it was time in late 1778 to establish winter camp, several units remained behind at Peekskill, Fishkill, and West Point, New York, and three brigades wintered at Danbury, Connecticut, but the bulk of General Washington's army marched south to winter camp at Middlebrook, New Jersey, in late November. A total of seven brigades spent the winter there, while an eighth camped at Paramus, New Jersey. Information on the precise nature of the hospital facilities serving troops in New Jersey during this winter is not plentiful, but it appears that some patients were housed in nearby churches, barns, and a courthouse, while others were sent to the hospital at Brunswick. There seem also to have been physicians caring for Middlebrook patients at Bound Brook.[6]

There was remarkably little sickness in the Continental Army north of Virginia in the years 1779 and 1780, perhaps as a combined result of inoculation for smallpox, a drop in the proportion of green to seasoned troops in the Army, and efforts to improve sanitation and discipline. Since the health of his army while it camped at Middlebrook did not demand all the time of the regimental surgeons there, General Washington was able to decide that it would be wise if they were to spend some of it improving their professional knowledge and skills. A series of lectures was planned, with the first to be conducted by Dr. William Brown, Physician General of the Middle Department, in February. The general observed that "All regimental surgeons are desired to attend." [7]

In May 1779, General Washington led his men out of winter camp toward West Point, New York, after ordering that the huts they had been using be left standing for the benefit of those too ill to keep up with their fellows. After the army reached West Point, the number hospitalized within the camp at any one time often ran higher than 300, with 20 to 30 percent of this number classified as convalescent. A comparable number might be described as lame. Well over 10 percent of the total in the hospitals within the camp were suffering from intermittent fevers, but putrid fever does not seem to have been a serious threat at this time.[8]

In the fall of 1779, Virginia and Carolina troops were sent south toward their own states, where enemy invasion was anticipated, and other units again camped for the winter along the Hudson River or in Connecticut, but the main body of the army left the Highlands of the Hudson in late November and arrived at the camp at Jockey Hollow, about three miles south of Morristown, early in December.[9]

These men were already in poor condition and without adequate food, clothing, or fuel, and now, since they were not using the site of the 1776-77 encampment, there were no huts available to house them when they arrived. With the snow lying two feet deep around them, they had to lie on the bare earth. For more than a week after their arrival at camp, there was no bread for them to eat.[10]

During the winter of 1779-80, rivers froze solid and temperatures reportedly dropped lower than they had been in decades. The four to six feet of snow which sometimes covered the ground interfered with the transportation and delivery of supplies and occasional thaws only turned roads into quagmires. Food had been hard to obtain even before the onset of winter because the drought of the previous summer had lowered both crop yields and the level of the water which powered flour mills. Now the frozen streams of winter again made milling impossible and, for a long period of time, adequate stocks of clothing were still unavailable. By spring, the army was near starvation and mutinies were beginning to break out.[11]

Surprisingly, however, in view of the conditions at the camp, there were relatively few patients in the hospitals serving Morristown in the winter of 1779-80. In February 1780, approximately 3.5 percent of the slightly more than 11,500 men at Morristown were reported seriously enough ill to be hospitalized and perhaps more than twice this number of the sick were cared for within their own quarters. Those men who did require prolonged hospitalization were sent to the nearby general hospitals at Basking Ridge (also spelled Baskinridge or Baskenridge) or Pluckemin, but in the period 1 March to 1 April 1780, 670 men, or 60 percent of the total requiring hospitalization, did not leave the care of the regimental and flying hospital surgeons. Only eighty-six died from 17 December 1779 to 3 June 1780. These patients were housed in regular huts rather than in especially designed structures, and the huts assigned during the winter to the Pennsylvania Line were taken over in June 1780 to serve as a general hospital for the patients who had to be left behind when the army left its winter encampment. Dr. James Tilton has been traditionally credited with having designed the Morristown hospital huts, but recent research has shown that Tilton's design was apparently used only once during this winter, not at Morristown but for an experimental general hospital building at Basking Ridge, near Morristown.[12]

The troops remaining along the Hudson during the 1779-80 winter apparently fared no better than those at Morristown. Severe snowstorms began late in November and alternated with freezing rain throughout December. The effects of the weather upon the men led Maj. Gen. William Heath to comment that among the men spending the winter there, the number who froze to death rivaled the number returning to the army after treatment at the New Windsor hospital.[13]

As far as the Hospital Department was

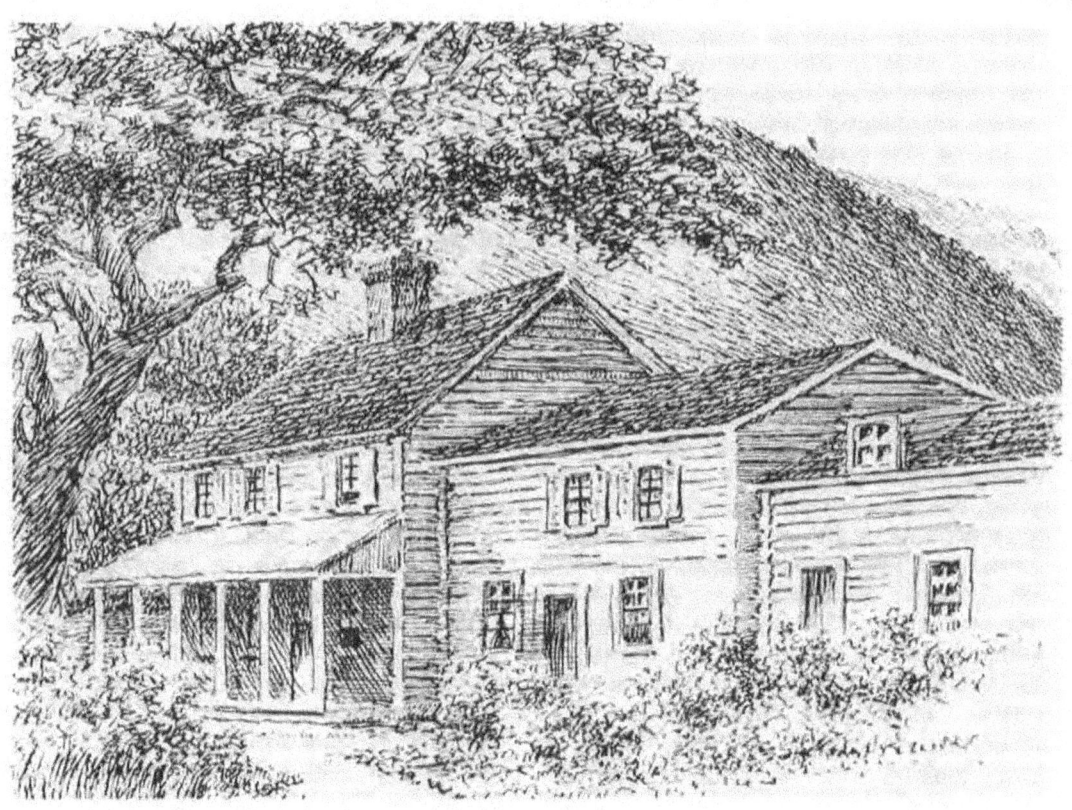

ROBINSON'S HOUSE. *From the number of patients reportedly cared for here, it might be assumed that other buildings in the same area were also used to house patients. (From Duncan,* Medical Men.*)*

concerned, conditions did not improve markedly with the coming of summer. In August, Dr. James Craik commented that "There is a large army without stores, surgeons or any thing comfortable for the sick & wounded." [14] The number of sick grew as the summer progressed, but there continued to be little for patients to eat. By early August, the hospital at Robinson's House, across the Hudson from West Point, held 126 sick and hungry men. Discipline and organization, furthermore, were so poor that, although Cochran urgently needed surgeons, doctors who could have helped him were in Philadelphia and, the Medical Committee was informed, had "no visible employment." [15]

The main part of General Washington's ragged army remained in New York for the winter of 1780–81. Conditions were so poor that mutinies began to break out once again in early January 1781. It was at this difficult time that Director General William Shippen resigned.[16]

Figures in the Hospital Department reports which have survived from this period do not agree with the corresponding Army monthly returns. Although at the end of March 1781, for example, the return of the new Director General, John Cochran, listed a total of 288 patients remaining in regimental and flying hospitals, the official monthly return submitted by General Washington listed only 251 "sick present." The

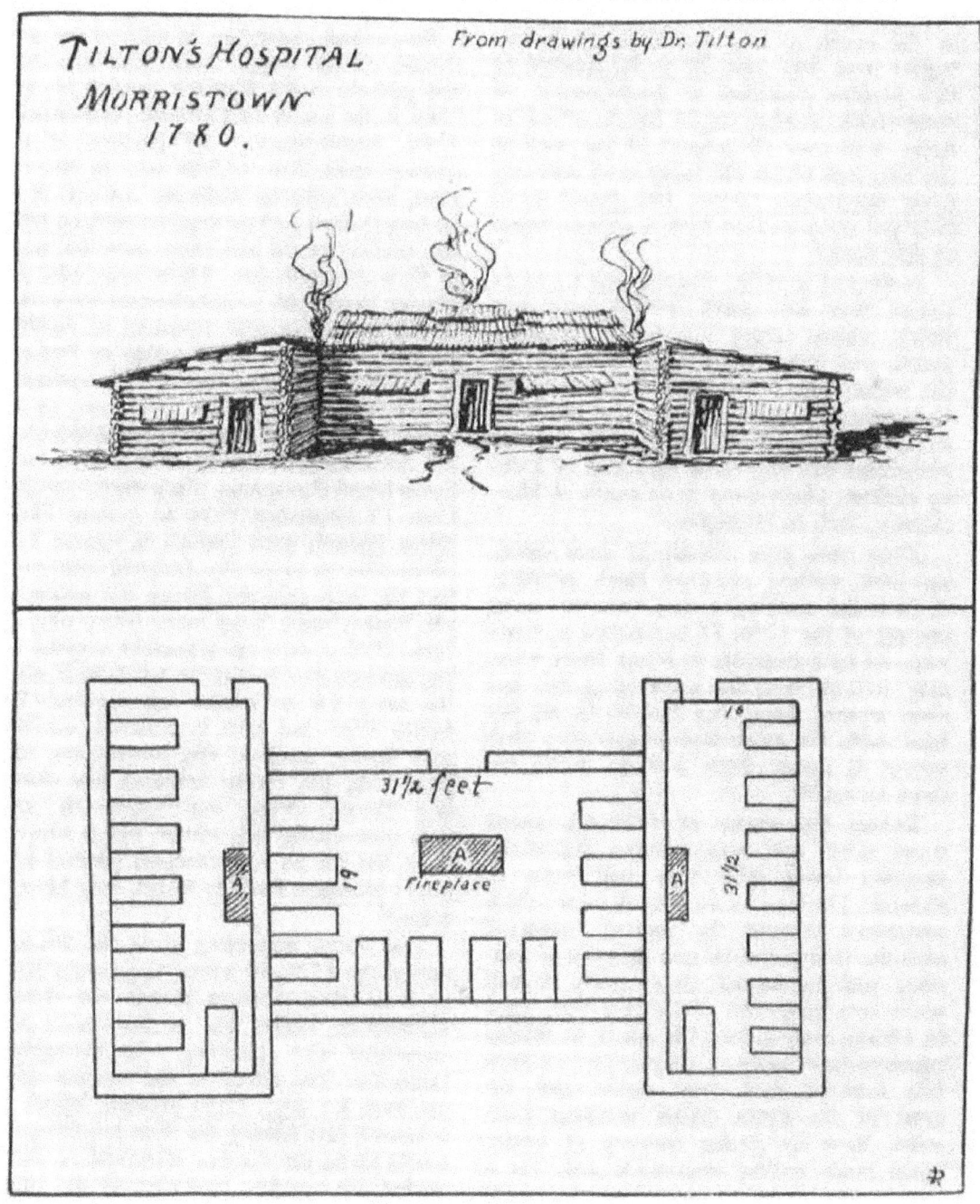

HOSPITAL HUT DESIGNED BY DR. JAMES TILTON. *(From Duncan, Medical Men.)*

following May, however, when Cochran reported a total of 398 men and 40 women and children being cared for by all of the Army's hospitals, the official return recorded a total of 723 under the care of surgeons, 406 "sick present," and 208 "sick absent" among the rank and file and 109 in both categories among the commissioned and noncommissioned officers. The official monthly report for June listed 566 sick in all categories, but the figure given by Cochran for June is 408, with 218 of these in the flying hospital. The discrepancies in the reports of any one given month may, of course, reflect differing base dates for the reports, inaccurate reporting at one or more levels, the inadvertent omission of one or more units from one of the overall monthly returns, or shifts in unit assignments between the times of composition of the different returns. Of the 288 listed by Cochran as remaining in the regimental and flying hospitals of the Army for March 1781, 43 were termed "lame," 18 "rheumatic," and 14 "venereal." In May, 41 of the 142 in the flying hospital were suffering from "casual hurts," 19 were convalescent, 16 suffering from intermittent and remittent fevers, and 6 from smallpox.[17]

In June 1781, while preparing for operations against New York City, General Washington ordered his regimental surgeons to send to the hospital at Robinson's House all patients unable to move with the army, except for those with smallpox, who were to be isolated in the huts used during the previous winter by New Hampshire troops.[18] It might be noted that this order for all practical purposes converted Robinson's House into a general hospital.

In July 1781, when the rate of sickness appears to have dropped below 11 percent, two flying hospitals were listed in Director General Cochran's records, without any description or commentary to distinguish between the two, one having forty-one patients remaining at the end of the month and the other twenty-one. In the August report, Cochran listed a flying hospital with 102 remaining at the end of that month and another 207 patients remaining with the "Army east" of the Hudson. Since General Washington, discouraged about operations against New York City, received word in August that he could have the support of the French force under Rear Admiral de Grasse for an attack on the British in eastern Virginia, by October there was a flying hospital at Yorktown. Reports from the army east of the Hudson continued to come in, however, since forty-four remained hospitalized there after forty-nine were sent on to a general hospital.[19]

Although the men camped along the Hudson saw no major action after the summer of 1778, Indian and Loyalist attacks on American settlements at Wyoming, Pennsylvania, on the Susquehanna River and at Cherry Valley, New York, on the Mohawk River in 1778, led in 1779 to a coordinated campaign under the overall command of Maj. Gen. John Sullivan against the perpetrators of these massacres. (*Map 7*) General Sullivan personally led 2,500 men based at Easton, Pennsylvania. Brig. Gen. James Clinton commanded 1,500 men from New York State and Col. Daniel Brodhead 600 men based at Fort Pitt, Pennsylvania. General Clinton's units left Albany in the spring of 1779 to establish a base at Canajoharie, New York, and then moved southwest to the Susquehanna River. They followed the river to Tioga, where they met General Sullivan's men. Colonel Brodhead, however, because of his inability to obtain adequate guides, failed to meet the Sullivan-Clinton force at Genesee, New York, as had been planned.

Before undertaking these operations, General Sullivan established a hospital unit at Easton and ordered his regimental surgeons to provide the necessary medicines for those whose health would not permit them to accompany the expedition. Many of these patients were ill with intermittent fevers which were blamed on the overly long baths they were accustomed to taking in the river.

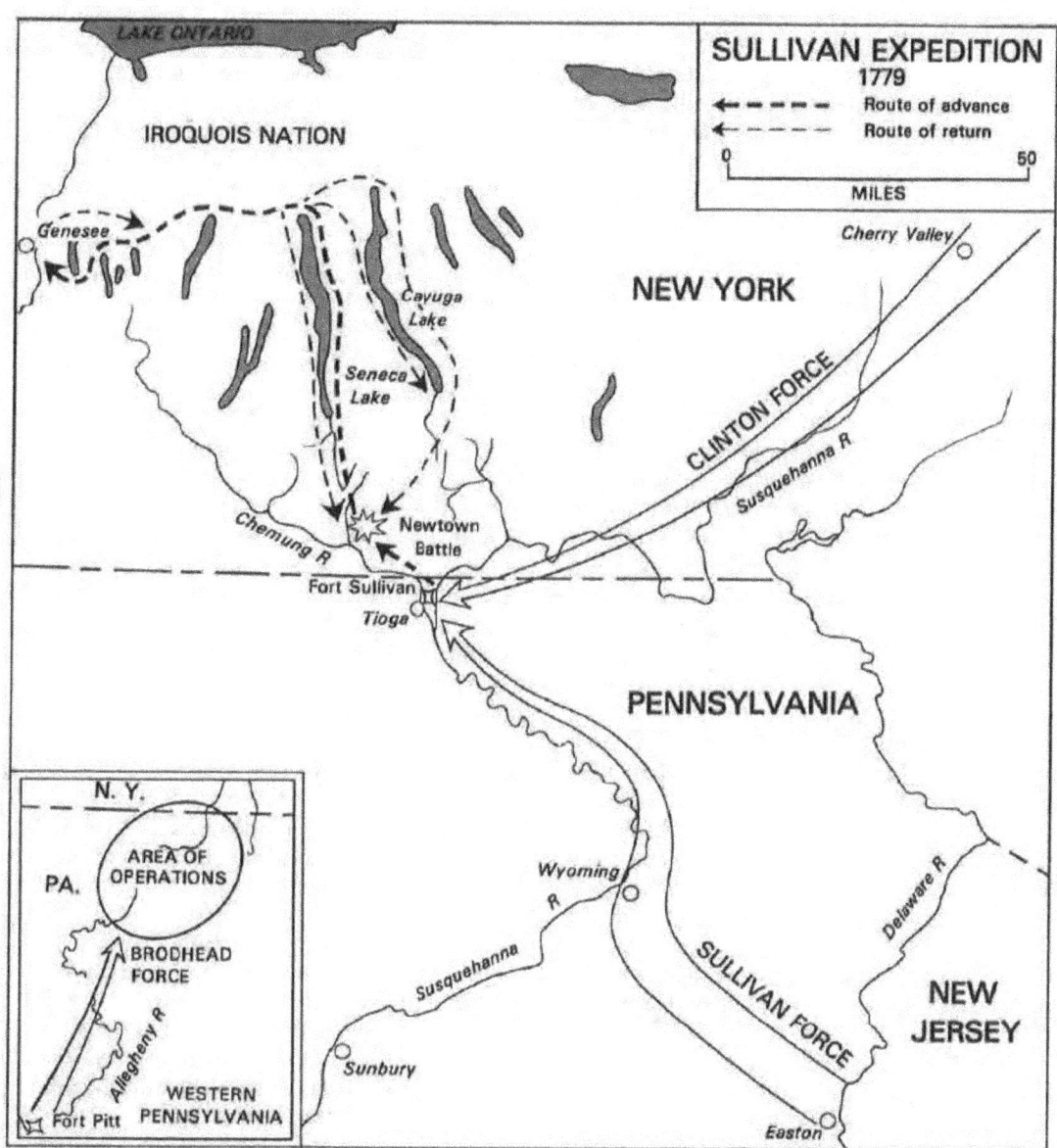

MAP 7

General Sullivan was among those whose health was precarious at this time, but although his condition seems to have gradually worsened, he continued with his men throughout the entire campaign.[20]

Leaving Easton, General Sullivan's men moved on to Sunbury, where Dr. Francis Alison was in the process of creating a general hospital to care for their casualties, arriving there on 21 June. Two days later they continued on up the Susquehanna River toward Wyoming. At Wyoming, General Sullivan ordered his regimental surgeons to report about their patients to the "Senr.

Surgeon to the Flying Hospital" once a week.[21] An officer noted while here that "A No. of the troops" were down with "the dissentary."[22] In mid-July, the sick at Wyoming were moved "to the genl Hospital under the Direction of Doct. McCrea," but whether McCrea's unit was the hospital which seems to have remained at Wyoming after General Sullivan's troops left is not clear.[23]

Both before leaving Wyoming to continue his northward march and after arriving at Tioga on 31 July, General Sullivan continued to plan the details of his order of march. He decided that the Surgeon General, by whom he presumably meant the head of the flying hospital, should remain by his side, the surgeons attached to the flying hospital, with their mates, should march at the rear of the entire army, and the regimental surgeons should remain at the rear of their respective brigades or regiments.[24]

While awaiting General Clinton's arrival at Tioga, General Sullivan's men built a small fort which was duly named Fort Sullivan. Here also plans were made for the operations of the next few weeks and regimental surgeons were ordered to obtain the supplies they believed they would need from McCrea. The problem of supplying milk for those staying at Tioga was among the difficulties most easily met; by a decisic worthy of Solomon, a cow whose ownership was being disputed by two officers was confiscated for the benefit of the hospital.[25]

On 26 August, after General Clinton's arrival at Tioga, General Sullivan, although he was by this time too ill to ride his horse, led the force north once again, leaving 250 able-bodied men behind to guard the hospital. Three days later, they defeated a combined Indian-Loyalist force near the village of Newtown and suffered about forty casualties. These men, along with those few who had fallen ill since leaving Tioga, were sent back to Fort Sullivan by water, along with the heavy artillery and ammunition wagons, all of which threatened the maneuverability of the force. As the expedition continued forward, this procedure was repeated, patients being sent back to Tioga each time, usually by water, with a small guard to ensure their safety on the trip.[26]

After reaching Genesee on 14 September and failing to encounter Colonel Brodhead's men, the expedition turned back toward Tioga, arriving there 30 September. On 3 October, the sick and wounded were sent on to Wyoming by water. When the main army passed through that town, a small group of officers was left behind to conduct them to Easton.[27]

An officer from the Sullivan expedition estimated that the total casualty list, including both the wounded and those dead because of enemy action or disease, did not exceed fifty. The total number of those who became ill at some time during the expedition, however, is difficult to estimate, although one authority suggests a figure approaching 450.[28]

Patients not only from General Sullivan's army but also from that of General Washington necessitated the opening or expanding of a number of general hospitals even when some of those in operation in the winter of 1777–78 were being closed down. In the fall of 1778, Shippen was confident that the few hospitals remaining in both the Middle Department and the Eastern Department were functioning well. Only six months later, however, a Hospital Department physician stated that while he agreed that the Middle Department was "really now upon a respectable footing," in the Northern and Eastern Departments, "everything is carried on, as in the beginning, with wild anarchy and uproar."[29]

In the Middle Department, by the fall of 1778, a number of the older units in Pennsylvania and New Jersey were apparently closed or on the verge of closing, but in the following three years, others within the department opened in response to the needs of the Army's operations.

The Schaefferstown, Pennsylvania, hospital was caring for seventy patients in early August of 1778 but does not appear in later records. A unit at French Creek, Pennsylvania, held 130 patients in September and 89 a month later. It is possible that this unit was later included in reports as a part of the Yellow Springs hospital, but it does not appear under its own name after October. There was also a unit at Downingtown, Pennsylvania, west of Philadelphia, in the summer of 1778, where in early August there were approximately seventy patients, but further information on this facility, too, is lacking. The Lititz, Pennsylvania, hospital was closed in late August 1778 and its patients were moved to Yellow Springs. The unit at Reading, Pennsylvania, was closed as of 1 January 1779, although hospital stores were apparently still being kept there the following spring.[30]

The facility at Yellow Springs was destined through the two years following 1778 to take in all the patients still remaining in other Pennsylvania hospitals outside of Philadelphia. In October 1778, there were 115 recorded at Yellow Springs; after this point, the number there began to decline. The unit continued to be highly regarded, however, and the Reverend Dr. James Sproat recorded his belief that "the hospitals [are] well provided for, and the gentlemen take good care of the sick," despite the fact that Dr. Bodo Otto, director of the unit, continued to find it necessary to plead for stores and clothing for his patients and salaries for his staff.[31]

By mid-1780 only fifty-one patients were still at the Yellow Springs hospital, all of whom were suffering from "chronic affections." In September 1781, when fewer than thirty patients could be found there, even before the victory at Yorktown, the Continental Congress finally ordered the Yellow Springs hospital closed and the remaining patients moved to Philadelphia.[32]

In July 1778, not long after the British evacuated Philadelphia, the Hospital Department reopened its facility in the Bettering House there. Dr. Jonathan Potts and Dr. Thomas Bond, Jr., then arranged with the managers of the privately owned Philadelphia Hospital to use that institution's "elaboratory" as a Hospital Department pharmacy. In September, Bond, whose father was one of the founders of the Philadelphia Hospital, also arranged to have some of the Army's convalescents taken in there, agreeing to give the hospital control over what cases could be admitted. The Army was to be held responsible for bedding and provisions as well as for the pay of nurses.[33]

The charity hospital in Philadelphia appears to have served as an emergency overflow facility for the department's Bettering House several times during the last years of the Revolution. In the spring of 1779, for example, the Bettering House was again overcrowded, and in late March a department spokesman asked the Philadelphia Hospital to take in more convalescents. On this occasion the hospital board refused to do so and referred scathingly to the "Inexpediency and impropriety of the request." The board maintained that it had been assured that the use of the laboratory was all that would be asked of it.[34] The behavior of soldier-patients appears to have been the principal cause of the board's wrath, since when Bond agreed to have a physician remain with Continental patients and to personally "do everything in his power to restrain the Soldiery, and prevent their committing damages and behaving irregularly," he was able to obtain a reversal of the adverse decision. Bond also agreed to try to have these convalescent soldiers out of the Philadelphia Hospital within six weeks and to guarantee that no patient with an infectious disease would be brought in.

On this occasion the department used only a garret and a lower ward and again provided bedding and food as well as firewood and other necessities. On 16 June 1779, having removed the Army's patients from the charity hospital, Bond was careful to thank the board for the use of the hospital's rooms. During the next year, the number of patients in the Hospital Department's facilities fluctuated, from a high of 130 in December 1779 to a low of 4 in May 1780. Once again in the summer of 1781, Hospital Department facilities in Philadelphia were so crowded that the department turned to the Philadelphia Hospital for help with its patients, who included about ninety sick British prisoners. This time it was the Superintendent of Finance Robert Morris who worked out an agreement with the hospital board which permitted the department to send soldiers to that institution. The department was to pay 15 shillings a week for each man and to agree that military patients would be required to obey the hospital's rules.[35]

In 1780, the Continental Congress urged its Medical Committee to move the department hospital out of Philadelphia to a site where the cost of living would be lower. Nevertheless, although by 1780 there were more hospitals in New Jersey than in Pennsylvania, Philadelphia remained the site both of a department hospital and of a hospital stores warehouse. The number of patients there may well have remained small, however, until the fall of 1781, when from the eight reported in July, the number rose in September to seventy-two and in October to eighty-five.[36] There was also a general hospital at Baltimore, Maryland, which stayed open through the summer of 1778. In August of that year, this facility began to dismiss its last patients, furloughing some and distributing the rest among relatives, so that by September it was no longer in operation.[37]

The old New Jersey hospitals at Trenton and Princeton appear only sporadically in reports dating from mid-1778 to the end of 1781. (*See Map 6.*) Twenty patients were at Trenton on December 1779, ten at the end of March 1781, and nine a month later. The Princeton hospital may have been open in the summer of 1778, at which time a typhus epidemic was reported raging there, but it does not appear in the reports of any later period. Also mentioned in the records surviving from 1778–79 was the unit at Brunswick which cared for some of the men who fell ill after the battle of Monmouth and served the Middlebrook camp the following winter.[38]

Among the new hospitals set up in the Middle Department in the last years of the war were three facilities in Pennsylvania, which cared almost exclusively for patients from General Sullivan's campaign against the Indians and Loyalists, and two in New Jersey which managed the care of General Washington's sick and wounded.

According to the 6 October 1779 report of Director General Shippen, the three fixed hospitals serving patients from the various units operating against the Indians and Tories in 1779 were at Fort Pitt, Pennsylvania, which presumably cared for Colonel Brodhead's casualties, at Sunbury, Pennsylvania, and at Fort Sullivan at Tioga, Pennsylvania. (*See Map 7.*) The records of the Fort Pitt and Tioga facilities are few, while those of the Sunbury hospital, more numerous, are not always entirely legible.

Shippen listed thirty patients at Fort Pitt and thirty-seven at Fort Sullivan on 6 October 1779. On 31 December he recorded thirty still at Fort Pitt but made no reference to any patients remaining at the Tioga facility, which was evacuated early in the fall at the conclusion of the campaign. The returns from the Sunbury unit began in the summer of 1779. They indicate that during the following months only a minority of Sunbury's patients were suffering from wounds. Of the 165 patients remaining there on 22 September 1779, for example, the diagnosis in 31 instances was bilious fever, in 11 diarrhea, and in 19 dysentery, but only 33 were listed as wounded. In the fall, with the campaign over, the number of patients at Sunbury began to drop, reaching 28 by mid-December 1779, and the proportion classified as convalescent to rise until it reached over 50 percent early in 1780.[30]

The conditions most frequently bringing sick men to Sunbury included a high proportion of dysentery and diarrhealike ailments, although by the autumn of 1779 this type of illness appeared less frequently. Other diseases seen in significant quantity were "lues veneria," bilious and intermittent fevers, rheumatism, and ophthalmia.[40]

By mid-April 1780, when the last report to be found among the papers of the physician who directed the Sunbury unit was prepared, only twelve patients remained there, four being convalescent, five wounded, and one each suffering from dysentery, asthma, and rheumatism. Precisely when this hospital finally closed its doors is not known, but since plans were being laid for its termination as early as October 1779,[41] we can perhaps assume it did not remain open much after the spring of 1780, when its patient load had become quite small.

The three new general hospitals opened in New Jersey first appeared in records dating from 1779. (See Map 6.) Two, those at Basking Ridge and at Pluckemin, were destined to care for patients during the grim winter spent by General Washington's men at Morristown. The latter unit was opened in the summer of 1779 when the general ordered that patients who were being cared for in barns in the vicinity of the Middlebrook camp be moved to the huts which had been used during the preceding winter by the artillerymen of Brig. Gen. Henry Knox at Pluckemin. By October 1779, ninety-eight patients were on the rolls of the new hospital.[42]

The second New Jersey hospital serving Morristown opened in the winter of 1779–80 at Basking Ridge, under Tilton's direction. Here a log building on a hill near a brook appears to have been Tilton's famed experimental hospital hut. It was apparently Basking Ridge's main building, since the facility could hold more than half of the maximum number of fifty-five patients reported being cared for at Basking Ridge at one time. Among the features of this structure were smaller units than those usually found, packed earth floors, walls without windows, and a fireplace in each section, the smoke from which left the room by means of a four-inch hole in the roof. As many as twenty-eight patients were placed here, with their feet toward the fire.[43]

While the number of patients at the Pluckemin facility increased throughout early 1780, that at Basking Ridge declined. The two hospitals, however, shared a common problem at this time in the form of patients who, upon recovery, chose to desert rather than return to duty.[44] By summer, the patient load at both hospitals had begun to fall off until on 1 July 1780 they held only fifty-three patients between them.

Beginning in the summer of 1780, the huts serving the Pennsylvania Line during the second Morristown encampment were taken over for a third New Jersey general hospital, established to care for the sick who were left in camp when the army returned to New York State. The huts at Morristown were small and in very bad condition, partially because of the "disorderly Behavior of the Patients." Only in a few instances were the individual compartments large enough to hold three men. Most of the huts did not provide adequate shelter from the rain and snow. Nevertheless, in the fall of 1780, patients from units in the area of Paramus, New Jersey, which was considered to be threatened by possible enemy action, were ordered moved to Morristown. In January 1781, Dr. Malachi Treat, reporting on the situation at the Pennsylvania huts, urged that the patients at Morristown be transferred to Trenton. He pointed out that, in addition to its thirty-five patients, the unit was encumbered by many women and children "who are a Nuisance at present." By March 1781, there were only nineteen patients in the huts, six of whom were classified as convalescent and five as wounded, and no new patients were being admitted. The number of patients continued to go down, and in June the hospital was closed.[45]

In theory, the setting of the Hudson River as the boundary between the Middle and Eastern Departments should have prevented any confusion over the extent of the authority of the head of the Eastern Department. The documents of the period, however, show Foster, the Deputy Director for the Eastern Department, exercising authority over storage facilities on the west bank of the Hudson. The hospital at Fishkill, to the east of the river, on the other hand, seems to have been in some ways independent of the Eastern Department. How much this confusion of authority added to the dissension which characterized this department in the years 1778–80 cannot be ascertained, but the personal antagonisms prevailing among Eastern Department physicians at this time were a matter of record.[46]

Named without indication of state on an Eastern Department return of the fall of 1778 were hospitals at Boston, Bedford, Poundridge, Springfield, Fishkill, and Danbury. It was a 1780 return, however, that listed Fishkill but maintained that no report had been received from the Eastern Department. Furthermore, a Middle Department physician, Dr. Charles McKnight, was in charge at Fishkill. This hospital had at least one small claim to fame; it was here that Cochran attended the Marquis de Lafayette while that nobleman was seriously ill with a fever.[47]

The Fishkill unit was still in operation in mid-1781 and its patients numbered as many as forty-five. The diseases found here included rheumatism and venereal diseases while the number of wounded in 1781 was low, apparently less than half a dozen. By July 1781, however, the decision to close the Fishkill hospital had been made.[48]

Two more Hudson River hospitals were those at New Windsor and at Robinson's House, but considerable confusion exists concerning both their status and the details of their operation. The New Windsor facility, located at this time in a church large enough to accommodate fifty patients, may have served as an administration center for some of the other units along the river, since Dr. Francis Alison, sent to the area in the fall of 1778, worked at Robinson's House, on the east bank of the Hudson, but sent his returns in to New Windsor.[49] The Robinson's House hospital was still referred to as a flying hospital, despite the fact that on a return of May 1781, it was listed separately from the flying hospital.[50] The overall capacity of the Robinson's House unit seems to have been comparable to that of the hospital at New Windsor, and in the summer of 1780, when it held 126, it was considered to be seriously overcrowded. This condition was relieved by sending some of these men to Fishkill.[51]

At some point in the winter of 1780–81, both the Robinson's House and the New Windsor units appear to have been closed, for in July 1871, before General Washington's army moved south to besiege Yorktown, Director General Cochran referred to new hospitals which he had only recently established at Robinson's House and huts formerly used by artillery units at New Windsor as well as in the barracks of West Point.[52]

Reports were again submitted for the unit at Robinson's House beginning in May 1781 and running at least through October of that year. The number of patients in that period varied from 60 to 142. A high proportion of these in the fall were suffering from bilious putrid fever, 57 percent, for example, in October. Reports from the New Windsor huts apparently began to come in by July 1781. The number of patients ranged from 96 in July to an estimated 250 in October. Here, too, the number of cases of bilious putrid fever rose sharply with the onset of autumn, as did those described as intermittent and remittent fevers. The West Point unit was in a barracks and served the garrison there. Of the 135 men hospitalized at West Point in the month of September 1781, more than half were ill with dysentery.[53]

Two other hospitals, both quite large and located not far from the Hudson River, appear on a single Hospital Department return, that of 6 October 1779, but are never mentioned again in the records which have survived from that period. The Otterkill facility, located quite close to New Windsor on the west bank of the river, held 112 patients at this time. (See Map 6.) It was not identical with the New Windsor facility, which was listed separately on the same report. There is no indication given as to why the existence of such a large facility as that at Otterkill should have been so brief. The second of these two units, at New Hackensack, on the east side of the Hudson, was comparable in size to that at Otterkill, and its origins and fate are equally mysterious.[54]

A large number of hospitals of varying size also operated in New England in the period 1778-81. Among the largest of these was the unit at Danbury, Connecticut, which admitted 938 patients in the course of September and October 1778. (See Map 6.) Of these, 69 died and 716 were dismissed as cured. Of the 294 remaining at the end of October, 208 were classified as convalescents. Some of the men at Danbury were probably those transferred there from smaller units to the west whose security was considered to be threatened by their proximity to the British in New York City.[55]

Although no returns exist from Danbury after that of 7 November 1778, when 162 of its 197 patients were convalescent, the hospital there continued in operation at least through the spring of 1780 and was quite possibly still functioning a year later. Like the patients at other hospitals in this period, those at Danbury suffered from the shortages afflicting the Hospital Department, particularly a lack of straw for bedding and vegetables.[56]

At least two other Eastern Department units reporting on their patients in the early autumn of 1778 seem to have been closed by the end of October. One of these was at Bedford, New York. (See Map 6.) During September and October, Bedford admitted 107 patients, 59 of whom were considered cured before the unit was closed. In August 1780, however, the Bedford hospital was open again and caring for 300 to 400 patients, according to Dr. William Eustis.[57]

Poundridge, New York, twenty miles northeast of White Plains, admitted seventy-four patients in the early fall of 1778, one of whom died and only one of whom was claimed to have been cured. It is possible that this hospital was also considered endangered by its proximity to New York City and its patients were moved elsewhere, perhaps to Danbury.[58]

There were at least two other general hospitals in Connecticut and one in Rhode Island during this period. (See Map 6.) The facility at Hartford, established for the sick and wounded of units stationed near that town, was short-lived. This hospital was closed in March 1779 and its patients were sent to New London. The latter unit may also have been closed not long after this time, for in the spring of 1780, the Continental Congress ordered Shippen to open a facility in New London to receive such sick prisoners as might be exchanged by the British and in so doing made no reference to any institution already existing there. This unit appears to have been little used and was closed in the spring of 1781.

Dr. James Thacher in his *Military Journal* also mentioned a hospital at Providence, Rhode Island, operating in 1779, and Dr. Philip Turner's 1778 return listed patients at a unit at Springfield, in an unmentioned state.[59]

There was a general hospital at Boston, Massachusetts, during this entire period, under the direction of Dr. John Warren, who, like Shippen, conducted classes while he served as a member of the Hospital Department. The hospital, like so many others, experienced severe supply shortages. Many returns in the period complain that no report had been received from the Eastern Department, or, specifically, none from Boston, and indications of the capacity of the Boston facility were, for this reason, scarce. A total of thirty-six patients were being cared for there at the end of October 1778 and thirty-seven in the spring of 1781.[60]

In the spring of 1778, the days of the Albany general hospital, the one remaining general hospital in the Northern Department, where Robert Johnston was acting as Deputy Director, had seemed numbered. (*See Chapter 4.*) Before the launching of the Sullivan expedition, many of the patients there were chronically ill or permanently crippled. Many of the other patients were ready to rejoin their units but unable to do so because of a lack of clothing. General Washington attempted to remedy this situation early in 1779 by ordering clothing sent north and requesting General Clinton to be most careful in its distribution. At the end of January 1779, Treat, Physician General in the Northern Department, maintained that all was going relatively well at the "out Post of God's Creations" where "your Eyes behold only Dutchmen" in spite of the continued lack of money and the fact that the clothing ordered for patients ready to return to their units had not yet arrived.[61]

When General Clinton set out to join General Sullivan in the campaign against the Indians and Loyalists, he decided to leave behind him in charge of the guard for the Albany hospital one Captain Gregg, the same officer who had earlier survived a scalping. Captain Gregg's wish to join the operations against the Indians was not granted by General Clinton, who commented that "if the Indians ketches him again they will Cut of [*sic*] his head as scalping Can't kill him." [62]

On 6 October 1779, only fifteen patients remained at Albany, but from that date to 31 December of that year, the patient load increased to 140. During this same period, the number of patients at Sunbury dropped markedly twice in close succession. The number at Albany slowly decreased after the end of 1779, reaching 86 by the end of February 1780, 62 at the end of March, and 35 by early July. By August 1780, it was being suggested that although there were six surgeons at Albany, one would suffice and the others should be sent to where they were more needed.[63]

All was not well at the Albany hospital in the summer of 1780, however, despite the plethora of physicians. Treat wrote the Medical Committee of the Continental Congress that "Our hospital is at present destitute of everything that can afford Comfort to a sick soldier" and that the hospital had no wine, sugar, tea, coffee, rice, or molasses and only a little rum, a state of affairs which was neither new nor unique.[64]

The patients at Albany still numbered more than thirty in the spring of 1781, and a report of May 1781 added that twenty-seven women and children were also being cared for by the hospital. Throughout the summer and early fall the number of patients at Albany fluctuated between sixty and ninety and the recorded diagnoses were scattered among many diseases, including intermittent and remittent fevers, dysentery and diarrhea, rheumatism, and "various chronic." [65] The shortage of supplies continued "and the sick suffer extremely at times for want of provisions," but by the summer of 1781 the staff at Albany had been reduced to one surgeon and four mates.[66]

Smallpox was no longer among the diseases most frequently listed by the Army's surgeons in any of the departments. The lesson taught by the devasting effects of smallpox in the early years of the Revolution was not forgotten in the later years and care was usually taken, north of the Carolinas, once the campaign season was out of the way each year, to inoculate those who were not already immune to the disease, especially if smallpox had already begun to appear among the men. The women and children accompanying the army might also be inoculated and although some of the men were not in good condition when subjected to this procedure, the death rate was still quite low, in one instance only four of 500.[67]

An added responsibility for the Hospital Department developed in July 1780, when 4,000 troops of the French Army under the Comte de Rochambeau arrived off New England to aid in the fighting against Great Britain. In anticipation of their arrival, General Washington and the Marquis de Lafayette began in the spring of 1780 to plan to acquire appropriate accommodations for patients from the French forces. The American general ordered Craik, as his personal friend and then Assistant Director General in the Middle Department, to take over responsibility for the establishment of a hospital near Providence, Rhode Island, for the new allies and urged specifically that Craik acquire sufficient space. These facilities were to contain room for a kitchen, an apothecary shop, storage, a bakery, and surgeons' quarters. There should also be enough meat and vegetables on hand to meet the initial needs of the French troops.[68]

Craik experienced considerable opposition from Rhode Island citizens, however, when he first tried to find the desired facilities. Local inhabitants apparently regarded hospitals as foci of infection and were of the opinion that the plague would arrive with the French fleet. At last Rhode Island College (now Brown University) in Providence surrendered its buildings for this purpose. In time, the French created their own hospital establishments at other sites, including Conanicut Island in Narragansett Bay. It was fortunate, indeed, however, that the initial housing problems were solved by 11 July, when the French fleet arrived off Newport, Rhode Island, because an estimated 1,700 to 2,600 Frenchmen of both the army and the navy were suffering from scurvy. The French, furthermore, had not been long in Rhode Island before their men began to show symptoms of dysentery as well. Fortunately, the French Army's medical organization was highly developed and the physicians were thoroughly capable of caring for their own men.[69]

SOUTH OF THE POTOMAC: BEFORE THE VICTORY AT YORKTOWN

As far as the care of sick and wounded soldiers was concerned, the South was, until March 1781, for all practical purposes divided into three sections, only one of which was a part of the Continental Hospital Department system. (*Map 8*) Although its position in relation to the position of Director General was at times in dispute, the establishment in Virginia was, from its inception, a part of the Hospital Department. (*See Table 1.*) In the Carolinas and Georgia, however, two separate systems, one centered about Charleston, South Carolina, and the other covering North Carolina, gradually emerged, independent both of the Hospital Department and of each other. The existence and the independence of hospitals south of Virginia were recognized, more or less in passing, by the legislation of Sep-

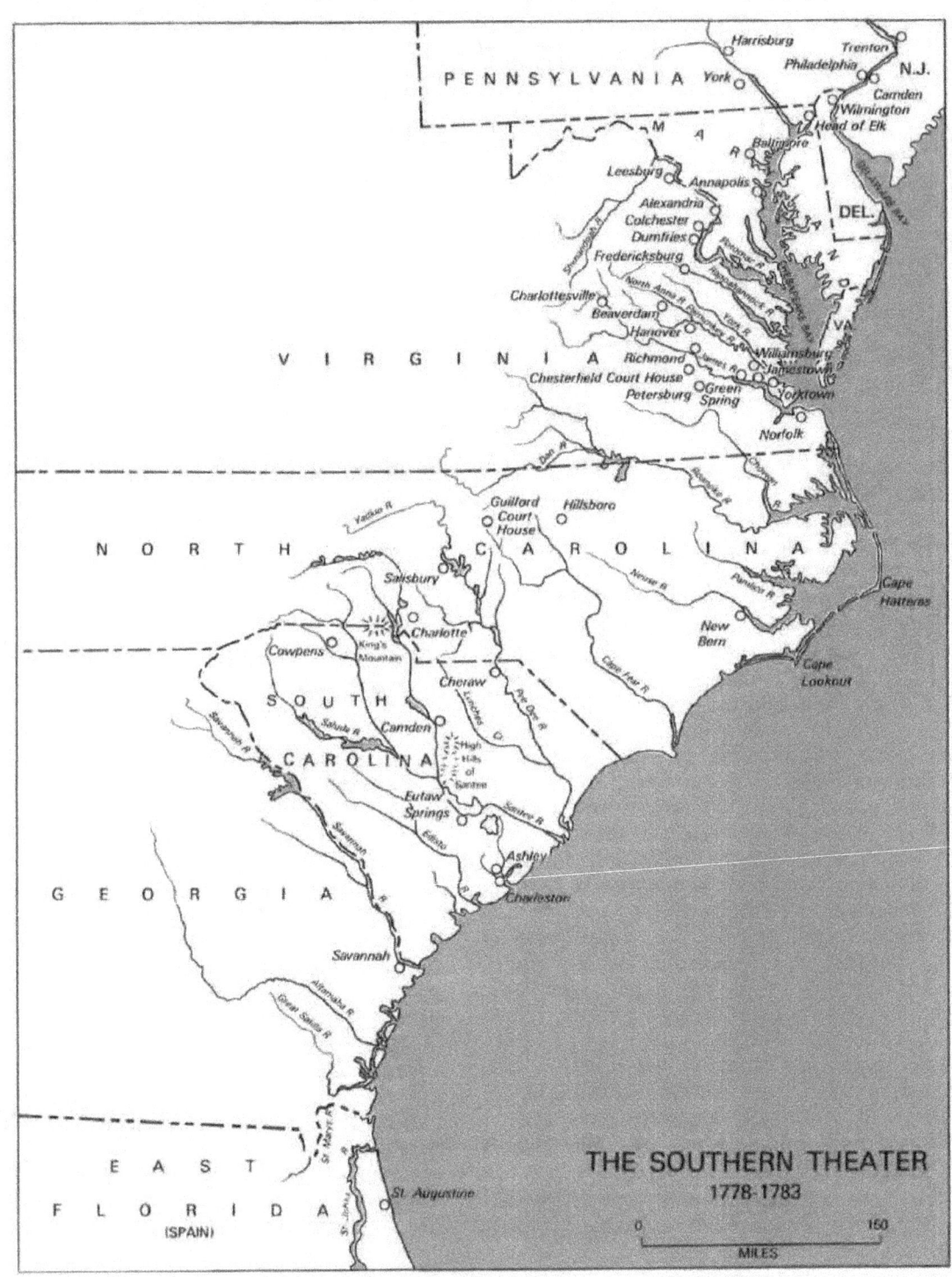

MAP 8

tember 1780, and the Director General of the Hospital Department did not formally assume responsibility for the operations of these institutions until 22 March 1781, at which time units from the North were moving into the South in ever greater numbers. Even under these circumstances, however, the congressmen from South Carolina opposed the subordination of the system in their state to the Hospital Department.[70]

The first general hospital established for American troops fighting south of Virginia was apparently that created in June 1776 in the Charleston area under Charleston's Dr. David Oliphant for "State troops, Militia, Sailors and Negroes in the public Service." Although some seem to have thought that Oliphant should have been responsible to the Hospital Department, he did not consider himself to be so and the post in which he served was not a creation of the Continental Congress.[71]

In time, as the tempo of the war in the South began to increase, Oliphant was encouraged to set up a medical organization which would include all of South Carolina and Georgia as well, a course of action which must have seemed particularly desirable because of the heavy toll which sickness was taking from the forces fighting the British in the South. At somewhat the same time, the sick and wounded in North Carolina (or perhaps only those of the militia of that state) were placed under the overall direction of Dr. Hugh Williamson. The operations of Oliphant's organization were severely impeded when its members were captured by the British on 12 May 1780, at the time of Maj. Gen. Benjamin Lincoln's surrender of Charleston. It was these men, nevertheless, who attempted, with little cooperation from their captors, to care for the sick and wounded among the American prisoners accumulated by the British at Charleston. Despite British denials, it appears that the general lack of cooperation these physicians received from

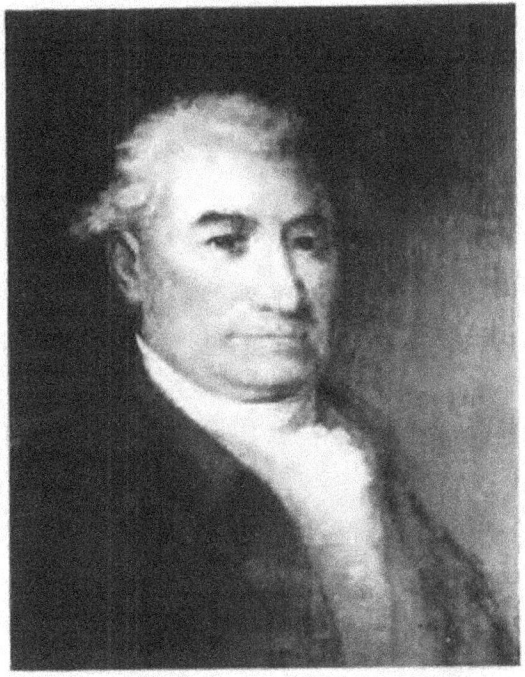

DAVID OLIPHANT. *(Courtesy of National Library of Medicine.)*

the enemy was matched by the experiences of Williamson when he crossed enemy lines to care for prisoners wounded at Camden, South Carolina, later that year.[72]

From the spring of 1780 onward, the medical care received by the troops south of the Virginia-North Carolina border seems to have been haphazard, lacking both organization and physicians, as well as nurses, food, and medicines. Despite the efforts of Maj. Gen. Horatio Gates to establish a general hospital and an appeal to Dr. William Rickman as "Director of the General Hospital of the Southern Army," for aid, care was almost, if not entirely, in the hands of regimental and militia surgeons. It appears, indeed, that, except for regimental surgeons, such representatives of the Hospital Department as were with units moved in from the North may have been required to stay behind when the troops crossed into

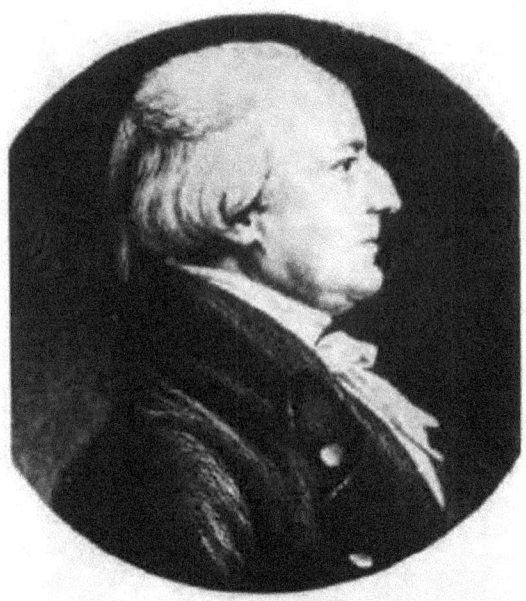

THOMAS TUDOR TUCKER. *(Courtesy of National Library of Medicine.)*

North Carolina. One authority reports, furthermore, that there seemed to be not a single American surgeon of any kind in attendance for the battle of King's Mountain in October 1780.[73]

The September 1780 reorganization of the Hospital Department officially recognized the existence of the hospitals south of Virginia, although it neither defined the relationship of these institutions to the Hospital Department nor affected the work of physicians south of Virginia. The growing pace of activity in this area, however, required that an attempt be made to impose some form of organization upon the physicians caring for the men under Maj. Gen. Nathanael Greene, who was appointed to command in the South in October 1780. A general hospital seems to have evolved at Charlotte, North Carolina, during the summer of 1780, but the care provided there, which was largely, if not entirely, in the hands of volunteer physicians, was very poor and, in General Greene's opinion, "shocking to humanity." In November, a Board of War meeting at Hillsboro, North Carolina, appointed Dr. James Browne director of the medical establishment in that state and assigned Williamson to the post of surgeon general. One author believes that Browne had been in charge of a hospital caring for General Greene's men at Cheraw, South Carolina.[74]

At about the same time, plans were also being made to transfer the Charlotte facility to Salisbury, North Carolina, where it was to be directed by Dr. William Read. Read, however, had barely established his hospital when General Greene began his retreat north into Virginia and the hospital had to be evacuated. Patients unable to ride on this occasion were, according to Read, moved on litters.[75]

In South Carolina, Oliphant was paroled by the British during the winter of 1781, but he remained in charge of the hospital for the American prisoners at Charleston. His chief assistant, Dr. Peter Fayssoux, as well as two junior hospital surgeons and four regimental surgeons, was exchanged in March 1781.[76]

In the spring of 1781, however, Dr. David Oliphant became Deputy Director for the area south of Virginia, with a deputy purveyor, chief physician of the hospital, chief physician of the army, and two hospital physicians under him. Despite the organizational change, inadequate care, as before, continued to add to the sufferings of men who were wounded or who became ill while serving in the South. Oliphant seems not to have been active on their behalf at this time and one of the physicians under him, Dr. Thomas Tudor Tucker, served as director of the Charleston hospital, which was still held captive by the British. The regiments which came in from North Carolina were in a particularly poor situation because they had neither physicians nor medicines of any kind.[77]

As the heat of summer began to settle

upon "a country as hot as the Antichambers of Hell," the incidence of disease mounted, triggering an increase in the number of desertions.[78] Fatigue and "frequent skirmishes" also added to the list of the disabled. The situation was made worse by the fact that a large quantity of the hospital stores was destroyed by the raids of the much dreaded British Lt. Col. Banastre Tarleton.[79]

Fighting in the summer months this far south was generally considered unwise, and so, as the temperature reached its peak, Maj. Gen. Nathanael Greene, now commanding in the Southern Army, led his men to camp for the summer in the High Hills of Santee in South Carolina. Dr. William Read, in charge of a hospital at Charlotte, North Carolina (a unit which had been reestablished there after having been moved earlier to Salisbury), was ordered to leave that facility in charge of a subordinate and to join General Greene to create and direct a flying hospital for his army. It appears that the chief physician of the hospital for General Greene's army was at this time Fayssoux, who joined him after being released from Charleston as the result of an exchange of prisoners in March 1781.[80]

The health of General Greene's men, while it may have benefited to some degree from the summer spent in the High Hills of Santee, was far from what might have been hoped for by the beginning of the autumn campaign season. Many hundreds were still sick, and supplies of bark, inadequate from the outset, were totally exhausted by mid-October. Oliphant was by now in Philadelphia, but the number of patients under Fayssoux, acting in his stead, increased after the engagement at Eutaw Springs, South Carolina, on September 1781, when more than 250 men were wounded, and physicians were themselves now falling ill. The burden of nursing fell on soldiers fortunate enough not to be seriously ill or wounded, few of whom had any real aptitude for this type of work. General Greene was profoundly distressed by the inadequate care his wounded were receiving and noted that "numbers of brave fellows who had bled in the cause of their country, have been eat up with maggots, and perished in that miserable situation."[81]

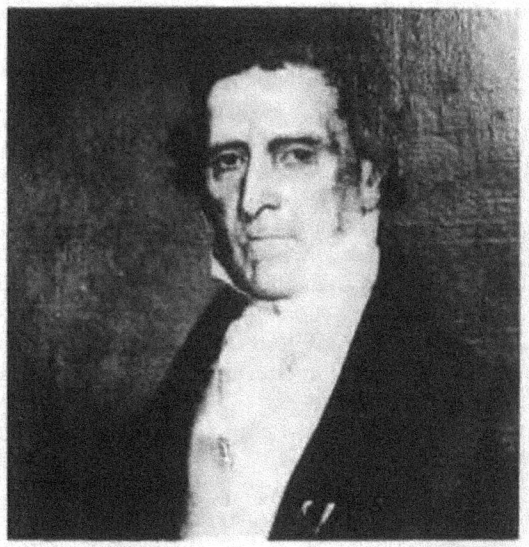

WILLIAM READ. *(Courtesy of National Library of Medicine.)*

The sick among those still imprisoned at Charleston in the late spring and summer of 1781 were many. Oliphant claimed, however, that the British were forcing ill prisoners to leave the hospital before they had completely regained their health and were feeding those still in the hospital a "salt diet," rather than supplying the type of nourishment considered necessary for sick men in a hot climate. Unfortunately, the Continental Congress, because of the shortage of funds, was unable to supplement this diet. That body did, however, retain in service the Continental physicians of the South Carolina system, who, in captivity themselves, were caring for the wretched men at Charleston.[82]

The hospital system in Virginia was

directed by Dr. William Rickman and was independent of that in the colonies further south. It is difficult to pinpoint exactly where Rickman's facilities were located in the summer of 1778, although he had apparently rejected the College of William and Mary because it had too many partitions which would interfere with the free circulation of air. Private homes had been deemed less than ideal because they implied a larger staff and higher operating costs. The palace at Williamsburg, used as a hospital during the siege of Yorktown, was seriously considered by Rickman several years earlier but was not taken over at that time.[83]

It is possible that a facility called the Vineyard Hospital, outside of Williamsburg on the road to Yorktown, was used for both Continental and Virginia militia patients beginning at least as early as May 1779, and that private homes, despite the disadvantages, were used before that time to house Army patients. Since recruits were at times inoculated in Virginia, special facilities were also set aside when needed as smallpox hospitals, such as those used in 1777 at Dumfries, Colchester, and Alexandria.[84]

A hospital was apparently in operation in the fall of 1778 near Fredericksburg, Virginia, at the time that units under the command of Maj. Gen. Benjamin Lincoln, newly appointed to command in the South, were passing through, since on 25 October, Cochran reported that 562 patients were being cared for in this area. Of these, 65 were described as flying hospital patients, 166 convalescent, 111 sick with either intermittent or remittent fever, 83 with bilious fever, and 34 "lame & rheumatism."[85] It is difficult to say whether this unit was serving as both flying and general hospital or whether those referred to as flying hospital patients were merely those transferred from the flying hospital.

In 1779, when General Washington began moving all Carolina and Virginia troops south, at least one of these units, that under the command of Brig. Gen. Charles Scott, was not accompanied by an adequate number of medical attendants. General Washington at first suggested that Rickman supply the deficiencies, but finally, since Scott was in "utmost distress" on this account, he turned to Shippen with the request that the Director General send two surgeons and two mates to join General Scott at Petersburg, Virginia. At least one surgeon and one mate joined General Scott in the summer of 1779, but twenty to thirty patients who could not move with his unit were left behind at Petersburg without a single surgeon to care for them. Despite the unhealthy reputation of that town, Continental hospital facilities were still there in the fall of 1780.[86]

Another Virginia hospital was established by Rickman in the spring of 1780 at Chesterfield Court House, which seems to have been along the route taken by troops moving into the Carolinas. This particular site was not the first choice of the Hospital Department but was urged upon it by the governor of Virginia. In early June, eighteen patients were being treated here, but by the end of the year, the log house which sheltered the unit was not finished and medicines, as elsewhere, were badly needed. The unit was still in operation in March 1781, with 55 patients on its rolls, 17 of them wounded and 25 convalescent.[87]

By the spring of 1781, however, Rickman was no longer in charge of the hospital in Virginia, having been dropped from the department at his own request the preceding fall. The identity of his successors is unclear. Dr. David Gould, who may have been his first replacement, died in July 1781. Either Dr. Goodwin Wilson, who supervised facilities at Beaverdam, Hanover, and Charlottesville at some time in 1781, or Dr. James McClurg may have followed Gould.[88]

In the spring of 1781, the British troops

under Lt. Gen. Charles Cornwallis marched north into Virginia and joined the units already in that area. Shortly after their arrival, reinforcements from New York joined them. The tempo of the war in that state, therefore, increased, and by midsummer, the hospital at Williamsburg was the main southern facility for the Hospital Department. This unit appears initially to have been under the direction of Tucker, who came up with his patients upon their release from Charleston.[89]

In the late spring of 1781, the men of Maj. Gen. Anthony Wayne's command began to move south. On 4 June, their sick were left behind them just south of Leesburg, Virginia, under the care of a surgeon. On 10 June, Wayne joined Lafayette on the North Anna River, and by 19 June, both units were in the vicinity of Richmond and "destitute of every necessary, both of life and convenience." Many of the physicians accompanying General Wayne did not have so much as blood-letting instruments.[90]

On 6 July, the combined forces of General Wayne and Lafayette met the British at Green Spring, Virginia, where General Wayne's men, who took the brunt of the action, suffered ninety-nine wounded. These men were cared for at a church nearby and on the 7th sent to an unidentified hospital.[91]

The number of sick from both Continental and French units in Virginia increased during the late summer, and wagons moved flying hospital patients from place to place in the heat. In early August, some of the sick from among General Wayne's men were sent to a general hospital located in a private home at Hanover, Virginia; the officers from this group were moved on to Pennsylvania later in the month. By late August, the Hanover unit was running short of almost all the stores it required, especially medicines, and the number of patients was so great that eight or nine buildings, some of them containing as many as eight rooms, were taken over. Untrained

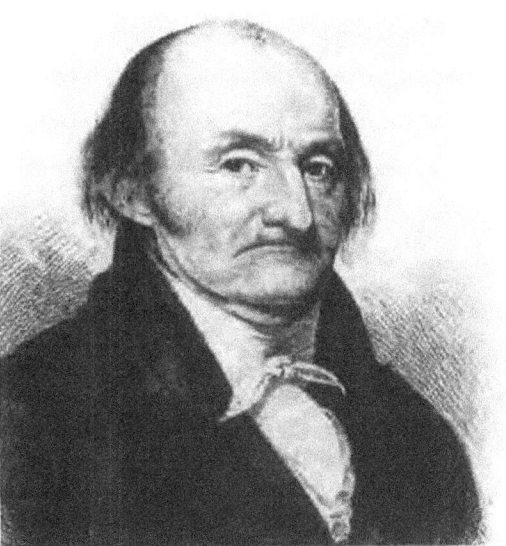

JAMES MCCLURG. *(Courtesy of National Library of Medicine.)*

soldiers, here as elsewhere, were pressed into service as nurses. In September, as preparations for the siege of Yorktown increased, the physician at the Hanover hospital himself died and the responsibility for the care of his fellows fell entirely upon one of the patients.[92]

A combined American and French force of 15,000 men was in place at Yorktown by the end of September, under the overall command of General Washington. Three or more hospitals were opened at Williamsburg, where Director General Cochran reported a total of 250 patients, and in Yorktown flying hospitals for both French and Americans settled down with the armies for the siege, the Continental unit under Craik's direction since Cochran had remained behind along the banks of the Hudson. Not all department reports identify the location of flying hospitals, but one report which still exists without question originated from the American Yorktown flying hospital. It is dated October 1781 and does not record the number of admissions and discharges,

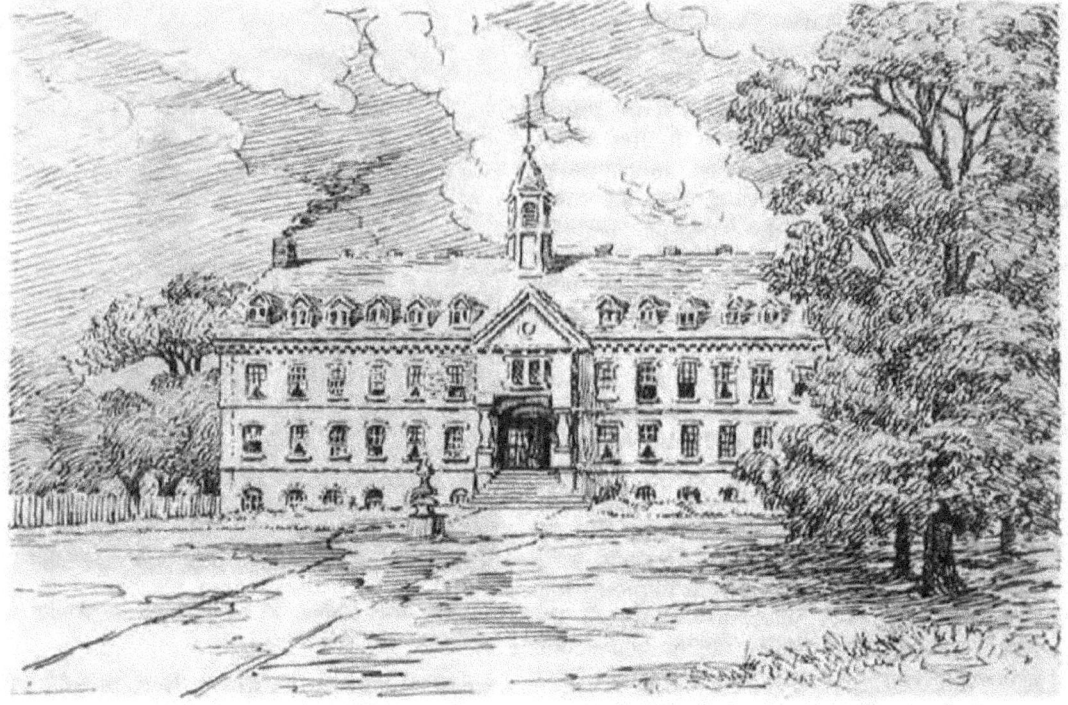

COLLEGE OF WILLIAM AND MARY: WREN BUILDING. *(From Duncan, Medical Men.)*

but it lists 6 dead and 147 convalescent, 209 with intermittent fever, 103 with diarrhea, and 646 remaining at the end of the month.[93]

In Williamsburg, the French took over the building belonging to the College of William and Mary which they, in contrast to Rickman, considered well suited for a hospital. They were particularly impressed with its size and sturdy construction, but in time found it necessary to take over the Capitol as well. Before they returned the college to its owner, one wing burned down. The Americans used the palace, which was not in good condition, and two churches to house their sick and wounded. A 200-man detachment from the forces besieging Yorktown stayed behind to guard hospitals and the stores left in Williamsburg while the main army moved against the British.[94]

Casualties for the allied armies during the siege of Yorktown were not great, but sickness, particularly malaria, took a heavy toll and an epidemic of smallpox was anticipated. The French experienced a rate of disease in their hospitals no better than that of the Americans even though their military hospital organization was elaborate and their physicians so much respected that Continental doctors were glad to have their aid and advice. Tilton blamed poor sanitation and a tendency to avoid the use of the medicines, including opium, popular among American physicians, for the limited success of French units.[95]

Early in the siege of Yorktown, the number of patients in American hospitals in the area rapidly increased. New England troops, especially, were suffering from the remittent and intermittent fevers considered endemic in that area. Craik noted that blankets were in short supply and that, unless action were taken at once, an unnecessarily high mortality rate could ensue. At the time of the

British surrender, 600 Americans were too sick or too severely wounded to be cared for by camp hospitals, approximately 400 of them at Williamsburg and more than 200 at Hanover. Thacher estimated that seventy-three Americans were wounded during the siege.[96]

AFTER THE VICTORY AT YORKTOWN

From November 1781 to the end of the war, an unofficial truce prevailed throughout the colonies. General Washington remained near New York City until the end of the war, while General Greene set up camp near Charleston, South Carolina, until the summer of 1783, when the last of the Southern Army left for home.[97]

The number of patients resulting not only from battle but also from the malaria-ridden environment was increasing at such a pace that even before the Articles of Capitulation were formally signed, General Washington himself was active in the attempt to find additional hospital space. He wished as many as possible to be cared for within the town of Williamsburg and emphasized the need for separate housing for those who came down with smallpox while in the area. He was distressed by conditions in the Army's hospitals there but apparently believed that captured funds would now make improvements possible. As soon as the Articles were signed, the general prepared to move his army out of the unhealthy climate as quickly as possible. The transports which were being loaded before the month was out sailed 4 November, but a sufficient number of officers was left behind to escort patients back to their units as they recovered.[98]

At the end of November 1781, 186 patients were still at Williamsburg, 23 of whom were suffering from smallpox and 49 each from wounds and dysentery. At Hanover there were another 114 patients who could not accompany the army when it moved north. Only 74 remained at Williamsburg and 32 at Hanover by the end of December, however. There is some question as to which physician was in charge of the Williamsburg hospitals at this time and no evidence to indicate who had charge of the Hanover facility. Apparently both Tilton and Treat directed the Williamsburg units at one time or another during or after the siege, but it seems likely that Treat, who was a Chief Physician and Surgeon of the Hospital at this time, held overall authority in Williamsburg during the siege and that Tilton, as a Hospital Physician and Surgeon, succeeded Treat.[99]

Despite General Washington's hopes, the sufferings of the patients in Williamsburg continued unabated after the siege, not only because of the lack of such fundamental items as wood and straw for bedding but also, in the opinion of at least one observer, because the surgeons there behaved in an irresponsible manner, failing to make the required purchases even when they had the money to do so. In December, matters were made even worse by a disastrous fire which burned the palace to the ground. Fortunately, there was only one casualty and the French took in those who would otherwise have been without shelter. In January, fifty-five Continental soldiers, nineteen of whom were wounded, were still hospitalized at Williamsburg. At last, in the spring of 1782, General Washington decided that there were so few patients remaining at Williamsburg that he could have the facilities closed.[100]

After the Yorktown victory, General Greene moved southeast toward Charleston. His men had been in poor health since the engagement at Eutaw Springs a month earlier and now many had to be left behind at the hospital in the High Hills of Santee under the care of Fayssoux. A second hospital was maintained at Charlotte, North Carolina, in late 1781 and early 1782.[101]

Many of the units which had been surrounding Yorktown, including those of General Wayne and Maj. Gen. Arthur St. Clair, were now sent south to join General Greene. These men were also in poor condition and inadequately fed and clothed. Some, at least, maintained themselves in good spirits by whatever means presented themselves, repeated references in at least one journal to the dire state of the author's health being followed by repeated references to "last night's carouse." As these troops neared Charleston, they came upon an area of very bad water with many stagnant swamps and ponds "full of little insects." [102]

When the troops of Generals Wayne and St. Clair reached the vicinity of General Greene's camp near Charleston early in January 1782, many were sick enough with fever to require hospitalization at the facility which had been established at Ashley, apparently in a private home. Although its physicians were "very kind" and it was "furnished with some stores, sugar, tea and molasses," the Ashley hospital was reputed to be a "very disagreeable place—all sick, and some continually dying." By March, although the health of the Southern Army had markedly improved, talk of mutiny was being heard.[103]

The journals kept during the spring and early summer of 1782 suggest that many of the men of the Southern Army did not lightly turn to physicians and hospitals for aid. The author of one account, for example, mentioned in his entry of 28 May 1782 that he was "loaded with sickness and distracted with toothache . . . almost dead with pain." He continued to make similar complaints for more than ten days without ever suggesting that he was seeking professional help, and on one occasion, apparently on his own initiative, took "a vomitt which almost killed" him.[104]

During the summer of 1782, General Greene's men again began to suffer from fevers, just as they had in previous summers, and matters grew worse as the summer progressed. By the end of August, they were "dayly experiencing instances of mortality . . . , soldiers dying fast," the hospital was crowded, many were sick at camp, and deaths were so frequent that funeral ceremonies were no longer conducted. By the second week in September, it was estimated that more than half of the men remaining in camp were ill, although there appears to have been at least some bark available.[105]

Treating oneself apparently continued to be an accepted practice in the fall of 1782. In one instance, for example, the victim's fever and aching began on 29 September. He first tried treating himself on the 30th, using an emetic. Still feverish on 2 October, he started taking bark and within the week felt very much better. He suffered a relapse ten days later, however, and again tried an emetic before turning to bark because of the "violent fever and pain" in his "head and bones." The fever returned once more for two days in mid-November, but the diarist unfortunately did not record his treatment on this occasion.[106]

This "cursed disorder," presumably malaria, which was still severely affecting the Southern Army in the autumn of 1782, led to the deaths of almost 100 men in September. Characterized by "ague and fever," it was blamed not on insects, despite the fact that their presence had been the subject of comment, but on the climate. General Wayne himself fell victim to it early in September and was treated with emetics and peruvian bark. He was still ill at Christmas and wrote Dr. Benjamin Rush that he was "broken down and nearly exhausted" as a result.[107]

In December, the British evacuated Charleston and, although General Greene remained there until the following August, the number of men in his command began to diminish. The Secretary at War ordered at the time that they be furloughed until peace was officially signed and some units were granted leave at once. Transportation difficulties interfered with the departure of others, and since it was July before the units from Pennsylvania and Maryland boarded their ships, the diseases which characterized the summer months in the South appeared again. One-third of those who were awaiting transport to their home states that summer were ill.[108]

There had been rumors during the siege of Yorktown that the British were trying to infect the Continental Army by sending out from the town "a large number of negroes, sick with the smallpox." Whatever the truth of the matter was, by January 1782, smallpox was spreading in the Continental Army in the North, and it was decided once more to inoculate all those who had not already had the disease. By the end of the month, approximately two thousand men had been immunized, and by May the process was complete.[109]

To care for men returning north from Yorktown who might become ill along the route and be unable to continue because of the winter weather, temporary hospitals were established along the route from Virginia northward. One such unit, at Head of Elk, Maryland, was opened no later than 22 November 1781. During December, 118 patients were admitted here, but only 38 remained at the end of the month, 60 having been discharged and 2 having died. Dr. Henry Latimer set up another such unit at Wilmington, Delaware, and 105 patients were admitted during December, of whom 23 died and 35 remained at the end of the month. General Washington decided to have the Head of Elk patients moved there, and late in January, thirteen convalescents from Head of Elk were moved to the Delaware unit. In February, plans were laid to move these patients and those at Trenton to Philadelphia.[110]

Upon their return from Virginia, the physicians of General Washington's army set up their flying hospital at New Windsor, New York. At some time before the fall of 1782, Dr. David Townshend became director of this unit. Regimental surgeons were required to report to him weekly about their patients and to receive their bandages and ointments from him. Obtaining wood was a constant problem here, and as early as 9 December 1781, patients were suffering as a result of the inadequate supply.[111]

Director General Cochran recorded that at the end of December 1781 there were 239 patients, including 25 women and children, in the New Windsor huts. Of this number, 27 were convalescent, 29 suffering from "ulcers," 23 from inflammatory fever, 27 from intermittent and remittent fevers, and 36 from diarrhea or dysentery. By the end of January 1782, however, the number of patients had dropped to 187, remaining below 190 until June 1782. In June and July, however, the number of patients again rose to 225 or more, with 38 of the men suffering from venereal disease, apparently the most common ailment at this time, although many cases of the various types of fever could also be found.[112]

The hospital at the New Windsor huts continued in operation at least until the end of December 1782, when the last of Cochran's reports which are still in existence was made up. By the last two months of the year, the patients were numbering well over 200, and as many as a quarter of them at any one time might be women and children. The incidence of malarial type fevers fell off rapidly until none was listed in the September, November, and December reports (there is no report for October), but "inflammatory fevers" afflicted thirty-three patients in the last two months of the year.[113]

Because of the rather casual use of nomenclature and the equally casual attitude toward reports, it is difficult from the documents of the period to separate one flying hospital from another and flying hospitals from regimental hospitals. In his report of

November 1781, for example, Cochran lists a flying hospital with the Eastern Army. Although it was obviously not the unit at New Windsor, no identification of it is available. In November, however, 17 were admitted to this unit, 24 were discharged, 2 died, 35 were sent to the general hospital, and 84 remained at the end of the month. The report of March 1782 lists "sick with the army," which was then broken down into two categories, the army at West Point and the army east of the Hudson. At the former, 100 were confined with smallpox, presumably, considering the time of the year, from inoculation, and forty-two with bilious fever. Eight died during the month there and 345 remained. East of the Hudson there were 35 patients with smallpox, 26 with bilious fever, 171 convalescents, and 367 remaining at the end of the month. February of 1782, however, was the busiest month for the hospital serving the army at West Point. During this month, 1,149 were admitted, and although 1,002 of these had smallpox, there were only 39 deaths. In the spring of 1783, an epidemic of measles struck the West Point area and General Washington urged that fresh meat, which was considered desirable for victims of this disease, be procured. The West Point unit was still in operation late in 1783.[114]

The total remaining sick with the Army at the end of each month throughout the year ranged from 370 in May to a high of 729 in July, when 216 were sick with intermittent and remittent fevers. Other diseases in the last eight months of 1782 were bilious and putrid fever, which hospitalized as many as 90 patients in the late summer before tapering off as the fall wore on to November's 34 and December's 26. As many as 170 men might be placed in the category of "casual hurts" each month.[115]

It was during the winter of 1781–82 that Cochran and Craik appear to have given some thought to improving the equipment of the Continental Army's flying hospital. They decided that dimensions of 15 feet by 26 feet were the most suitable for the tents which the hospital apparently used while the army was on the march. They should also either "have fly's to them" or "be made of the best stuff." Their idea pleased General Washington, who passed it on to the Secretary at War.[116]

It is difficult, however, because of the relatively imprecise information given by eighteenth century documents, to be sure of the number and type of the hospitals in the vicinity of General Washington's army after the Yorktown victory. One unit is listed as located at New Boston on the Hudson River and, according to some sources, under the direction of Eustis in December 1782. Thacher, however, also mentioned that both Townshend and Eustis were at the New Windsor hospital in December 1782. Eustis himself wrote of being Hospital Surgeon at New Boston in the autumn of 1782. General Washington referred in November 1782 to "the Hospital of Dr. Eustace," thus distinguishing it from Townshend's unit, but did not further identify it.[117]

The returns submitted by Director General Cochran in the last half of 1782 called the New Boston unit the "New Boston huts," where the August 1782 population of 216 gradually dwindled to 34 at the end of December 1782. The number of wounded here was always small, no more than four according to the records available today, but in the summer, fevers of both the intermittent-remittent and bilious-putrid types accounted for a large proportion of the sick, almost half in August. General Washington was particularly concerned about the fuel supply for Eustis's unit, presumably New Boston, as the winter of 1782 approached, but believed that it could be kept adequately supplied because no more patients were being sent there.[118]

Several of the oldest general hospitals in the department's organization were still in operation when General Washington's victorious army left Yorktown. The hospital at Trenton, New Jersey, for example, was still in operation as General Washington's men made their way north. Cochran recorded 72 American patients and 23 British prisoners at Trenton at the end of November and 38 Americans at the end of December.[119]

The number of patients at the department's Philadelphia hospital, already rising before the battle of Yorktown, reached a peak of 314 in November 1781. Only 30 of these men were listed as wounded, however, while 43 had inflammatory fevers, 40 diarrhea, 52 "various chronic," and 63 smallpox. Early in December, there were approximately 100 smallpox patients at Philadelphia, although no differentiation was made between those who had acquired the disease by inoculation and those who had contracted the disease naturally. The patient load decreased markedly, to 107, in December 1781 and vacillated between 94 and 146 until June, when only 68 patients remained. Bilious-putrid fevers do not appear to have posed a serious threat in the winter and early spring of 1782, although other fevers afflicted from a quarter to a half of the patients there. This unit was apparently sufficiently crowded in the spring of 1781 to cause the Hospital Department once more to contact the privately run Philadelphia Hospital to request the use of its facilities for Continental patients and sick British prisoners, but the appeal was denied.[120]

The total number of patients remaining at the military facility in Philadelphia continued to be less than 100, except for August, and until late fall a sizable proportion was afflicted with intermittent and remittent fevers. Women and children at that time formed a third of the facility's patients. Sick British prisoners were a responsibility of the department in Philadelphia throughout 1781 and 1782, and their number ranged from twenty-eight to seventy. Reports concerning them are less detailed, however, than those on American patients in Philadelphia, and in many reports they are all lumped together under the heading "various diseases." Despite the strain on the Philadelphia unit, it was only in 1783 that the department was successful in placing some of its patients in Philadelphia's civilian facility.[121]

The Albany unit, like that in Philadelphia, was still open when the Hospital Department was disbanded, even though its closing had been ordered two years earlier. In November 1781, fifty-four patients were at Albany. This unit seems to have been closed early in 1782 and then reopened in the spring, since forty-five patients were reported to be there in May. From forty-four to fifty-four patients, as many as half of whom might be women and children, were cared for at Albany through November 1782, beyond which time there apparently are no further reports still in existence. The staff there in late 1783 consisted of one surgeon and his mate.[122]

By the spring of 1782, General Washington had come to regard the continued operation of the general hospital at Boston as an unjustifiable expense, especially since the Corps of Invalids was no longer stationed there. As a result, the general ordered Cochran to close that facility at once.[123]

Although there was no major action after the victory at Yorktown and Congress had forced the closing of some of the major hospitals even before the end of 1781 (see Chapter 2), the concern of General Washington and, until its termination in the fall of 1783, of the Hospital Department for those soldiers who were still suffering from wounds and sickness did not diminish. The general continued to inspect such hospitals as still remained open and to urge that they be "amply Supplyed with Medicines, refreshments and accomodations."[124] Even under the adverse conditions of the last two years of the Revolution, therefore, there were patients for whom the Hospital

Department was still responsible who could praise "the humane treatment and comfortable accommodations they . . . invariably experienced." [125]

In 1783, although they did not realize it, physicians were unable to offer their patients anything better than humane treatment and comfortable accommodations. Although the often cold, half-starved, poorly clothed men of the Continental Army suffered more from disease than did their disciplined and seasoned opponents, eighteenth century medicine was everywhere helpless against disease and infection and had little to offer against pain. The time had not yet come, furthermore, when an understanding of the importance of scientific observation to medicine would make it possible for those physicans who cared for the victims of war, regardless of the army in which they served, to contribute significantly to the progress of medical science. Administrators may have learned much about the management of a military hospital system in the course of the Revolution and individual surgeons undoubtedly added to their skills while confronting diseases and injuries which they would never otherwise have encountered in such numbers, but no significant insights into the prevention, diagnosis, or treatment of disease appear to have resulted from the American Revolution. Indeed, although they did not know it, physicians would continue for many decades after the signing of the Peace of Paris to be unable to offer their patients anything of a value to rival that of their compassion and concern.

6

Between Wars, 1783 to June 1812

The period between the end of the Revolutionary War and the spring of 1812 was a low point in the history of the medical service of the U.S. Army. The very concept of a regular standing army was suspect to the leaders of the new nation, who believed that the Army should be strictly limited to as small a force as was compatible with the protection of westward moving settlers and the magnitude of the threat from abroad. Much reliance was placed upon militia and volunteer units which were employed as more appropriate to the defense of a republic than the Regular Army. A force of as limited numbers as that initially maintained in this period did not require the establishment of a formal medical department, and, indeed, there were no top management posts in the Army at this time.[1]

The strength and organization of the Army, however, fluctuated with the threat to the nation as perceived by its leaders. The resultant instability was increased by the inadequate size, organization, and leadership of the Department of War, which was created in the summer of 1789. Despite the fact that three Secretaries of War in the interwar period, Henry Dearborn, James McHenry, and William Eustis, were physicians and that the number of men actually in the Army had greatly increased by 1794, no central organization was established for the medical services. (*Table 7*) Even for those brief periods before 1812 when laws calling for a central organization were on the books, the medical department, like the Army itself, existed largely on paper. (*See Appendix H.*)

The organization created on paper by the legislation of 1799, a medical department for both Army and Navy, indicated that the lessons of the Revolution had not been entirely lost. A purveyor, for example, was specifically called for, to handle the buying of medicine and the other requirements of the projected department, and the regimental surgeons were fully under the control not only of the physician-general, or head of the department, but also of the senior hospital surgeon of an army or district. The relationship of medical officers and line officers was in some instances carefully outlined. A regimental surgeon could be temporarily reassigned away from the care of the patients of his regiment, for example, only by the physician-general or a senior hospital surgeon with the consent of the commander-in-chief or of the commander of an army. In addition, the rules which the department was to draw up for hospital discipline and camp sanitation were to be subject to the approval of the commander-in-chief or the commander of a separate army or district as well as, ultimately, to that of the President of the United States. Provision was also made for the calling of medical boards to examine candidates for positions within the department, but the establishment of these boards was to be at the discretion of the physician-general.[2] (*See Appendix H.*)

Initially it was only the constant threat of Indian attack that made the maintenance

TABLE 7—ORGANIZATION OF MEDICAL SUPPORT OF THE REGULAR ARMY, 1784–1813

Date	Regular Army	Medical Personnel
1784, June:	All but 80 men from Continental Army to be discharged	....
	700 men called up from state militias to form regiment for 1-year service	....
1785, April:	700 men called up from state militias for 3-year service	1 surgeon, 4 surgeon's mates
1789, August:	1 infantry regiment: to consist of 560 men	1 surgeon, 4 surgeon's mates
	1 artillery battalion: 280 men. Dept. of War established	1 surgeon's mate
September:	Army's organization accepted under new Constitution	....
1790, April:	Infantry regiment expanded: to include 1,216 enlisted men and non-commissioned officers	1 surgeon, 2 surgeon's mates for infantry regiment; 1 mate for artillery battalion
1791, March:	Second infantry regiment authorized: 912 more men	Ratio of 1 surgeon and 2 surgeon's mates per regiment maintained, but President may take on more mates
1792, March:	3 more infantry regiments authorized, plus 1 squadron light dragoons	1 surgeon, 2 surgeon's mates per regiment, plus a surgeon's mate for the dragoons
December:	Army reorganized into form of Legion: composed of 4 sublegions, 1,280 men in each	1 Surgeon-General for the Legion plus 1 surgeon and 3 surgeon's mates per sublegion and 6 mates for garrison duty
1794, May:	Corps of Artillerists and Engineers established: 4 battalions	1 surgeon, 4 surgeon's mates
1796, May:	Legion organization abolished: Army reorganized into 4 regiments of infantry, 2 companies of light dragoons, and the Corps of Artillerists and Engineers	For each regiment, 1 surgeon, 2 surgeon's mates; no medical attendants for dragoons; 1 surgeon, 4 surgeon's mates for Corps of Artillerists and Engineers; up to 10 more surgeon's mates could be appointed by the President
1798, April:	Second regiment of Artillerists and Engineers authorized	1 surgeon, 3 surgeon's mates
May:	Increase in size of Army up to 10,000 men authorized	President authorized to appoint a Physician-General if he believed it advisable, to serve until dismissed by President
July:	12 infantry regiments authorized; 1 dragoon regiment created	1 surgeon, 2 surgeon's mates per regiment: more if President believed it advisable, to serve until dismissed by President; James Craik appointed Physician-General
1799, March:	Additional 24 infantry regiments authorized, as well as 3 cavalry regiments, another battalion of Artillerists and Engineers, a regiment and a battalion of riflemen	Medical Department created by Act to Regulate the Medical Establishment [a] Each regiment, regardless of type, to have 1 surgeon, 2 surgeon's mates
1800, May–June:	All but 4 infantry regiments, 2 regiments of Artillerists and Engineers, 2 troops of dragoons, to be mustered out	Only 6 surgeons and 12 surgeon's mates retained in Army; Craik mustered out
1801, March:	....	Only 7 mates still in Army
1802, March:	Army reduced to 2 infantry regiments, 1 artillery regiment	2 surgeons and 25 surgeon's mates authorized, all to be attached to garrisons and posts

TABLE 7—ORGANIZATION OF MEDICAL SUPPORT OF THE REGULAR ARMY, 1784-1813—Continued

Date	Regular Army	Medical Personnel
1807, December:	....	2 surgeons in Army, only 1 on duty; 31 surgeon's mates, only 27 on duty
1808, April:	Army of 9,900 authorized, to include 3,300 already serving	Addition of 5 surgeons, 15 surgeon's mates for hospitals, plus 1 steward and 1 wardmaster per hospital authorized
1812, January:	Increase of 10 infantry regiments, 2 artillery regiments, and 1 dragoon regiment authorized	Ratio set of 1 surgeon, 2 surgeon's mates per regiment of any type plus hospital surgeons and mates as needed and 1 steward per hospital
18 June:	When war declared, authorized strength of Army was 35,603 men in 17 infantry regiments, 4 artillery regiments, 2 dragoon regiments, a Corps of Engineers, and 1 regiment of riflemen	....
26 June:	Army reorganized: size of infantry regiments set at 900 men and authorized number of infantry regiments raised to 25	Each infantry regiment to have 1 surgeon, 2 surgeon's mates, dragoon regiments 1 surgeon's mate each
1813, January:	Raising of up to 20 more regiments authorized	Each new regiment to have 1 surgeon, 2 surgeon's mates

NOTE: For actual strength of Army, see Weigley, *Army*, p. 566.
SOURCES: Emory Upton, *Military Policy of the United States* (Washington: Government Printing Office, 1904) pp. 69, 75–76, 78, 80, 82, 83, 85–86, 89; U.S. Congress, *American State Papers: Documents, Legislative and Executive of the Congress of the United States. Class V: Military Affairs*, 7 vols. (Washington: Gales and Seaton, 1832–61), 1: 5, 40–41, 154–55; Callan, *Military Laws*, pp. 212–13, 230, 238; Weigley, *Army*, p. 118.
[a] See Appendix H.

of any regular military force acceptable. Periodic expeditions with small numbers of regulars and their surgeons serving as a nucleus for larger numbers of untrained militia and volunteers were sent into the Northwest Territory to forestall large-scale Indian attacks. Forts were also established to protect the settlements going up in these areas formerly held by the Indians. In time, however, the defeat of poorly organized campaigns such as those of Brig. Gen. Josiah Harmar in 1790 and Maj. Gen. Arthur St. Clair in 1791 led to increases in United States military strength which, because of the growing fear of war with either France or England, were maintained even after Maj. Gen. Anthony Wayne's defeat of Tecumseh and the Shawnee Indians at Fallen Timbers in 1794.[3]

As the threat from France waned, the Indian menace once more became uppermost among the Army's concerns, although the northwestern campaign of Maj. Gen. William Henry Harrison against the Shawnee in 1811 was the only active move against the Indians after 1800 and before the War of 1812. In 1802, the organization of medical support was changed to center it around the garrisons which were now being established as a line of defense along the nation's perimeters. The President, after congressional approval, assigned surgeons and mates by fort rather than by regiment. To meet the new approach, the number of mates was increased, but it was not until 1808 that the need for physicians other than garrison surgeons was recognized and a plan was created which authorized the assignment of both medical and administrative personnel specifically to hospitals. Ap-

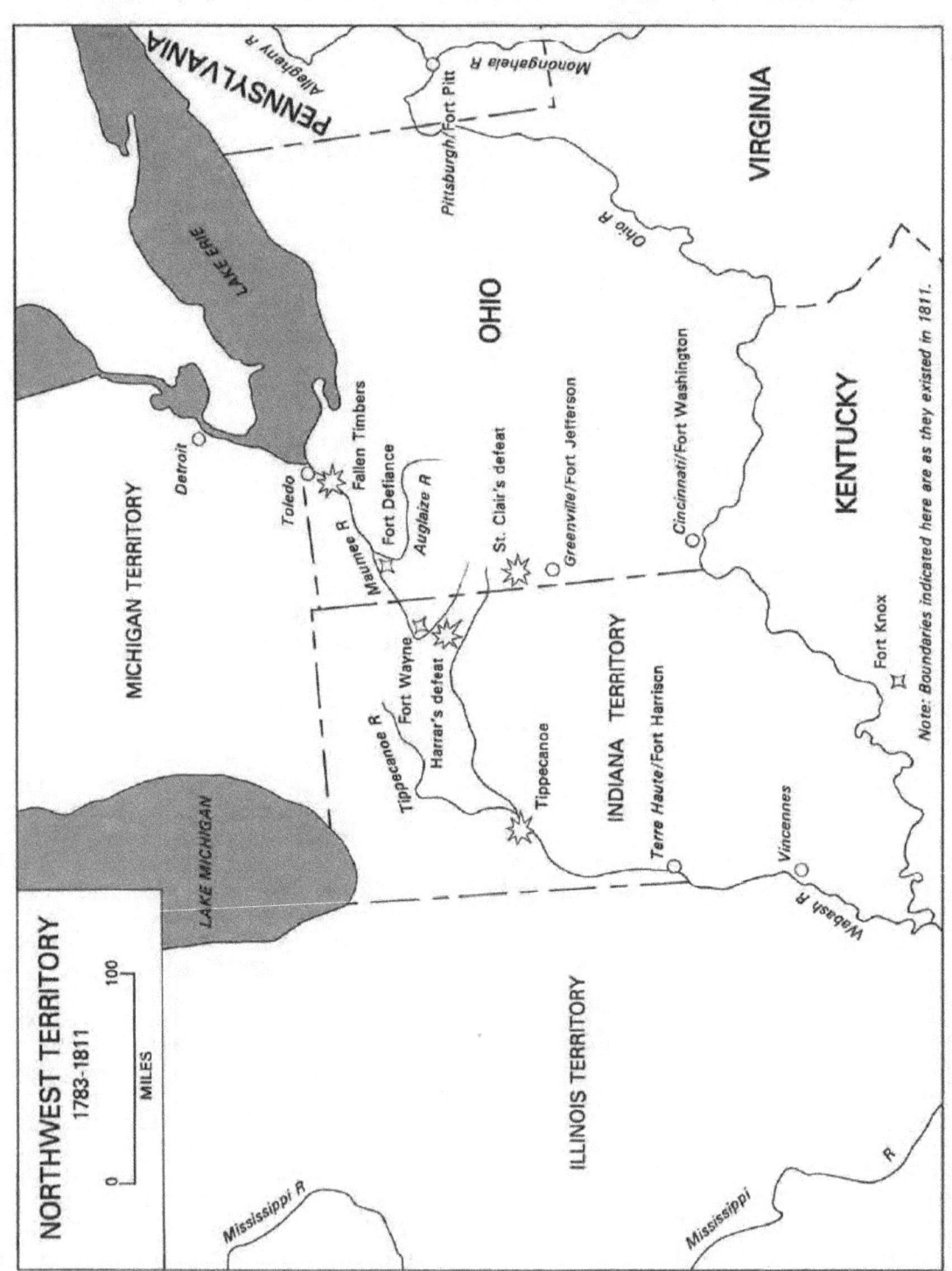

parently only one hospital surgeon and one hospital mate were actually appointed at this time. It was only six months before the outbreak of war that provision was once again made for the assignment of surgeons and mates directly to individual regiments.[4] (*See Table 7.*)

The prestige of the military surgeon at this time could not have been high. He still had no official rank and was paid a salary lower than that of major. Lewis and Clark apparently did not consider the services of a surgeon to be necessary for their famous expedition to explore the lands beyond the Mississippi River, and only two years before the beginning of the War of 1812, a group of surgeons complained to the Secretary of War that they were "the mere menial drudges of camp."[5]

CONTINENTAL ARMY PATIENTS REMAINING IN HOSPITALS

After the peace treaty of 3 September 1783 brought the formal end of the American Revolution there was no further reason to delay the final closing of those hospitals which were still caring for patients from the Continental Army. Presumably the medical board which was formed in the summer of 1782 to decide whether to transfer the "invalids and debilitated men" remaining in the Army to the Invalid Corps or to discharge them from the Army, as well as to determine their eligibility for a pension, continued in operation until all in this category had been processed. For a time, however, the remnants of the Continental Hospital Department functioned as a peacetime organization dedicated to the care of these men at West Point, Albany, and Philadelphia. In the summer of 1783, however, Gen. George Washington predicted that it would be possible to close this establishment completely by the following summer. The staff of the former Hospital Department was gradually dismissed as the need for its services diminished.[6] Since, except for fewer than 100 men assigned to guard stores and magazines at such places as West Point and Fort Pitt, the men still remaining in service from the Continental Army were dismissed on 2 June 1784, one can only assume that by this time all former Continental Army patients, including those in the Corps of Invalids, had also been discharged.

CAMPAIGNS AGAINST THE INDIANS

The first major operation involving the U.S. Army was that led by General Harmar in 1790 against the Indians in the Northwest Territory, near present-day Fort Wayne, Indiana. (*Map 9*) At this time the Army consisted of one infantry regiment, to which was assigned a surgeon and two mates, and an artillery battalion with its surgeon's mate. (*See Table 7.*) Serving as the Army's top physician was Dr. Richard Allison, of whom a contemporary said, "none were more brave, humane, and benevolent."[7] Allison was assisted by surgeon's mates John Elliott and John M. Scott, while the mate assigned to the artillery battalion was Nathan Hayward. Little is known of the medical care received by the 320 regulars who accompanied the 1,100 militia men on this expedition, but the sick rate was high and Allison complained long before the campaign began that the medicines provided for his use constituted an "injudicious assortment" of "the refuse of the druggists' shops" and were of such poor quality that he was unable to determine proper dosages.[8]

The governor of the Northwest Territory during this period was Arthur St. Clair. In 1791, St. Clair was assigned the rank of major general in the Army, which had been enlarged for a second attempt to subdue the Indians in the Northwest. It is interesting to note that General St. Clair, like so many

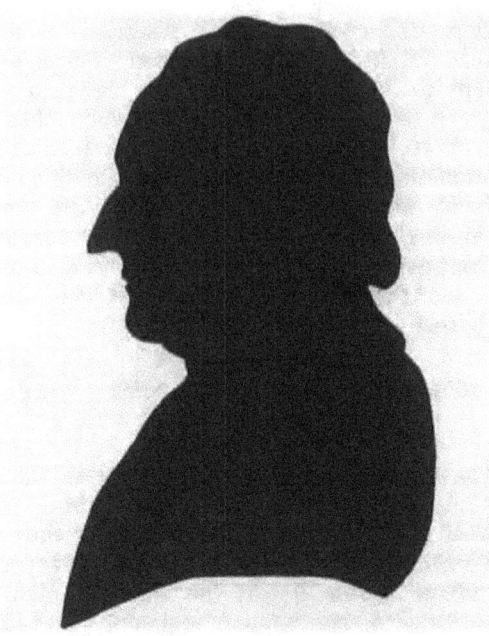

RICHARD ALLISON. *(Courtesy of National Library of Medicine.)*

other men in prominent positions with the Army at this time, had had some medical training. Among the members of his expedition who served as physicians were Allison, as chief surgeon, and Elliott, who continued to function for a time as Allison's mate and then, with Allison's full approval, was promoted to surgeon of the 2d Regiment. This latter post had first been offered to Eustis who, destined for greater things, turned it down. Among other medical attendants was Victor Grasson, a surgeon's mate attached to a volunteer unit.[9]

General St. Clair's force of 1,500 militia men and volunteers and 600 regulars was larger than that of his predecessor, but the general himself was in poor health and so badly afflicted with gout that he could not walk without aid. Before the expedition was over, he was unable to so much as mount his horse without assistance. His men, furthermore, were "badly clothed, badly paid and badly fed." Since they were for the most part recruited from cities and large towns, they were also reputed to be "enervated by idleness, debaucheries, and every species of vice." [10]

By the fall of 1791, General St. Clair's surgeons were faced with severe problems. Hospital stores, particularly wine, were in very short supply and the number of men who were sick had risen so high that the general decided to remain at Fort Jefferson, near present-day Greenville, Ohio, until the end of October, hoping that both health and supply problems might improve. By the end of the month, however, when they resumed their march, 120 men were so ill that they could not continue any further.[11]

Considering the nature and condition of his force, it is not surprising that on 3 November, General St. Clair was soundly defeated by the Miami Indians, who attacked him about thirty miles from Fort Jefferson. Of a total of 1,400 effectives, 632 were killed and 264 wounded. Surgeon Grasson was among those killed, but Allison distinguished himself in the desperate confusion by aiding the officers in rallying their men. Even before the battle was over the Indians were scalping their victims. A witness noted: "I saw a Capt. Smith just after he was scalped, sitting on his backside, his head smoking like a chimney & he asked me if ye battle was not a most over." [12]

The retreat which followed was so rapid that those among the sick and wounded who were fortunate enough to be taken along by their fellows were deposited at Fort Jefferson, twenty-nine miles from the battleground, less than eight hours after the flight began. Having settled the disabled there, however, the able-bodied set out again and reached Fort Washington, where Cincinnati now stands, on 8 November. The wounded continued to straggle in to Fort Jefferson for days after the battle. "Some soldiers have come in with ye Skin & Hare taken clean off of their Heads," an officer

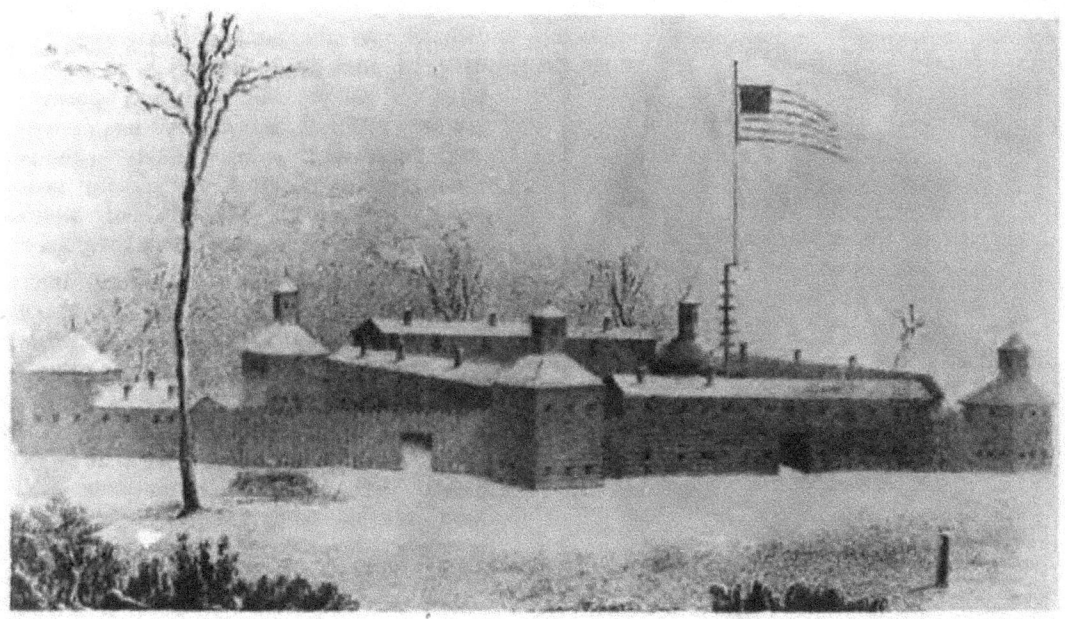

FORT WASHINGTON. *(From a drawing by Maj. Ebenezer Denny, reproduced in Wilson, Bradley.)*

wrote his brother,[13] and one had not only been scalped but also had "a tomehawk stuck in the head in two places."[14] Although two medicine chests were lost in the defeat, every possible effort seems to have been made to establish hospital facilities and to obtain all the provisions needed for the wounded, whose situation was "truly distressing."[15]

The failure of two attempts to subdue the Indians in the Northwest led to a reassessment of the approach to the problem. The leaders of both expeditions were officially exonerated of any major blame, which was placed upon the War Department, the Quartermaster's Department, and contractors. Maj. Gen. Anthony Wayne was given the Army's five regular infantry regiments and cavalry and artillery to establish the Legion for a new effort against the Indians. General Wayne was also granted the time to train his men thoroughly near Pittsburgh before taking them into action, but although Congress had by this time authorized a ratio of one surgeon and two surgeon's mates per infantry regiment as well as a mate for the light dragoon squadron, there was only one surgeon actually with the army when it began its training.[16] (*See Table 7.*)

General Wayne regarded "the health and comfort of the soldiers" as "objects of the first consideration" and was personally concerned with the maintenance of their health and the proper care of those who became ill. The general ordered the single surgeon, Dr. John F. Carmichael, with his men to begin at once to set up a tent hospital.[17] When, in addition to "a virulent Veneri," smallpox broke out, General Wayne ordered Carmichael to begin inoculating all men who had never had the disease.[18] Shortly thereafter he also ordered Carmichael to locate "two industrious humane and honest *Matrons* to assist in nursing and cooking for the Sick." Although he had little control over the shortage of hospital supplies, General Wayne decided to deal with the severe

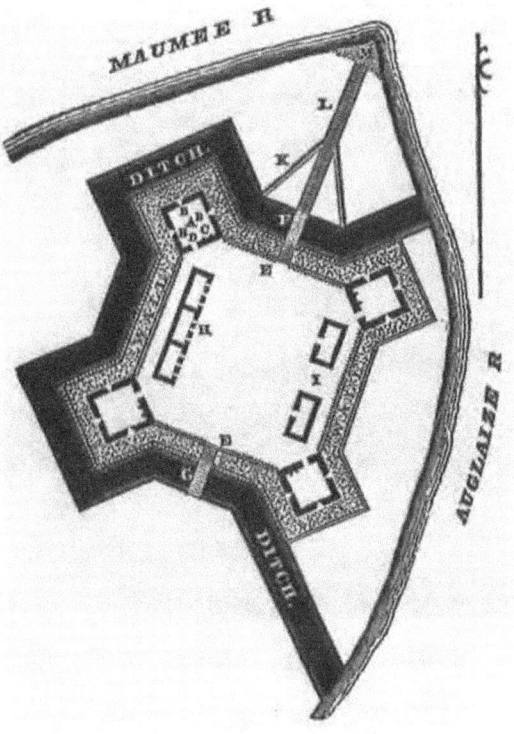

FORT DEFIANCE. *(Courtesy of Library of Congress.)*

and prolonged shortage of vegetables by offering the whiskey ration of his men, both sick and well, to the local inhabitants in exchange for their produce.[19]

Discipline within the hospital also concerned General Wayne even after the arrival of a second surgeon to help Carmichael. On at least one occasion, the general was required to court-martial a sergeant "for riotiously beating a Woman kept by him as a Mistress to the injury of the Sick in the Hospital . . . for abusive language and using Menancing [sic] words and gestures to Doctor Carmichael, when requested by him to desist from the above purpose."[20]

General Wayne began his active campaign in the spring of 1793, moving first to Fort Washington (Cincinnati) and then slowly westward, establishing forts as he went. He was now accompanied by at least four physicians, including his chief surgeon,

Allison. As the summer progressed, however, his men began to fall ill in increasing numbers, fevers and influenza posing the greatest problem. Supplies of hospital stores and medicines were quickly exhausted. Finally, in desperation, the general ordered Allison to buy the needed items wherever he could find them, regardless of price.[21]

The decisive action of General Wayne's campaign against the Indians was the Battle of Fallen Timbers, which took place on 20 August 1794 not far from the new British fort near the site of present-day Toledo and shortly after the building of Fort Defiance. The wounded, a total of approximately 100, eleven of whom later died of their injuries, were considered fortunate to be moved from the battlefield in a carriage, but at least one witness believed that the evacuation could have been better managed. "The wounded of the third sub-legion are under obligations to doctor Hayward for his attention and humanity to them in this distress," he wrote, but "Doctor Carmichael through neglect had the wounded men of the artillery and cavalry thrown into wagons, among spades, axes, picks, &c." and as a result, they had to endure "extreme pain, beside the frequent shocks of a wagon on the worst of roads." By 27 August, however, the wounded had reached Fort Defiance and were "happily fixed in the garrison, and the doctors say there is no great danger of any of them dying."[22]

Even before Fallen Timbers, General Wayne himself had become gravely ill with gout; Allison reported him to be "in agony." The sick rate among his men, already high in the early summer,[23] was still increasing in September, the principal ailment being "the fever and ague." An officer explained that "The number of our sick increase daily, provision is nearly exhausted, the whiskey had been out for some time. . . . Hard duty and scanty allowance will cause an army to be low spirited, particularly the want of a little of the *wet*." General Wayne may have believed it advisable to trade whiskey for vegetables, but not everyone agreed with him; "the troops would much rather live on half rations of beef and bread, provided they could obtain their full rations of whisky" than enjoy the ample supply of vegetables now available at Fort Defiance. Unfortunately for the whiskey lovers, however, their favorite beverage was in very short supply by that time.[24] Shortages continued until a member of General Wayne's staff commented of the wounded that "no set of men in the like disabled situation ever experienced much more want of conveniences &c." and from time to time the general still found it necessary to have Allison make purchases on an emergency basis.[25]

September was a bad month for malaria in many areas of Ohio in this period, and in September of 1795 the number of sick was again growing rapidly. The burden of the hospital at Greenville, moved from its initial location in a blockhouse to huts, grew from 120 to more than 300 patients in the space of a month. Patients from General Wayne's army had been "totally destitute of any kind of Hospital stores . . . since last Winter, except a little occasionally purchased from the Merchants at this place & Cincinnati in cases of the last necessity." Finally the general moved the entire hospital into the open woods in an attempt to stem the onslaught of disease. Since Allison was no longer able to find either opium or peruvian bark in adequate quantity locally, his surgeons began trying substitutes for peruvian bark, fearing that if the tide were not turned, they might soon be facing an epidemic of putrid fever. October found General Wayne once again pressing the War Department for supplies, pointing out that he was "totally destitute of . . . Medicine & Hospital stores," but only in mid-November did even a portion of the desperately needed hospital stores begin to arrive at General Wayne's camp.[26]

Supply shortages occurred yet again and to an alarming degree in 1796, at a time when the number of physicians available to care for General Wayne's men was also inadequate. Secretary of War McHenry seems to have believed this situation hopeless, for he suggested that the area of present-day Toledo be abandoned because of the prevalence of the disease there. The supply of peruvian bark was exhausted, and in the garrisons the general had assigned to posts from Fort Washington to Detroit, more than 400 officers and men were sick, most of them with malaria.[27] General Wayne, however, was not required to contend with these problems much longer. His health had continued poor, and in December 1796, on his way home from Detroit, he died.

The last campaign against the Indians in the Northwest to be undertaken before the outbreak of the War of 1812 was launched in 1811 when it seemed that the Shawnees under Tecumseh were becoming an ever greater threat to settlers. At Vincennes, approximately 300 regulars and twice that many militia men were placed under the command of the Indiana Territory's governor, William Henry Harrison, who was in time commissioned a brigadier general. General Harrison, who had studied briefly at the Medical School of the University of Pennsylvania, was another of the Army's leaders who had received some training as a physician.[28]

General Harrison established a general hospital at Vincennes under the supervision of two physicians from the 4th Infantry Regiment. The head of this hospital, Dr. Josiah Foster, was a man whom Harrison knew and very much admired. Militia units appear to have, as usual, provided their own surgeons for this campaign.[29]

Although during the summer his men were in generally poor health and suffering particularly from "bilious autumnal fever,"[30] in September 1811, General Harrison moved his men from Vincennes up the Wabash River to erect Fort Harrison near the site of Terre Haute, Indiana. At this time, he ordered that the sick from his force, many of whom were afflicted with the painful disease then called "the fever and ague," or intermittent fever, be sent to Fort Knox, where a surgeon's mate supervised their care.[31]

By late October, General Harrison was ready to move directly against the Shawnee in their village on the Tippecanoe River near the site of present-day Lafayette, Indiana. At this time the 900 to 1,000 men under his command were accompanied by three physicians, a surgeon, and two mates, two of whom appear to have been attached to the Regular Army. The health of the regulars had improved, but that of the militia was apparently deteriorating. The sick, among whom were presumably both militia and regulars, were left behind at a small blockhouse built for their use, with a sergeant's guard to protect them.[32]

The Indians, led in Tecumseh's absence by his brother, launched a surprise attack on 7 November 1811 upon General Harrison's camp near their village, but the level of discipline which the Americans had attained was such that they were able to resist the attack and mount a counterattack of their own which culminated in the destruction of the Indian confederacy Tecumseh had formed. General Harrison's men suffered total losses of fewer than 200. Of this number, 37 were killed in action and more than 150 were wounded, among whom was a militia surgeon's mate. Despite the relatively primitive conditions under which he was forced to work, among the operations which Foster apparently performed were two amputations at the shoulder, a type of surgery not often undertaken at the time.[33]

General Harrison's force returned to Vincennes on 18 November, moving the wounded much of the way by boat, but by the time they reached that post, the injuries of twenty-five of them had proven fatal. By 4 December, three more men had died in the general hospital at Vincennes and so many wounds were proving unusually slow to heal that Foster suspected that the Indians had used poisoned ammunition. Examination of the balls found in wounds revealed that they had been "chewed before they were insertd into rifles for the purpose of enlarging the wound and lacerating the contiguous flesh." [34]

FORTS AND THEIR GARRISONS

The defense policy of the new nation called for the establishment of forts or fortifications at strategic points both in areas where Indians and settlers were likely to come into conflict and along the coast, to guard against attacks from European nations. Among the concerns of the Secretary of War in 1794, for example, was the completion of fortifications on three islands in New York harbor, at eight New England ports, at eleven towns and cities from Philadelphia south to Georgia, and at West Point on the Hudson River.[35]

One such coastal fort was Fort Jay, on Governors Island in the Harbor of New York City, constructed in 1794 in anticipation of war with France. A surgeon's mate was sent there in the spring of 1802, when the policy of assigning medical support by garrison rather than by regiment was adopted. (See Table 7.) A difficulty which was by no means unique to the New York City garrisons arose, however, when the Army surgeon assigned to the area allowed other concerns to distract him from his Army duties. About eight years after this physician was sent to Fort Jay, testimony at a court-martial revealed that the only Army physician then assigned to care for the New York garrisons was living and practicing medicine within the city and on occasion unavailable to these men when they needed him.[36]

Fort Adams on the Mississippi River south of Natchez seems to have served as a supply distribution center for lesser outposts in the area. So important had this fort become by 1802 that it was assigned to the care of Carmichael, one of the two surgeons still remaining in the Army at that date. Carmichael had previously spent some time at Fort Adams and was, therefore, familiar with the climate and the problems associated with it. In 1803, a surgeon's mate was sent to work under Carmichael, a move which could have been necessitated either by unexpectedly heavy demands upon Carmichael's time or by the fact that this surgeon, too, had found other duties to keep him busy. He functioned as a customs collector during part of his stay at Fort Adams, for example, giving up this position only in the spring of 1803. The Secretary of War commented on this particular occasion, "I trust in the future his whole attention will be paid to his medical duties." By the spring of the following year, however, Carmichael was preparing to resign.[37]

The character of the forts in the Northwest Territory varied greatly; some were simply stockades while others were relatively complex installations where life was not entirely devoid of luxuries. At Fort Washington, for example, a physician owned a summerhouse which stood in the midst of the extensive gardens lying just beyond the walls of the fort.[38]

Particularly detailed records which provide insight into the work of a garrison surgeon were left by the surgeon's mate at Fort Defiance in Ohio in 1795. Here Dr. Joseph Gardner Andrews was responsible for the health not only of the garrison of approximately 160 officers and men, but also of a small number of civilians, including five women and a child. In addition, Andrews, like other Army physicians during this period, cared for the ill among neighboring Indians.[39]

In the course of fulfilling his duties in 1795, Andrews confronted diseases which were undoubtedly familiar to most of the surgeons serving with the U.S. Army. On 1 January, he had thirty-seven patients, all members of the garrison, twenty-five of whom were wounded. Four of the remainder were suffering from what he diagnosed to be rheumatism, three from diarrhea, one from dysentery, and one from intermittent fever. A month later, although one of his earlier patients was dead, the total number had dropped to twenty-seven, three of whom were convalescents and fifteen wounded. By 1 March, the doctor had lost another patient and a child was among those listed as sick. By April, although the child was well again and Andrews's patients numbered only twenty-one, intermittent fever had made its appearance among them.[40]

Both the total number of patients and the number with intermittent fever gradually dropped as spring and summer wore on, however, despite the fact that in July there were "musketoes plenty" in the area between Fort Defiance and Fort Wayne. By late August, Andrews was himself acutely ill, and by 1 September, all nine of his patients were sick with intermittent fever. Ten days later, despite his own condition and the fact that he had "not a particle of Hospital Stores," he was attempting to care for fifteen patients, all of whom had intermittent fever. Less than a week later, when he himself still "Had the Ague & fever extremely severe," he turned to "the Dogwood bark in simple decoction" in an attempt to treat his intermittent fever patients, who now numbered twenty-one.

The situation as far as hospital supplies were concerned had come to the attention of the officers at Fort Defiance, who finally managed to obtain eight gallons of liquor for the fort hospital by promising to pay for it themselves should the government refuse to do so. By the end of September, Andrews had also received a keg of wine and 30 pounds of brown sugar, items which were sorely needed by the time they actually began to arrive. By 1 October, sixty-one of the total population of Fort Defiance were sick. Of this number, fifty-eight were listed as having intermittent fever and three remittent fever. Andrews observed that "The Intermittents in this place are extraordinarily rapid in depriving the patients of strength." The prevalence of fevers was not limited to Fort Defiance, 500 having been reported sick with the two types of fever at Fort Jefferson.

By 7 October, Andrews was feeling well enough to pronounce himself recovered, but two weeks later his fever recurred, fortunately, it seems, for a brief time only. Others were also recovering at this time, and his report of 1 November records only thirty patients, one of whom was suffering from wounds and two, one of whom died a short time later, from typhus. By December 1795, Andrews's patients numbered only eleven, two of whom were convalescent and seven afflicted with "debility."

Although the Indians Andrews treated included even a Delaware chief, it was an American who seems to have caused him the most trouble. Ensign Frothingham was, to the surgeon's great disgust, much given to treating himself and brought with him to Fort Defiance "a quantity of medicines, lotions & unguents almost equal to the contents of my Chest, like a person who has dabbled sufficiently in medicine to render it a dangerous tool." With the aid of an Indian squaw, this officer "induced a dropsy, or rather a very dangerous relapse, as . . . he had the anasarca last year." Although he at last promised to follow Andrews's advice exclusively, two weeks later, on 6 December 1795, "after a tedious illness wch he did not endure with that christian fortitude, that his affectation of religion seemed to induce an expectation in the minds of his Brother Officers," Ensign Frothingham "died . . . without a pang." Andrews stated that an autopsy revealed that his kidneys had ceased to function.

WILKINSON IN THE LOUISIANA TERRITORY, 1809

In 1808, fear of a possible attack by the British upon the newly acquired Louisiana Territory led to the assignment of Brig. Gen. James Wilkinson, another physician who had abandoned the active practice of medicine and an officer who moved successfully from one scandal, including the Aaron Burr conspiracy, to another, to command the troops to be sent to strengthen the defenses there.[41]

The units assigned to General Wilkinson in 1809 included three regular infantry regiments and elements of a fourth, in addition to companies of dragoons, light artillery, and riflemen, for a total which at times approximated 2,500 regulars. It is difficult to ascertain precisely the number and status of the physicians on duty with General Wilkinson's forces in 1809, but records surviving from this period indicate that among their number were the surgeons for two or more infantry regiments and one for a regiment of riflemen, in addition to a surgeon and a mate assigned to the general hospital at New Orleans as hospital physicians; there were probably others there as well. General Wilkinson, however, believed that there should have been more physicians with his men.[42]

A general hospital was established at New Orleans to care for the sick of General Wilkinson's command, but exactly how many patients this facility could handle is not clear. The general maintained that two empty barracks next to the hospital would be used to add as many as 500 places to the hospital's capacity. During the summer of 1809, the immediate supervision of this unit was the responsibility of the hospital surgeon's mate. The hospital surgeon reportedly had a large private practice in the New Orleans area.⁴³

As far as the Army's health was concerned, the situation was building up to disaster by the spring of 1809 in New Orleans. General Wilkinson's troops were undisciplined, his officers inexperienced, and hospital stores short. In mid-April, only two surgeons, one of whom was ill himself, and two mates were actually on duty to care for the 550 regulars who were ill in the New Orleans area, and General Wilkinson finally believed it necessary to hire private physicians to help care for his men. Although the fevers which were expected in the summer in this area had not yet appeared, the health of the men continued poor, the diseases most frequently seen being "mostly of the bowels, and ascribable to a change of diet, and the water of the Mississippi." Eustis, Secretary of War at this time, expressed great concern for the future health of General Wilkinson's men and agreed with him that the Army should leave the city of New Orleans.⁴⁴

Although on 30 April, Eustis suggested that General Wilkinson move his men north up the Mississippi River to Fort Adams and Natchez, in the late spring the general moved them to a location twelve miles south of New Orleans, on the west bank of the Mississippi, an area known as Terre aux Boeufs; he later claimed that he did not receive Eustis's communication of 30 April until after the move to Terre aux Boeufs had been completed.⁴⁵

Terre aux Boeufs had a reputation for pools of water which stagnated long after a rainfall, but General Wilkinson maintained that the site he had chosen was a healthy one with good water. Although he had found it necessary to order drainage ditches dug there, he claimed specifically that the area was dry.⁴⁶

The sick rate at the new campsite continued very high, although General Wilkinson, in defense of his decision, pointed out that Terre aux Boeufs was an improvement over New Orleans. In an eight-day period at New Orleans in early June 1809, ten men died and nine more deserted, but in the last twenty days of the month, when the army was at Terre aux Boeufs, only eleven men died and three deserted. He also stated that on 14 June, shortly after the move, 565 of the 1,662 men present at camp were sick, but that on 27 June, only 429 were sick of a total of 1,690.⁴⁷

The summer was a grim one. General Wilkinson claimed that hospital tents were set up for each regiment at Terre aux Boeufs and eventually an eighty-man hospital as well, but, even so, at times the sick had to remain in their own tents. The supply of medicines was inadequate and the surgeons in attendance were often sick themselves. The flour was at times moldy, worm-infested, and so hard as to challenge an ax. It was suspected that the general was in collusion with the contractors who were responsible for supplying his force.⁴⁸

The supply problem was not alleviated, however, by either the management of Secretary of War Eustis or the custom of allotting supplies by company without reference to hospital requirements. Eustis alternated between forbidding the purchase of the expensive eggs, poultry, and wine physicians wanted for their patients and maintaining that he could not understand why all things necessary for the health of the troops had not been purchased. The general himself blamed the youth and inexperience of the contractor's agent and finally resorted to the step of authorizing his hospital surgeon to buy personally whatever the sick needed.⁴⁹

General Wilkinson did not initially move his men upstream when he finally did receive Eustis's suggestion because, he maintained, those familiar with the area told him that such a move at that time would endanger the health of his men. The general stated to Eustis that since the trip would have to be made by water, it could lead to the deaths of as many as nine-tenths of his men. On 22 June, however, Eustis specifically ordered an immediate move to Fort Adams and Natchez.[50]

Despite General Wilkinson's misgivings, the voyage up the Mississippi River was undertaken, albeit not as soon as Eustis wished. Dr. Alfred Thruston, surgeon for the 7th Infantry Regiment, had officially protested the idea of moving the men during the heat of summer, but in September, the sickest men having been sent back to the general hospital at New Orleans, 1,542 men began the journey. All of them were taken across the river to the east bank in boats, and then the 982 men able to do so were put on shore to proceed north on foot. The remainder, 382 of whom were convalescents still too weak to march, stayed in the boats for the entire trip.[51]

Although there seems to have been no lack of both medicines and such staples of the diet of the sick as tea, sugar, chocolate, brandy, and wine during the voyage, it was soon impossible to provide the sick with proper medical care. Their number multiplied rapidly and the boats were soon so crowded with the ill that the surgeons could move among them only at night, when camp was set up on shore.[52]

The trip from Terre aux Boeufs to Natchez was completed in approximately 45 days. By early October, however, there were so many ill among the men that two groups of patients, each accompanied by a physician, were left off before they reached Natchez. The officers took up a collection to buy supplies for the hospital which was set up for 100 patients south of Fort Adams, and another 120 sick officers and men were landed at Fort Adams itself. An estimated 300 more men died on the journey.[53]

General Wilkinson himself, however, was not with his men for this tragic voyage. At the time of the departure, being seriously ill with "remittent fever, attended with very violent paroxysms," he remained at New Orleans. In November, he set out for Natchez, where a short time later he was relieved by Brig. Gen. Wade Hampton.[54]

It seems reasonable to assume that several diseases were to blame for the devastation of General Wilkinson's army in the spring, summer, and fall of 1809, when at least 500 and possibly as many as 1,000 died. The surgeon for the 5th Infantry Regiment, Dr. William Upshaw, reported that the most prevalent diseases in the early summer were "chronic diseases, bilious and intermittent fevers, some cases of scurvy." The chronic ailments seem to have been diarrheas, which were blamed on changes in food and water despite the fact that some cases predated the arrival at New Orleans, and a violent dysentery.[55]

General Wilkinson himself noted that the heat was usually blamed when the number of sick was high and that although June and July were wet months, the disease rate among his men did not peak until later. If one were to assume that malaria was one of the principal diseases afflicting the men along the southern Mississippi River, however, the late summer peak would not be unusual. More recent records indicate, for example, that the number of admissions to Army hospitals in the continental United States because of malaria in 1921 was greatest in August and September and that the peak month during both world wars generally came no earlier than July and at times as late as the early fall.[56]

General Wilkinson and the others concerned with the health of his troops, however, appear to have had no real suspicion that mosquitoes were related to the high disease and death rate in 1809, even though they did try to protect the troops from them. In August of 1808, the Secretary of War suggested to the military agent for New Orleans the purchase of "a reasonable supply of musquitoe nets for the troops." In April of the following year, General Wilkinson ordered 100 mosquito bars specifically for the field hospital serving his sick and still more for the rest of his men. It was noted at the time, however, that since the diarrhea common in his army caused non-hospitalized men to leave and reenter their tents frequently in the course of an evening, mosquito bars did not always solve the mosquito problem.[57]

At least one attempt was made by a surgeon familiar with the sufferings of General Wilkinson's men to find a single disease which could be blamed for most of the illness. Dr. Jabez Heustis chose scurvy as the culprit, but admitted that not all of the symptoms he had recorded were those usually associated with it.

This disease first made its appearance among the soldiers in the form of an intermitting fever, which, by degrees, assumed a more malignant aspect, acquiring the character of the bilious remitting, or yellow fever; becoming more malignant as the season advanced, and the heat increased. In some instances this fever was of a violent inflammatory character, in others, typhoid symptoms marked both its invasion and progress.... Towards the end of July the epidemic malady appeared among the troops in a new form, of such an anomalous aspect, as at first to occasion doubts as to its nature.[58]

Before the more obvious symptoms appeared, according to Heustis, the "features became sad ... and the face assumed a sallow hue." In time the joints became stiff "and the tendons in the arms rigid and contracted." The patient then began to experience "pain in the parotid glands," and, in time, "buboes ... in the groin," petechiae, loose teeth, and bleeding gums. From this point onward the disease progressed rapidly, according to Heustis, "destroying the whole inside of the mouth in twelve hours, and frequently in less than half that time." In one case, a patient was so severely affected that he took "hold of his tongue ... deliberately drew it from his mouth, and threw it on the table, for the contemplation of his companions."[59]

Heustis was not entirely satisfied with scurvy as an explanation for the illnesses which afflicted General Wilkinson's men. The symptoms he observed reminded him in some ways of descriptions of "the Eastern plague," which, as he understood it, was also characterized by enlarged glands, "feotor of the breath," buboes in the groin, and petechiae. Furthermore, he noted, scurvy was not usually accompanied by diarrhea and dysentery. Officers did not often contract this illness, a phenomenon which Heustis attributed to their custom of buying fresh food from local inhabitants, something enlisted men could not afford to do, but he concluded that "The efficient cause of this pestilential distemper was undoubtedly the use of unwholesome and corrupt provision" such as "old, rancid" pork and beef which was "poor, lean," and that air "highly impregnated with noxious miasmata" was undoubtedly a contributing factor.[60]

Heustis blamed 1,000 casualties upon the disease he was attempting to define. He estimated that 150 of that total had been "destroyed at Terre-aux-Boeufs," 250 during the journey upriver, and 600 at the new campsites. He believed, however, that the chief physician caring for General Wilkinson's men in the Natchez area had contributed to the high mortality rate with his "injudicious use of mercury, which was prescribed as a general remedy by the superintending physician .... A few doses of this medicine relieved the patient of his misery, and put an end to his earthly sufferings." He added that other physicians with General Wilkinson's men did not share the faith of their superior in mercurials and in his absence omitted his prescriptions in favor of "vegetable remedies," such as sorrel and wild peppergrass.[61]

Management of Supplies

Army physicians had no supply system of their own in this period, and for much of the time, no physician was directly involved in the purchasing and distributing of hospital supplies and medicines. Attempts were made to control the use of these items and to increase the efficiency of the supply system by such steps as establishing separate lists of medicines to be purchased for southern and northern areas, but complaints of shortages and poor management continued to come in from the field, and physicians were forced to exercise what ingenuity they could. To augment their supplies of medicines, they turned to such locally available remedies as the barks of wild cherry, sassafras, willow, and other trees, using them for conditions ranging from fevers to consumption. It should be noted that in spite of the fact that it was so difficult to keep its physicians adequately provided, the War Department at times permitted some of them to use government supplies for their own private patients.[62]

Complaints were heard involving both the quantity and quality of medicines bought, according to Secretary of War Eustis, by the "Purveyor of Public Supplies." Eustis, apparently determined that something be done to give a physician a role in the purchasing and distributing of medicines and hospital supplies, finally turned to Dr. Benjamin Rush for advice. He also asked for the name of someone who could work with the men who had the overall responsibility for purchasing. Rush recommended Dr. James Mease, who worked at this task during the winter and spring of 1810. With Rush's aid, Mease composed a list of the necessary supplies and then personally inspected and packed the items to be distributed to the surgeons.[63]

Mease's services seem to have been rendered on a temporary basis, for in February 1812, Dr. Francis LeBaron was given the task of managing the "selection, inspection and putting up of the medicines and hospital stores." LeBaron's position was not an official one, a fact which seems to have very much concerned him. He urged that Congress create the official position of "Inspector of Medicine & Hospital Stores," but by the end of 1812, nothing had been done about the matter.[64]

LeBaron's duties included the composition of standardized lists of drug needs and the solicitation of bids on them from the leading druggists in Boston, New York, and Philadelphia. He was also responsible for constructing and outfitting of medicine chests, each of which was intended to serve 500 men and to be carried on a baggage wagon three and one-half feet long.[65]

LeBaron's center of operations appears to have been Philadelphia, but he was also expected to establish storage depots elsewhere. On 8 June 1812, a few days before war was officially declared, he was ordered to set up a depot at Albany, "for an Hospital Establishment for the Northern Army." [66]

Throughout the entire period from 1783 to the outbreak of the War of 1812, the medical support of the units composing the Regular U.S. Army lay, for all practical purposes, entirely in the hands of individual surgeons. Separated from one another by vast distances, frustrated by shortages of medicines and supplies, they struggled with the health problems of soldiers who were poorly trained, poorly clothed, poorly fed, and only too often poorly led as well. It was of physicians caring for the Army's sick and wounded under just such circumstances, however, that a soldier who had witnessed their efforts wrote "too much cannot be said in their praise." [67]

"ESTIMATE OF MEDICINE, HOSPITAL STORES, ETC. FOR EIGHTY MEN [FOR] ONE YEAR." (Courtesy of National Archives.)

Estimate of Medicine &c. Continued

	Northern Posts		Southern Posts	
	℔	oz	℔	oz
Ol. Ania		1		1
Flor Sulph	4	"	8	
" Chamomil	1	"	2	"
" Benzoin	"	½	"	½
Ungl. Mac. Sub.	2	"	8	"
" Byst. flav.	4		10	
" Sativa	4	"	8	"
Emp. Vesicus	"	8	1	
" Diaprlon	1	"	2	"
Cantharis in a Sep. Bott. pulverized	"	8	"	8
Magnesia Alba	"	4	"	4
Sac. Saturn	2	"	4	"
Tart. Emet.	"	2	"	4
Vitriol. Alb	"	2	"	4
" Antimon.	"	1	"	1
Pol. Digitalis	"	4	"	4
Caust. Lunar	"	1	"	1
Suc. Glycer	2	"	2	"

Hospital Stores and Furniture

	Northern Posts		Southern Posts	
Brandy	Gallons	10	Gallons	20
Sherry Wine	"	10	"	20
Vinegar	"	10	"	20
Molasses	"	10	"	20
Sugar Brown	℔	25	℔	75
Chocolate	"	24	"	50
Bohea Tea	"	14	"	20
Tapioca	"	4	"	4
Sago	"		"	4
Pearl Barley	"	8		
Rice			"	100
Cinnamon	oz	2	oz	4
Allspice	"	3	℔	1
Ginger	℔	2	"	4

Hospital Stores &c. Continued

	Northern Posts	Southern Posts
Matrasses	N° 4	N° 8
Sheets	" 4	" 8
Blankets	" 8	" 16
Essence of Spruce	Potts 4	Potts 8
D° glass wide mouth qr. pt. Bottles	N° 4	N° 6
D° " fine d° d°	" 4	" 6
Pint wide mouth Gr? St. Vials	" 6	" 10
Half pt. fine vials	" 6	" 12

Instead of furnishing Matrasses, strong linnen might be purchased for the purpose, sufficient to make them 6 feet in length and 2½ feet wide, a sheet should measure 7 feet long and 4 feet wide—

In purchases of Medicine to be supplied, regard should be had to the number of Companies which compose the Garrison; where it consists of from two to five Companies it is presumed that a deduction may be made from the articles generally of 25 pr. cent. The same remark will apply with equal propriety to Hospital Stores.

Instruments necessary for one Military post

Sufficient for one year	Amputating Sett	1	For one year	Sponge oz	2
	Trepaning "	1		Lint No	1
	Pocket "	1		Pins p.	1
	Teeth "	1		Tape piece	1
	Male Catheters	1		Sheep skins N°	2
	Scales and Weights	1		Wrapping paper 2"	6
	Bell metal mortar & pestle	1			
	Glass d° d°	1		In addition to the foregoing specified articles, each post ought to be furnished with Stationary, as follows Northern posts 6 quires of writing paper, Southern Posts 12 quires of writing paper, with proportionate allowances of quills &c.
	Crown Lancets	6			
For one year	Penis Syringes Doz	2			
	Vials assorted	3			
	Corks d°	6			
	Pill Boxes papers	1			
	Flannel yards	5			
	Muslin	5			

7

Administration of Medical Support, June 1812 to January 1815

Largely because of British impressment of American seamen and their aid to the Indians, the United States had been anticipating war with Great Britain for several years before the actual declaration on 18 June 1812, but neither the Army nor the organization of the Army's medical support was ready for open hostilities when they came.[1]

OPENING MONTHS OF THE WAR OF 1812

The direction of the nation's armed forces at this crucial time remained in the somewhat inept hands of Secretary of War William Eustis. It was Eustis who sent Brig. Gen. William Hull orders hours before war was formally declared but did not inform him that this step was imminent. It was also Eustis who assigned Maj. Gen. Henry Dearborn to command in the North without telling him that his command included Detroit, leaving General Dearborn to assume that Detroit was not his responsibility. Eustis resigned in December 1812, however, and was replaced by John Armstrong.

Initial preparation for war involved little in the way of organizational change for the Army despite the increase in size from slightly more than 6,500 in 1812 to 19,000 in 1813. The nation's leaders had little enthusiasm for centralization and staff offices; the medical department which had been established in anticipation of war with France at the turn of the century had been disbanded when the threat abated. The enrolling of surgeons and mates to be directly attached to hospitals had been authorized in 1808, however, and the assignment of surgeons and mates directly to regiments was revived in January 1812. (See Table 7.)

Eustis continued LeBaron in his informal position as inspector of the supplies needed by the Army's surgeons in their work but supervised his work closely. With the coming of war, however, it became necessary to establish depots beyond the one already planned for Albany, which Eustis was planning to turn into a major medical supply center for troops all along the Canadian frontier. Late in August, the Secretary of War sent LeBaron a series of orders requiring him to send at once to Pittsburgh "medicine & apparatus for five Regiments, in small chests; also to Annapolis, medicine, surgical instruments &ca, for four hundred militia on duty at that place."[2] Only a few days later, Eustis also ordered LeBaron to send "the necessary medicine & Stores for an Hospital Establishment at New York."[3]

Although the militia called into federal service supplied its own surgeons, it looked to the Regular Army for medical supplies. LeBaron was, therefore, required to send sufficient hospital stores and medicines from his Albany warehouse to Niagara for the 5,000 militia there and to be prepared, should there not be a sufficient quantity on hand at Albany to meet this requirement, to send more north from Philadelphia at once. Supplying the militia, however, made anticipation of needs much more difficult. Although militia and volunteer units played an important role in the War of 1812, the accurate prediction of how many such units might come in or when they might appear was impossible. Should unexpectedly large numbers come in during the autumn or spring, the "sickly seasons," shortages could occur very rapidly.[4]

Eustis directly supervised the financial management of medical supply and ordered LeBaron in October 1812 to prepare estimates on projected expenses for 1813. He also informed LeBaron that the Quartermaster believed that money could be saved by purchasing supplies where they were to be used, thus avoiding shipping expenses. LeBaron, however, explained that local sources of supply, even for such easily obtained items as vinegar and cornmeal, were uncertain and that he could not be sure of obtaining these items locally when they were needed.[5]

Eustis also personally made decisions such as the one involving the size of the medicine chests to be constructed for the Army's use. LeBaron was ordered to have small chests made, despite the fact that surgeons could not seem to agree about what medicines were absolutely necessary to such a chest. LeBaron pointed out that when large chests were used, he could include adequate amounts of all the drugs which might be required without being forced to try to predict what each individual surgeon might use in every possible situation. It was not until the following spring that the discussion was finally resolved in favor of small chests.[6]

LeBaron himself criticized the lack of system and organization which made "wanton waste" possible and noted that the surgeons themselves were complaining that they were unsure as to the nature of their responsibilities. He cited an instance when a militia surgeon reported for duty at a site where three months' allowance of hospital supplies was stored for militia use, then invited in his friends, "and eat, & drank them up," returning home before the hospital surgeon for the area could discover what had happened.[7]

WORK OF THE MEDICAL DEPARTMENT

Nine months of the War of 1812 passed before the offices of Physician and Surgeon General and Apothecary General were created in March 1813. Although demands upon the Army's physicians were heavy, it was June before appointments to these positions were actually made, and the additional regulations necessary to complete the central organization of the Army Medical Department and to define its functions were issued at irregular intervals throughout the remainder of the war.

It was on 3 March 1813, in an act reorganizing the general staff of the U.S. Army, that the Congress also created in a few brief words the positions of Physician and Surgeon General and Apothecary General, both of which were to be filled by civilians. (See Appendix I for texts of those portions of major legislation which affected the Medical Department.) Unlike the department designed in 1799, this new organization involved only the Army, and rather than detailing the responsibilities of both officers, it made the President responsible for outlining the specific duties of both.[8] In May 1813, therefore, President Madison issued his "Rules and Regulations of the Army of the United States."

The new regulations forbade private practice to all Army physicians and outlined the duties of the Physician and Surgeon General, who was made responsible for the specific assignments of individual surgeons. The Physician and Surgeon General was also responsible for the appointment of stewards

TABLE 8—PAY AND ALLOWANCES FOR THE STAFF OF THE MEDICAL DEPARTMENT, MAY 1813

Position	Monthly Salary	Forage Allowances	Rations
Hospital Surgeon	$75	2	6
Hospital Surgeon's Mate	40	2	2
Steward	20	0	2
Wardmaster	16	0	2
Surgeon	45	2	3
Mate	30	2	2

SOURCE: *American State Papers: Military Affairs,* 1:435.
NOTE: The Physician and Surgeon General received a straight salary of $2,500 a year without allowances, the Apothecary General $1,800 without allowances.

and nurses and for the management and use of the stores, instruments, and medicines bought for the Medical Department by the Purchasing Department, with the Apothecary General serving as his assistant. A scale of pay and allowances was also established for the department and, in addition, every hospital and regimental surgeon was granted the privilege of a private room at whatever facility he was serving. (*Table 8*) Another passage in the May 1813 regulations prescribed a uniform for the Physician and Surgeon General, the Apothecary General, and hospital surgeons and mates. It was to resemble that of the general staff, but was specifically characterized by an embroidered gold star on the high collar of the black coat, "pocket flaps, and buttons placed across the cuffs, four to each, and covered buttons in all instances, of the color of the coat." [9]

The following December, further regulations were issued to govern the department's operations. The senior surgeon assigned to each of the nine military districts into which Secretary of War Eustis had divided the military organization of the country in 1812 was to be the director of the medical staff of that district, including regimental surgeons. The specific assignment of each physician was to be based upon his personal ability and training. All Army surgeons had to be either graduates of approved medical schools or capable of passing an examination administered by an Army examination board. In the spring of 1814, one such board consisted of the Inspector General of the Army, the Physician and Surgeon General of the Medical Department, two hospital surgeons, and three regimental surgeons.[10]

The areas covered by the military districts in the spring of 1813 were as follows:

1: Massachusetts, New Hampshire
2: Rhode Island, Connecticut
3: New York to the Highlands, part of New Jersey
4: Part of New Jersey, all of Pennsylvania and Delaware
5: Maryland, Virginia
6: North Carolina, South Carolina, Georgia
7: Louisiana, Tennessee, Mississippi
8: Kentucky, Ohio, Northwest Territory
9: New York north of the Highlands, Vermont

SOURCE: Marguerite McKee, "Service of Supply in the War of 1812," *Quartermaster Review* 6 (1927): 49–50, 50n.

Modifications and additions to these regulations continued to appear during the course of 1814. In March, for example, two rations a day and forage for two horses were added to the salary already allowed the Physician and Surgeon General, and $15 a month was added to the pay of regimental surgeons and mates. The President was now also permitted to hire as many assistant apothecaries as he believed necessary. In December 1814, yet another set of regulations for the Medical Department was issued and policy limiting the number of patients admitted into general hospitals was officially stated; unless the movements of an army required leaving its patients behind, only the wounded or the chronically ill should be sent to the general hospital. The Apothecary General and his assistants were at this time made directly responsible to the superintendent general of military supplies for the disbursement of all hospital supplies bought for the Medical Department by the Commissary General of Purchases.[11] (For a detailed description of the duties of various members of the department as understood at this time, see Appendix J.)

By the end of 1814, the departmental structure included hospital surgeons, who were assigned responsibilities according to their seniority, and their mates, as well as post or garrison surgeons and regimental surgeons and mates. The senior hospital surgeon in an army or district served as its medical director and was responsible for the medical staff of that army or district. Although regimental surgeons and mates seem to have been identified with their regiments more closely than with the Medical Department and the reports of the Physician and Surgeon General did not even mention them, they were nevertheless required to submit monthly and quarterly reports to the medical director of the army or district in which they were serving. These reports were consolidated with those from hospital surgeons and post surgeons by the senior surgeon in charge and forwarded on to the Physician and Surgeon General.[12]

The precautions necessary to ensure high standards of cleanliness and sanitation were officially spelled out in the December 1814 directives. The wardmaster, for example, was responsible for seeing that closestools were cleaned at least three times a day and that either water or charcoal was kept in them. Beds and bedclothes were to be aired each day and exposed to sunlight when possible. The straw in each bed sack was to be changed at least every month. When a patient was discharged or died, the straw from his sack was to be burned. Each patient was to be washed every day and his hair combed. At least one female attendant was to be assigned to each hospital or infirmary to perform such menial tasks as the cleaning or washing of bunks, floors, bedding, and cooking utensils, for which she was to be paid no more than $6 a month plus one ration a day.

The regulations of December 1814 also went into detail concerning the housing of regimental and post surgeons and mates. Although the latter were regarded as having a lower status than their colleagues assigned to regiments, they were, like the regimental and hospital surgeons, assigned to single rooms. To heat each room, regardless of occupancy, a half a cord of wood was allotted in the May–October period and three times that amount during the colder months of the year.

Regimental surgeons were made responsible for the continued training of their mates and private practice once again was forbidden in this last set of instructions. Should medical care be required at any time for units unaccompanied by an Army surgeon, however, provision was made for the officer in command to hire a civilian physician and pay him according to the patient load. Should there be more than thirty patients involved, the civilian doctor would be paid a salary identical with that of the surgeon's mate.

It was not until 11 June 1813, however, that the position of Physician and Surgeon General of the Medical Department was filled with the appointment of Dr. James Tilton. Tilton, who has been described as "one of those American eccentrics who had that combination of erudition and native radicalism which has provided this country with some of its most engaging characters," had become familiar with the problems of military medicine during the Revolution and had already expressed some distinct ideas on the best approach to some of them.[13]

At this time, however, Tilton himself was not in the best of health. In the summer of 1814, he commented often on his "frail condition," citing his "anthrax," which was "still an open wound of some extent," and the "rheumatic swelling of my knee that is not a little inconvenient."[14] The growth on his knee was "threatening to make a cripple of me" in September 1814 and apparently later proved to be malignant, his leg being amputated within less than a year and a half of these references to it. There is no specific

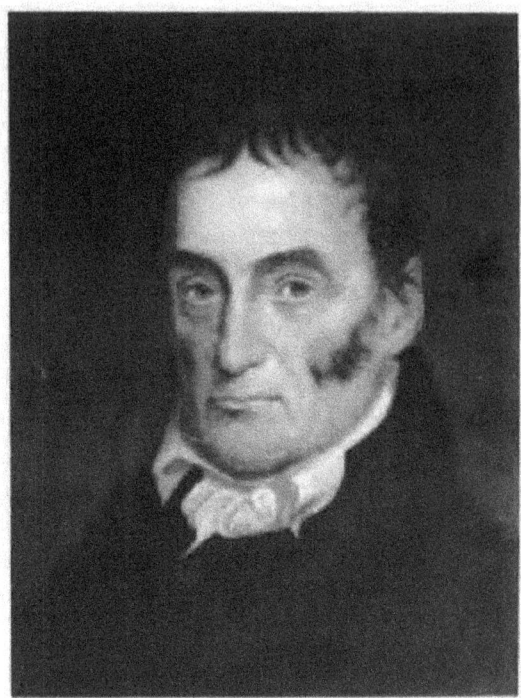

JAMES TILTON. *(Courtesy of National Library of Medicine.)*

evidence, however, to indicate that his poor health and the fact that he spent much of his term of office at his home in Wilmington, Delaware,[15] interfered with his effectiveness as head of the Medical Department.

Serving under Physician and Surgeon General Tilton was Apothecary General Francis LeBaron, officially appointed to this position on 11 June 1813, although he had been managing the supplies since before the outbreak of war. Not long after he became Apothecary General, LeBaron requested the appointment of assistant apothecaries, but fourteen months elapsed before the first two assistants were hired. By the end of 1814, however, there were nine assistants working under LeBaron, assigned to Philadelphia, Norfolk, Charleston, New Orleans, Williamsville, Sackett's Harbor, New York City, New London, and Boston.[16]

There was confusion, however, as to the whereabouts of many of the other members of the Medical Department. In the spring of 1814, for example, the Adjutant General wrote Tilton to request from him a list of the assignments given his surgeons and commented that "with your list and by the help of the records in this office, probably we shall be able to account for and where the officers of your department are."[17] In responding to this request, however, the head of the Medical Department pointed out that, although the list he was enclosing was accurate concerning hospital surgeons and mates, "The garrison surgeons and mates may be defective, as they are a species of Surgeons that I have had but little to do with."[18] There was also apparently some confusion about which surgeon was in charge in each area. In his final report for 1814, for example, Tilton commented of the 8th District that he had been told that a Dr. Turner, who was only a regimental surgeon, had "very improperly assumed the directing."[19]

The difficulty experienced in establishing the locations of members of the department can be illustrated by the wanderings of one of its members, Dr. John R. Martin, who was ordered in June 1813 to join Maj. Gen. William Henry Harrison in Ohio. In February 1814, however, Martin was in Washington, D.C., but was ordered to go to Pittsburgh, Pennsylvania. This order was rescinded two days later and he was ordered to remain where he was. The next month he was ordered to Erie, New York, but two months after this he was apparently located in Ohio and was sent a letter which ordered him to go to Buffalo. His presence in Buffalo, however, was by August considered to be "likely to interrupt the harmony which subsisted" there and his assignment was changed to Sackett's Harbor, New York. One cannot be sure of where Martin was actually located while his assignments were being changed.

It seems likely, for example, that the "Dr. Martin" who assisted another physician in caring for wounded Americans taken captive by the British in late August north of Washington, D.C., at a time when John R. Martin had been ordered to upstate New York was none other than this same John R. Martin.[20] The length of time it must have taken Martin to go from one place to another would only have added to the confusion, and it is possible, of course, that some of these changes of assignment never caught up with him.

The relationship of the staff of the Medical Department to the numerous militia and volunteer units which served at various times against the British in the War of 1812 appears never to have been specifically outlined. In practice, the surgeons reporting for service with these units usually cared for their own sick and wounded. On at least one occasion, at the time of the British raid on Washington in 1814, a separate hospital was established for militia wounded.[21] When necessary, however, the hospital staff of the Medical Department cared for these men within the general hospital system.

Despite the criteria established in December 1813, the caliber of the physicians serving in the Regular U.S. Army at this time was by no means uniform. While some surgeons earned enviable reputations among their colleagues, others were less fortunate. According to the outspoken Tilton, a garrison surgeon's mate at Detroit, for example, was "not only incompetent in medical knowledge, but so sottishly abject in his conduct, as to be utterly unworthy of trust or confidence." A surgeon with the 18th Infantry Regiment was "not only incompetent, but deranged to such a degree as to make it unsafe & improper to trust patients in his charge." The much-transferred Martin, his superior noted, had been "accused of purloining the rations of the sick." Martin and another surgeon were, indeed, "nothing more than disorderly excrescenses . . . that had better be lopped off."[22]

In the opinion of at least one experienced Army physician, it was difficult to retain the surgeons who served on the regimental staff because of the inadequate pay they received. Costs along the Canadian frontier were particularly high, he pointed out, and regimental surgeons and their mates tended to serve a year because of "Curiosity alone" and then leave.[23] It should be noted, however, that well over half of the surgeons on the regimental staff in 1813 returned the next year to serve either in the same capacity as they had been serving in 1813 or in a different one within the regimental framework.

By the end of 1813, the staff of the Medical Department had become quite large and the several documents issued since the spring of 1813 had to some degree outlined the way in which the department should operate, but the policy concerning the hiring of additional personnel appears to have remained unclear. A question which arose in the summer of 1814, however, was answered in the December 1814 additions to the regulations. Dr. Benjamin Waterhouse, hospital

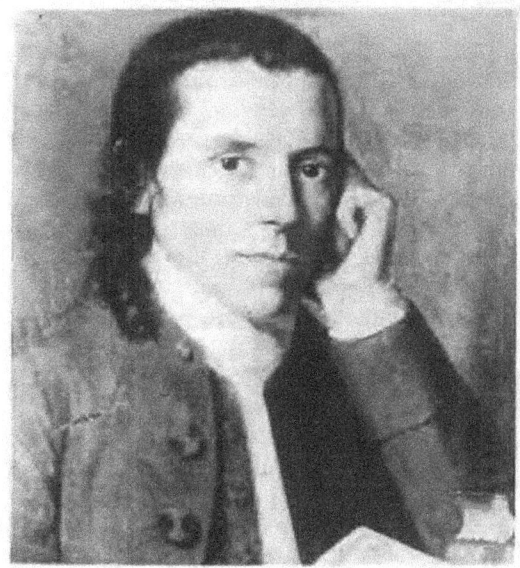

BENJAMIN WATERHOUSE. *(Courtesy of National Library of Medicine.)*

surgeon in Boston, commented that he was not sure whether nurses should be allotted rations in addition to their salaries of $6 a month. The rules of the department as he then understood them stated that nurses should receive no more than $6, but nurses of the necessary caliber could not be hired at that rate, in his opinion. Waterhouse also posed another question. Young men were being actively sought to work in the department, but he wondered whether those "of a family, habits & connexions notorious for opposition to the Administration, the war, & the loaning of money to the government" should be hired. He himself believed "that no man should eat the bread of the government who throws himself into the scale of the opposition," especially since the Army was already "sadly encumbered by people of this class" who were "afraid or ashamed to wear even the cockade." [24]

During the less than two years he was in office, Physician and Surgeon General Tilton attempted to initiate a system of reporting from Army surgeons around the nation. He wished to accumulate not only data on the numbers of hospitalized patients, their diseases, and the number who died, but also other information of value to medical science concerning weather, climate, and the siting of hospitals. The department was still in such a state of confusion, however, and the surgeons were so accustomed to working independently that in August 1814, when Tilton turned in his report for the department to the Secretary of War, he was forced to point out that his subordinates had provided him with little of the requested information. Six months later, furthermore, the situation had changed very little. [25]

On the basis of the reports he did receive, however, Tilton concluded in the summer of 1814 that in general the health of the Army was good. He believed that while improved discipline and the resultant greater personal and hospital cleanliness played a major roll in the Army's health, the effort to avoid crowding general hospitals was also an important factor. [26]

In February 1815, the Physician and Surgeon General submitted his second report, which included all but the last weeks of the hostilities of the War of 1812. There was so little improvement in the response of the various surgeons under him that he pointed out to the Secretary of War that "The negligent habits, which had gained footing, in the medical department before anything like system was attempted to be established can hardly be reformed, without further legislative & executive aids." Only one report had come in from the 1st District, for example, there was no report whatever from the 8th, and even in the 3d District, where the senior hospital surgeon had apparently gone to considerable trouble to collect data from the physicians under him, the reports were not complete. [27]

Because of the attitude prevalent among his subordinates at the time he became head of the Medical Department, it is difficult to assess Tilton's performance as Physician and Surgeon General fairly. He proposed measures, among them the creation of examining boards and the submission of regular reports from the field, which would in the hands of his successors make it possible for the department to operate with notably greater efficiency and effectiveness than it had ever done before 1815; but Tilton was not in office long enough to achieve any significant success along these lines himself or to leave any clear indication whether his health was seriously limiting his ability to enforce the orders he issued. Years of effort would have been required to effect the necessary improvement in discipline, and his attempts to exercise effective supervision and control over the selection and assignment of Army surgeons under the relatively rapidly changing conditions of war were also frustrated by the inevitably slow communications of the period.

During this period, purchasing was still,

in theory, handled on an Army-wide basis, by the Commissary General of Purchases. This system has since been evaluated as a total failure, with the work of the contractors who supplied rations receiving particularly heavy criticism. Except where a specific contract had been arranged, the Army's purchasing department was assigned the responsibility for buying such hospital stores as the Medical Department needed and turning them over to the Apothecary General's department. In practice, the situation was not so simple and the management of supply for the newly appointed Apothecary General was also complicated by poor roads, the long distances which often separated garrisons and armies from supply centers, the shortage of specie, and a general distrust of paper money.[28]

Having been ordered on 21 June 1813 to "establish" himself at Albany, LeBaron arrived in upstate New York at the end July. Surgeons were ordered to send him their estimates there, where he was to requisition his needs from the deputy commissary of purchases and turn for transportation to the Quartermaster General. Apparently these three gentlemen as well as the Army contractor for the area all experienced particular difficulty in meeting militia needs, and in October 1814, the Adjutant General ordered them to design a form which would include the pertinent regulations and which could be used in an effort to improve the management of supply for these units.[29]

LeBaron's role was never an easy one; he came under fire not only for the quality of some of the stores he provided, which suggests that he may have actually been doing his own buying directly, but also for the way in which medicines were packed. The Secretary of War complained in the spring of 1813 that the medicine contained unnecessary ingredients which made "the preparations elegant" [30] and in the fall of the same year that LeBaron's chocolate was "a vile cheat and highly pernicious to the sick," and his port wine was "vile stuff," "the worse and weakest kind." The secretary maintained that LeBaron, who at the time complained about high prices and a lack of funds, could afford stores of a better quality if he acquired them locally wherever possible, thus avoiding high transportation costs.[31] To follow this suggestion, however, LeBaron would have had to do his own purchasing.

The problem of the size of the medicine chests which he distributed continued to plague LeBaron. Some surgeons were refusing to take chests with them because of the difficulties involved in moving such large containers when the Army was on the march, and one physician was so impressed by their size that he referred to them as "the most astonishing things." LeBaron, however, maintained that the larger chests were used because there had been a requirement that no regiment have more than two chests. Since initially neither he nor the surgeons had had enough experience to predict precisely what types or quantities of drugs would be needed, he had found it necessary to supply a greater variety and a greater quantity than might actually be needed.[32]

The Secretary of War finally ordered LeBaron to reduce the size of the chests he issued in the future, and the Apothecary General began to prepare smaller ones, weighing approximately 160 pounds, in addition to storage chests, weighing from 120 to 200 pounds, from which they could be replenished. He was actually, however, faced with the problem of disposing of at least eight of the large boxes which he now could no longer send out to the Army's surgeons. He hoped that the Navy would take them, since size would not be a handicap on shipboard, but the Navy had no need for more chests. LeBaron then suggested sending them to New Orleans, using water transportation as much as possible, to serve there as a source of supply for new posts which might be opened in that area. The Secretary of War pointed out that it would be wise to send these containers to posts which could not be easily supplied and where there would also be no need to move them about.[33]

LeBaron tried to emphasize planning as a method of preventing unnecessary distribution problems and urged such steps as the establishment of a distribution center for the South at New Orleans. Despite his efforts, however, events he could not foresee added to his troubles. On one occasion, while he was away on an inspection trip, supplies which had been accumulated at Pittsburgh for two divisions were all sent to the single division under General Harrison. On another occasion, in the Niagara area, stores which had been at Sackett's Harbor simply disappeared, "mostly lost, destroyed, or stolen." The troops at French Mills were in need at this time, but Maj. Gen. James Wilkinson's men had already used up all the stores which had been stockpiled at Burlington, Vermont.[34]

In December 1814, a third difficulty arose when Dr. James Cutbush, Assistant Apothecary General, arrived at Philadelphia to take up his duties. LeBaron had placed all the medicines stored there in the hands of a civilian apothecary following the death of an otherwise unidentified Dr. West, but the retail druggist made up into medicines some of the simple drugs which had thus fallen into his hands and proposed that the Army pay the retail rate to get them back.[35]

Many of the problems experienced by LeBaron and other members of the new Medical Department resulted from the fact that the outbreak of the War of 1812 found the Army's system of medical support unprepared to meet the suddenly escalating demands placed upon it. Congress, however, appeared relatively unimpressed by the seriousness of the situation and assigned to the executive the task of establishing guidelines for the management of a Medical Department which it created only nine months after the declaration of the war. Hastily and casually conceived and staffed for the most part with men unaccustomed to the demands of military medicine, the Medical Department was severely handicapped in its attempts to provide adequate care for the Army's sick and wounded.

8

Early Campaigns in the North, 1812 to 1813

During the first campaign season of the War of 1812, the physicians caring for the regular soldiers of the U.S. Army were forced to work under a decentralized, peacetime organization. During the second season, the effort required to meet the unpredictable demands of war at the same time that the Medical Department was being reestablished made it difficult for Army surgeons to give their patients the best care available even by nineteenth century standards.

SEASON OF 1812

American plans for the early months of the War of 1812 called for a three-pronged attack on Canada by means of thrusts from the Lake Champlain–St. Lawrence River area, from Niagara, and from the Northwest Territory. (*Map 10*) By the end of 1812, all three moves had failed.[1]

For the attack against Canada from the American side of the St. Lawrence River, six thousand to eight thousand men were gathered in the fall of 1812 at Greenbush, near Albany, under the personal command of Maj. Gen. Henry Dearborn. In November, the army marched from Plattsburg, New York, to launch an attack against Montreal. The militia, however, stood on its right not to fight on foreign soil. Those who did cross into Canada managed to fire on one another in the confusion. After the fiasco, the militia returned home and the light artillery and dragoons returned to Greenbush. Three regiments of regulars went to Burlington, Vermont, for the winter, while three more spent the season at Plattsburg.

Maintaining the health of the troops in this area was a problem from the outset. The season was rainy and the ground was wet. Although the camp at Greenbush was often moved, diarrhea and dysentery took a considerable toll. Not only intermittent fever but also typhus and rheumatism were prevalent even as early as mid-September. Despite the threat to the army posed by the high disease rate, when Dr. James Mann, placed in overall charge of the medical services for the forces in upstate New York, arrived at Greenbush the second week in August, he found that the physician who was to have preceded him had not arrived and that the troops were without medical care.[2]

Since no preparations had been made to care for those of the men at Greenbush who might fall ill, upon his arrival Mann had to go over the hospital supplies, which, fortunately, he found to be in good order, as well as to care for the ill with the aid of but one other physician, a regimental surgeon's mate who arrived a few days after Mann. There were no buildings prepared to receive the sick and Mann did not wish to erect new tents because of the wet ground, so the sick were left in the tents they shared with their healthy comrades. An average of 100 men fell ill each week at Greenbush, and by the

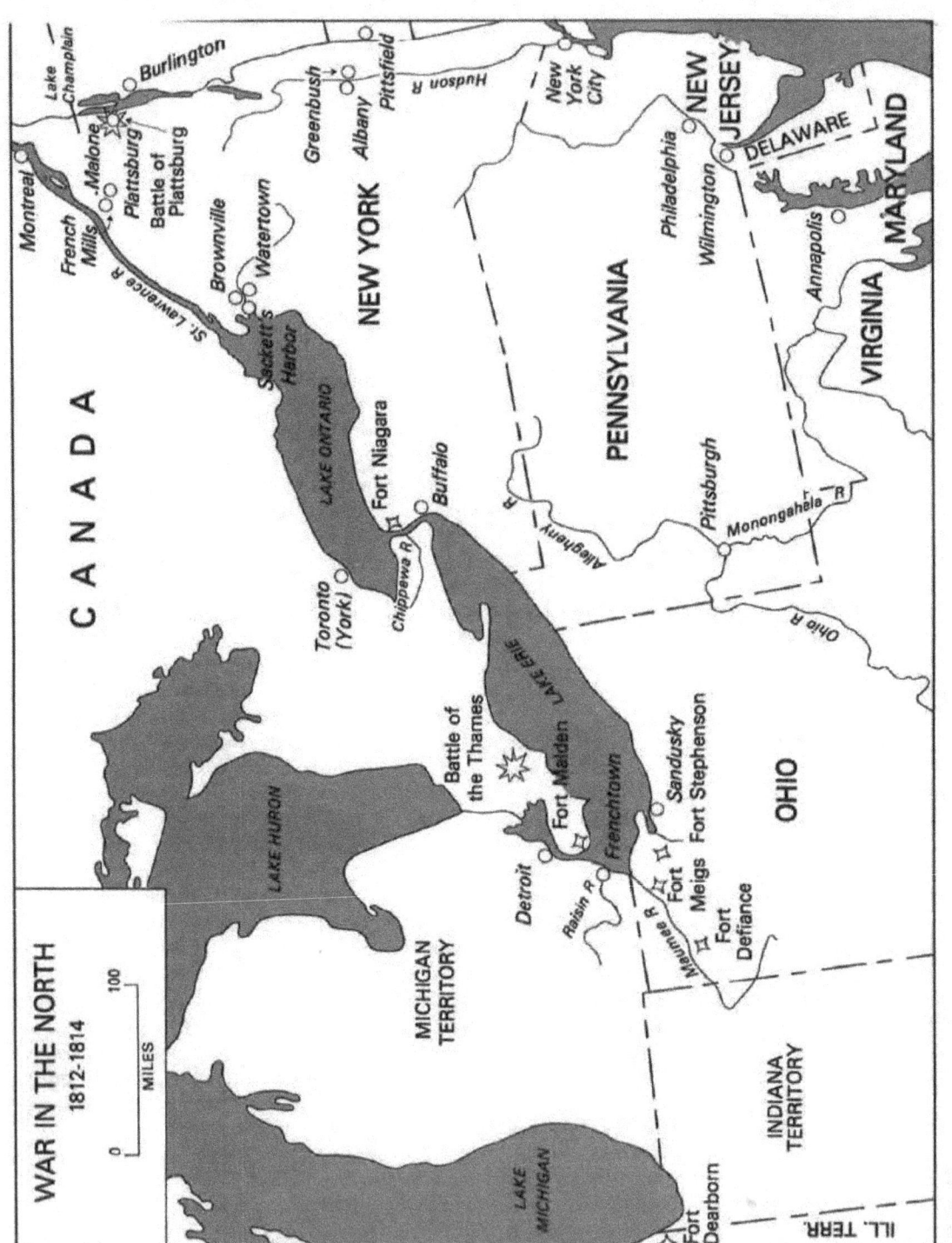

time the last units of the army left for the abortive attack on Montreal, a total of 200 men had been left behind because of poor health. Nevertheless, Mann believed that the health of the men at Greenbush was good when considered in the light of the fact that most of them were new to the military life.[3]

Mann believed that the basic problem which underlay all others as far as medical support of the Army was concerned was the lack of overall organization. He himself worked on an outline of rules and regulations for a hospital department when he could find a spare moment, but he had difficulty finding the time to complete it. He was not sure of his authority; although he had hired a wardmaster and steward, for example, he had not taken on nurses or orderlies because he was not sure that he was entitled to do so. He also noted that conflicts with line officers were made almost inevitable by the ill-defined nature of the role of the hospital surgeon.[4]

Among the varied duties which Mann was required to perform in the fall of 1812 was the distribution of hospital supplies from the Greenbush area to Niagara and Plattsburg, New York, and Pittsfield, Massachusetts; the administration of medicines to the ill of the rifle corps who did not have a regimental surgeon to care for them; and the revision of diets for hospitalized patients. He decided that the convalescents in his care did not need the full diet required by the healthy and active soldier. Mann suggested that the convalescent receive 12 ounces of meat and 12 ounces of bread a day. The "half diet" should consist of 6 ounces of meat and 10 ounces of bread, with the addition of a gill of rice or a half pint of meal plus half a gill of molasses. Those on a "low diet" should receive only bread, rice, or barley with sugar, without any meat. Although chocolate or tea with sugar was to be permitted from time to time, Mann opposed the use of whiskey.[5]

Mann regretted being so busy with his responsibilities as hospital surgeon that he had little time to study the diseases he encountered and to record his observations. During the fall and winter of 1812–13, however, he saw many cases of rheumatism, pneumonia, measles, dysentery, and intermittent fever. When he first arrived at Greenbush, he also found that a few of the men had fallen ill with what he diagnosed as typhus before they reached the camp. Four of the seven men who died in the period from mid-August to the end of September were from among this group of typhus patients, and two others who died had long been afflicted with what we would today call tuberculosis. Mann had expected to encounter what he called spotted fever, which had been prevalent in the East in earlier years, but this disease never became a problem in the Northern Army.[6]

On the basis of his observations during the first fall and winter of the War of 1812, Mann concluded that rheumatism afflicted men older than 40 more frequently than younger soldiers and was quick to recur after exposure to wet, cold weather in those who had previously suffered from it. Mann preferred to reserve venesection for the treatment of the acute form of rheumatism, using calomel, opium, blistering, and the application of warmth for chronic cases.[7]

Among the other conditions studied by Mann were pneumonia and dysentery. In some cases of pneumonia, death could occur within 24 hours of the appearance of the first symptom, which was usually a sensation of weight upon the chest. The convalescent from this form of pneumonia, Mann noted, often had a jaundiced appearance. The type of dysentery seen by physicians in the North at this time "was attended in most cases with a fever of the synochal type, accelerated action of the arteries, and heat increased considerably above the healthy standard." Mann favored treating it by bleeding, preferably a single bleeding of 16 ounces followed by a "full cathartic of

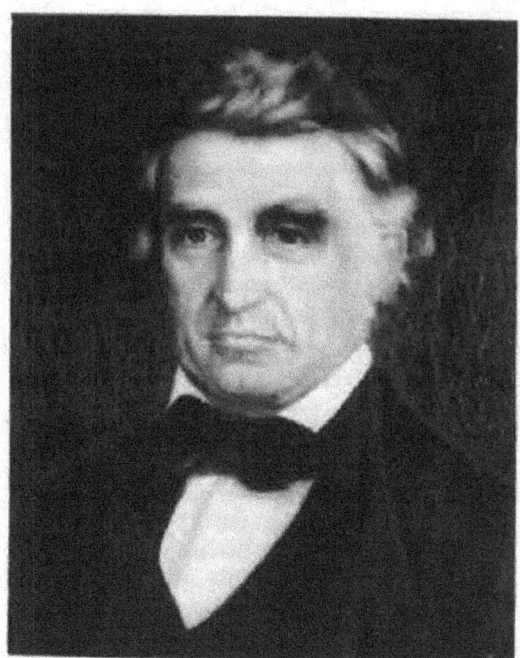

WILLIAM BEAUMONT. *(Courtesy of National Library of Medicine.)*

calomel and jalap." "Anodynes," or painkillers, might be administered after the "intestines were well evacuated." Mann also discovered that "There were cases when calomel and opium, in small doses, at intervals of 4 or 6 hours, were found beneficial." Emetics were generally used only when all else had failed, but dysentery could take on "a typhoid form" which made the administration of wine or diluted brandy, up to two pints of the former, as well as purgatives, advisable. Milk was also recommended, especially for the convalescent from this variety of dysentery, but meat and broths were strictly forbidden.[8]

Intermittent fevers apparently appeared at Greenbush only in men hailing from south of the Hudson River who had had the disease before. These men were treated with emetics when the "cold stage" was about to appear and then, during periods when there was no fever, with cathartics, bark, and wine in addition to the emetics. A disease which was more common than intermittent fever was measles, which, at one time or another during the winter, afflicted as many as one-third of the entire army.[9]

Among the physicians who eventually served under Mann was Dr. William Beaumont, a surgeon's mate, who later was to gain fame through his studies concerning digestion. At this time, Beaumont was particularly concerned with the respiratory diseases he was encountering with great frequency. He commented that the men were making "the very woods ring with coughings & groaning." Pleurisy was a common affliction among his patients and was handled, in its earliest stages, by bleeding followed, as the symptoms subsided, by the administration of opium, digitalis, and "Glyc. Snn Tart. Atn," a combination Beaumont found to be "very efficatious [*sic*] in relieving the Cough." For patients who could not otherwise be relieved, Beaumont favored the raising of blisters.[10]

Mann believed that attention to certain precautions could lower the incidence of disease within the Army. Soldiers should, for example, wear woolen shirts. "Spirits" should be eliminated from the rations of the healthy as well as from those of the sick, since "Immoderate potations of spirits by weakening the sensorial powers, and inducing general debility" were a "predisponent cause of disease." The presence of alcohol in hospitals would constitute a threat to the health of the soldier who was "habitually intemperate," who would always be "industrious to procure the means of indulging his appetite." Mann observed also that some of the men were convinced that "ardent spirits" were good for bowel complaints and were, apparently, dosing themselves to the point of inebriation.[11]

No matter how successful Army surgeons might be with their patients, however, there would always be those who, for political reasons of their own, in Mann's opinion, would be willing to exaggerate the Army's rate of death and disease "with design to render government and its officers odious." Furthermore, Mann maintained that this rate would always be higher than the public might expect it to be because young and healthy men did not join the Army.[12]

Early in February 1813, Mann made an inspection tour of the hospitals caring for General Dearborn's men at Plattsburg and Burlington. He was favorably impressed by the way in which Dr. Joseph Lovell, later to become Surgeon General of the United States Army, was managing the hospital at Burlington, although the number of deaths there from November to February approached 200. The death rate at Plattsburg, where the surgeon's mate who was in charge of that unit kept the wards clean and in good condition and supplies were more than adequate, was comparable to that at Burlington.[13]

When Mann returned to Greenbush, however, although the progress being made on a new building was encouraging, he discovered that the surgeon he had left in charge had been seriously neglecting his patients and that a pneumonia epidemic was growing. Mann was so angered by what he found that he considered placing formal charges against his subordinate but finally decided against taking so drastic a step. Despite the situation which had developed in his absence at Greenbush, only eighty-nine patients had died there from 1 August 1812 to February 1813, with the highest rates occurring in December. Mann attributed the improvement which followed in January to a change from using "stimulants .... employed as medicine" to "evacuating and antiphlogistic" remedies.[14]

The American forces in the area between Lakes Ontario and Erie, slightly less than half of whom were militia, numbered about 6,500. They were divided among Lewiston, Buffalo, and Fort Niagara. It is not sur-

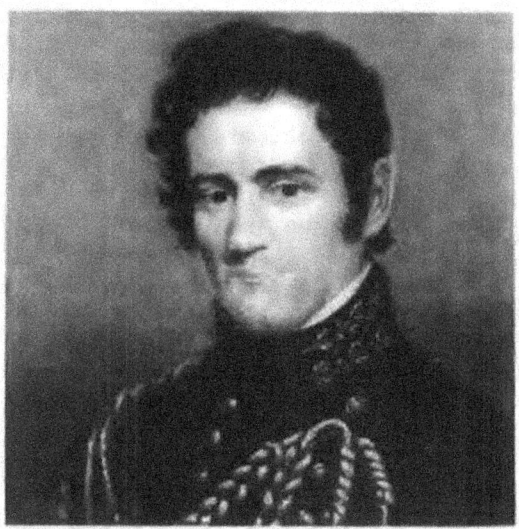

JOSEPH LOVELL. *(Courtesy of National Library of Medicine.)*

prising that the campaign here was also a failure; the militia exercised its right not to fight on Canadian soil whenever it wished, the commander of the militia was totally lacking in military experience, the commander of the regulars was unreliable, and the two commanders were apparently incapable of cooperation.

The health of the men on the Niagara frontier appears to have been no better than that of their fellows in northeastern New York State. A letter written in early November 1812 from Buffalo reported that three or four of the Regular Army there were dying each day and that more than 100 of those wounded in an attack on British-held Queenston on 13 October later died. The high death rate there was blamed on a lack of "proper surgeons." The most common diseases afflicting the men at Buffalo were measles and dysentery, the latter being blamed on the fact that the men were eating fresh meat. At Lewiston, some units reported one-third to one-half of their men sick in November, and it was noted that the hospital tent of one regular infantry regiment held the bodies of five men who had been dead more than 24 hours but had not been buried because of a shortage of coffins.[15]

The 1,300 regulars at Fort Niagara were cared for by three physicians. One was attached to the fort's regular garrison and two were from regiments newly stationed there. The situation of the surgeon of the 14th Infantry Regiment may well have been indicative of that faced by others near Niagara. In early October, he was without medicines, hospital stores, or surgical instruments. There were, unfortunately, not only sick but also wounded needing care at Niagara because the fort was bombarded at times by the British guns across the Niagara River.[16]

Brig. Gen. William Hull was in command of operations in the Detroit and western Great Lakes area in the first few months of the War of 1812. He arrived at Dayton, Ohio, early in the spring of 1812 and marched northward from there, reaching the Rapids of the Maumee River by the end of June. Here, since his horses were exhausted, he hired a schooner, the *Cuyahoga*, and a small boat to carry his sick and wounded and a major portion of his baggage, including his medical supplies and a trunk full of confidential military records, the rest of the way to Detroit.[17]

The British, however, controlled Lake Erie, and to reach Detroit the *Cuyahoga* had to pass under their guns at Fort Malden. Since General Hull had not been officially informed that war had been declared, he was unaware of the magnitude of the risk he was taking. The enemy, having learned of the declaration of war, captured the *Cuyahoga* on 2 July, but the small boat, carrying some of the sick, seems to have escaped to arrive safely at Detroit.[18]

There is some confusion as to what happened to the small boat and its occupants. A few patients and the surgeon's mate from the Ohio volunteers who was sent along with them apparently were in this craft. Although the diary of a physician captured by the British at this time has been attributed to this mate, Dr. James Reynolds, by its editor, others have disagreed with him. The preponderance of the evidence seems to indicate that the physician in the small boat and, presumably, the patients with him, reached Detroit safely on 3 July 1812 and that Reynolds was killed just before General Hull's surrender of Detroit in August by a nearly spent ball which tore off one leg and mangled the other.[19]

After their hospital supplies were captured, the providing of medical support for General Hull and the bulk of his army after their arrival at Detroit by land on 5 July posed a problem. New supplies were to have come in from Fort Fayette, located near Pittsburgh, but Fort Fayette itself was short on these items also. Further difficulties, according to General Hull, were caused by the fact that the hospital surgeon originally assigned to the units at Detroit, Dr. Josiah Foster, died before he had progressed far in the organization of medical services there. Foster's place was taken by Dr. Abraham Edwards, a former surgeon's mate who had also had experience as a line officer.[20]

The British deliberately played upon General Hull's fears. Rumors were circulated about huge numbers of Indians who were presumably thirsting for American blood. Canadian militiamen were clothed in the red uniforms of British regulars and paraded where the Americans could see them. On 16 August 1812, in what one historian has termed "one of the most disgraceful episodes in the military History of the United States," [21] General Hull surrendered not only Fort Detroit but other forts in the area as well.

Among those included in General Hull's surrender was a detachment of fifty-four men with their families at Fort Dearborn, where Chicago now stands. The physician caring for the population of this fort was

Dr. Isaac Van Voorhis of the 54th Infantry Regiment. At the time of the surrender, General Hull ordered Fort Dearborn evacuated and, despite warnings from friendly Indians that they would be ambushed, the occupants obeyed. An estimated 1,500 Indians set upon the small group, which included 9 women and 18 children, after it left the shelter of the fort and killed 30 soldiers, 10 male civilians, 2 women, and 12 children. Among the dead was regimental surgeon Van Voorhis.[22]

Not long after General Hull's surrender at Detroit, Brig. Gen. William Henry Harrison was appointed commander of all forces, regular and militia, a total of approximately six thousand men, in the Northwest. Several expeditions were sent out against the Indians during the fall, and by December, General Harrison's men held a line across northwest Ohio from Fort Defiance to Sandusky.

By November, however, typhus had appeared among General Harrison's men, the weather was cold and wet, and proper shoes and clothing were lacking. Three or four men were dying each day. On Christmas, one of General Harrison's officers reported that, of the approximately six hundred men in his unit, recently returned from an expedition against the Miami Indians, more than three hundred were suffering such severe frostbite that they were unfit for duty.[23]

Near the ruins of old Fort Defiance in the fall of 1812, where militia units and detachments from two infantry regiments were stationed under Brig. Gen. James Winchester, the burden borne by the Army's physicians was great. Hospital stores were being stolen before they could be delivered at the camp, and typhus was raging among the men. By winter, although the new fort, including its hospital, had been completed, supplies were exhausted and the suffering from cold and hunger was increasing. One of Winchester's men noted on Christmas Eve that "Our sufferings in this place have been greater than if we had been in severe battle. More than one hundred lives have been lost, owing to the bad accommodations. The sufferings of about three hundred sick at a time, who are exposed to the cold ground and deprived of every nourishment, are sufficient proof of our wretched condition."[24] Wrote another soldier, "We now saw nothing but hunger, and cold, and nakedness, staring us in the face."[25]

Having been ordered by General Harrison to move from their new fort to the Falls of the Maumee River and to build huts there for the winter, General Winchester and 1,200 men set out, arriving at the rapids on 10 January. Shortly thereafter, upon learning that the Americans at a small settlement called Frenchtown (now Monroe, Michigan), thirty-five miles away and only eighteen miles from British-held Fort Malden, were being threatened by the enemy, General Winchester sent an advance party of his men to help them.[26]

After an indecisive engagement on 18 January when more than fifty Americans were wounded and twelve killed, these men set up camp at the village. The officers took over some private homes and the hospital was set up in a tavern at some distance from the main camp. On 21 January, however, after General Winchester and the main body of his force had joined the men already at Frenchtown, the enemy attacked and overwhelmed the Americans, killing 397, wounding 27, and capturing more than 500, including General Winchester. Among the dead were the senior surgeon for the entire force and the surgeon of the 17th U.S. Infantry Regiment. Another physician had taken up the weapon of one of his patients while the struggle was still taking place and set out to join the fighting; he was never seen alive again. A volunteer surgeon and his mate were captured when they elected to remain with about sixty to sixty-five wounded men at the hospital.[27]

On accepting the surrender of the Americans who were still fighting, the British promised to assign a guard for the wounded to keep them from being killed by the Indians before they could be moved to Malden. The promise was ignored, however. No guard was posted, and so, after enjoying the liquor they found stored in the tavern-hospital, the Indians tore the blankets away from the wounded and then set fire to the buildings. Those who tried to escape were shot and tomahawked.[28]

General Harrison attempted to aid General Winchester, but his relief party was unable to reach the scene of the battle in time.[29] General Harrison then fell back on the Maumee River and, abandoning any further thoughts of a winter offensive, passed the rest of the winter constructing the fort to be known as Fort Meigs.

Season of 1813

Although there was military activity both in the North and the South during the campaign season of 1813, the United States forces involved in the South were for the most part either those of the Navy or of the Tennessee units of Andrew Jackson which he led against the Creek Indians of the Mississippi Territory. General Wilkinson's expedition of Army regulars into West Florida which culminated in the occupation of Mobile met with no opposition. In the Northwest, the campaign season of 1813 was so successful that by the onset of winter and after young U.S. Navy Commander Oliver Hazard Perry's victory over a British fleet on Lake Erie, the entire area was under American control. General Harrison was thus able to move 700 of his regulars from the Northwest to Buffalo and Sackett's Harbor. Although the general himself resigned from the Army at this time, these men took part in the campaign in western New York State.

In the Northwest in 1813, there do not appear to have been any general hospitals, at least not of the size and caliber of those in northern and western New York State. There were garrison facilities at some of the posts,[30] but presumably most of the ill and wounded of General Harrison's army were the responsibility of regimental surgeons and mates or even of militia physicians.

During the spring and early summer of 1813, General Harrison's army was in unusually poor health and his hospital stores and medicines were being consumed not only by the sick but also by the wasteful habits of militia surgeons and mates at the various small posts scattered throughout the Northwest. Hospital supplies of liquor were apparently a source of particular concern to General Harrison, who noted that a "dry Barrell" should be "put over that which contains" hospital liquor because "Experience has long since convinced all those in the Western country who are desirous of having their Liquors secured from plunder and adulteration that it is the only way of affecting it." [31]

In May 1813, the enemy attempted to take Fort Meigs before the reinforcement expected by the troops there could arrive. Although the siege was abandoned after nine days, the defenders suffered 81 killed and 189 wounded at a time when the medical support available for them was "extremely deficient in almost every respect." There was "no head to the Hospital Department," and the surgeons were young and inexperienced and, for the most part, from the militia. One officer noted that the militia was content to look for its physicians "wherever a person could be found with a lancet in his pocket, or who had by some means or other *obtained the title of doctor*." Although there had been a "man of skills and talents" in charge of the medical services at this fort before the siege began, this otherwise unidentified gentleman was no longer in the Army by May of 1813, having left both the fort and the Army, it would seem, in disgrace, considered to be "alike destitute of honor and reputation." [32]

There was no place to put the wounded at Fort Meigs while it was under siege; they lay in trenches "on rails barely sufficient to keep them up out of the water, which in many places from the bleeding of the wounded, had the appearance of puddles of blood." There were even times when there was nothing available with which to cover these unhappy creatures, since the same supply shortages experienced by other camps also afflicted Fort Meigs. The force there was so shorthanded that men could not even be spared to give adequate care to the wounded,[33] several of whom died "of a lock-jaw," brought on, General Harrison believed, by "their great and unavoidable exposure to the cold." [34]

Once the siege was over, blockhouses were cleared of guns and stores and turned into temporary hospitals, but the men were still "but badly provided with the little necessaries and comforts which belong and afford so much relief, to the brave soldier who has recently lost a leg or an arm, or had his side pierced with a bayonet." [35] General Harrison took it upon himself to forward an urgent order worked up by a hospital mate for medicines and stores in their behalf. (See Chapter 1.)

General Harrison's operations in the summer and early fall of 1813 in the Lake Erie area were successful and culminated in October in the defeat of the British and their Indian allies in Canada at the Battle of the Thames River and the death of the Indian leader Tecumseh. However, apparently little had been done in advance to prepare for the care of the sick and wounded. One of the men with this expedition described coming down with "the Ague" on board a boat because of the wet, cold weather. He had, apparently, no alternative but to continue the march once on land. The only help available to the sick was that which their fellows could provide by carrying their weapons and packs for them and, when crossing small streams, by carrying the sick themselves on their backs.[36]

After the final battle in October, General Harrison reported that five of his men had been killed and twenty-two wounded in the engagement and that five of the wounded died shortly thereafter. Although there does not seem to be any record of where these men were initially cared for, after Detroit was recaptured a hospital was opened under Dr. Cornelius Cunningham, a garrison surgeon's mate, in the house formerly occupied by Governor William Hull. For a brief time before moving on to New York State, General Harrison and his men returned to Detroit, and in November of 1813, four hundred of the regulars who had been with him in Canada were left behind in the Detroit facility. By this time, the sick rate was again soaring and the men were both tired and hungry. Some of the illness was blamed upon the large quantities of bad bread they had reportedly eaten. A month later, however, the situation had not improved. "The troops . . . . still Continues to be very much sick and many have Died since we came to this place." [37]

In the Northeast, troops under Maj. Gen. Henry Dearborn left Sackett's Harbor in April 1813 to take Toronto, then called York, and Fort George. (See Map 10.) They then held off an enemy attack on Sackett's Harbor itself, but in December 1813, the British launched a successful attack, retaking Fort George and capturing Fort Niagara as well. A series of enemy raids which included the burning of Buffalo and Black Rock brought the hostilities of that campaign year along the Niagara to a close.

Farther east, a two-pronged American move against Montreal in the autumn of 1813 was a complete failure. After replacing the ailing General Dearborn at Sackett's Harbor, General Wilkinson moved east along the St. Lawrence River, intending to join Maj. Gen. Wade Hampton's forces

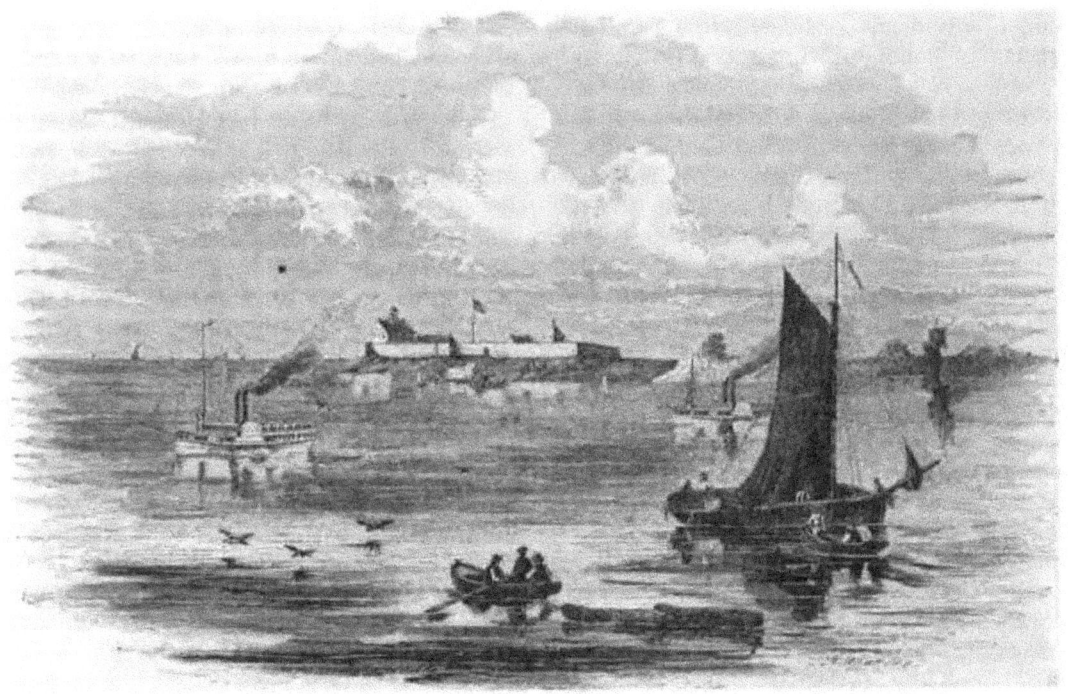

FORT NIAGARA. *(Courtesy of Library of Congress.)*

moving north from the Lake Champlain area. Both generals, however, retreated after separate defeats by the enemy. General Hampton returned to Plattsburg and General Wilkinson fell back on French Mills. General Wilkinson was accused at this time of excessive drinking and of attempting to blame his condition on illness.[38]

In New England and the states south of New York in this period, where there was little if any military action involving the Regular Army, there were at least one or two garrison or regimental physicians in each military district, caring for the men of small Army units scattered among small posts. In the 1st District, which included Massachusetts and New Hampshire, for example, there were eighty-seven patients at such posts as Forts Independence, Constitution, Sullivan, Preble, Seammel, and Sumner.[39] *(See Chapter 7.)*

Although hostilities in the North and Northwest involved both the 8th and 9th Military Districts, the greatest amount of action during the entire period was concentrated in the 9th District, or upstate New York and Vermont. Hospitals here were relatively numerous and during the campaigns of the summer, in response to demand, could be quickly set up in barns or tents. Finding attendants for these facilities, however, was difficult and they were initially selected from the line. Such men often turned out to be those "of incorrect habits, and bad dispositions" and eventually it was realized that it was better to choose attendants from among convalescents, some of whom could always be found who had "happy dispositions, who were kind to the sick." [40]

When it was necessary to move the sick and wounded, a number of forms of transportation could be used to negotiate the notoriously poor roads of the area. Some patients were moved in litters made of blankets hung between poles, others in wagons or sleighs, according to the weather, while still others avoided the roads altogether when they were moved in boats. The concept of the ambulance also appeared during this period; Mann referred to the "flying machines, called *volantes*" developed in France during the Napoleonic Wars,[41] and Winfield Scott, in that section of his memoirs which concerned the War of 1812 but which was written many years later, actually used the term *ambulance*.[42]

The forty-ward general hospital at Burlington, Vermont, with its staff of eight hospital surgeons and mates, had as fine a reputation as any facility in the 9th District. Its site, sixty to seventy feet above the level of the lake and on sandy, well-drained soil, was healthy. Rules requiring high standards of sanitation were firmly established. Floors and walls were kept scrupulously clean with soap and limewater, and all bunks were removed and thoroughly washed when they fell vacant. The straw in each bed sack was removed every two weeks and burned. When the weather permitted, windows were kept open all day; when it was cold, they were opened frequently for short periods of time. Closestools, bedpans, and "urinaries" were removed as soon as used. Although there could be as many as seven hundred to eight hundred patients at Burlington at any one time, infectious diseases did not pose a major problem.[43] The responsibility for the good record of the Burlington facility in the first two years of the War of 1812 was shared by two surgeons, Dr. Joseph Lovell, who opened the unit in 1812, and Dr. Walter W. Wheaton, who succeeded Lovell some time in 1813.[44]

Another general hospital was in operation late in 1813 at Malone, New York, about thirty-one miles from Sackett's Harbor and near the northern border of the state, where General Wilkinson had set up his headquarters. An academy, an arsenal, and two private homes which seem to have been located near the borders of a millstream "surrounded by a fine country of land" were taken over for this purpose. Within ten days, these accommodations, with a total capacity of 250 men, were prepared to house the sick comfortably, each man in his own bed, under the supervision of hospital surgeon Mann, who arrived in December.[45]

There was at least one general hospital in the vicinity of Sackett's Harbor throughout most of 1813. At Sackett's Harbor itself there was a facility which in 1812 had been occupied by the militia's patients and which was, by the spring of 1813, when Mann first saw it, "in filthy condition." Dr. William Beaumont arrived with his regiment at Sackett's Harbor in March 1813 and joined Mann in reporting the prevalence of respiratory diseases, diarrhea, and intermittent fevers, among the ill there.[46] Beaumont described a type of pneumonia characterized by "universal pain in the bones & musseles [sic], cold chills, nausea & pain in the head and breast,—sometimes accompanied with acute local pain in the side, with cough & other evident Pneumonia symptoms" which appeared among his patients.[47]

General Dearborn, however, believing it impossible to care for the sick within the line of defense at Sackett's Harbor, ordered a temporary hospital established at Watertown, New York, twelve miles from Sackett's Harbor. Within ten days, Mann had prepared accommodations for 100 there and moved the sick into them. Among those so moved were twenty men whose feet had been badly frozen in the course of a march from Plattsburg under Brig. Gen. Zebulon Pike. On 23 April 1813, however, Mann was ordered to leave Watertown and to return to Sackett's Harbor to be ready to accompany the 1,600-man expedition preparing the move against Toronto. A surgeon's mate was left behind at Watertown to care for the patients there.[48]

It was fortunate that the patients had been

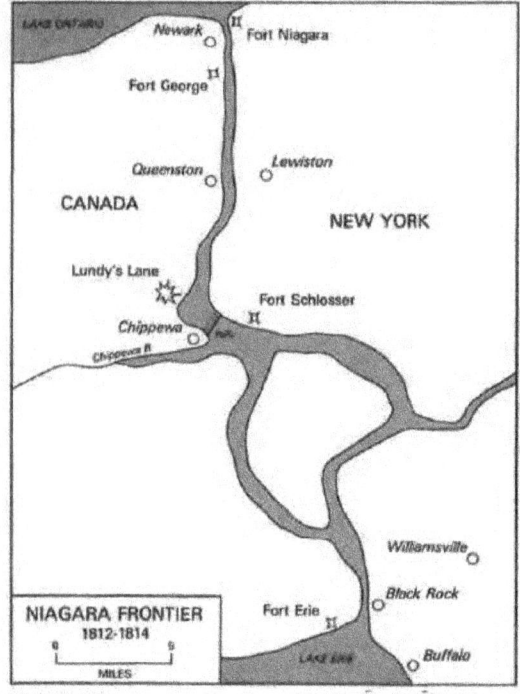

MAP 11

urged that camp be moved to a drier site for winter quarters before autumnal diseases made their appearance in full force.[49]

Further confusion exists concerning the nature of the facilities in the Fort Niagara-Fort George area. (*Map 11*) Mann described a tent hospital located two miles east of Fort Niagara where the wounded from the attack on Toronto were cared for beginning on 8 May 1813 and also noted that about two hundred wounded were moved from Fort Niagara to Lewiston in mid-June 1813. It is not clear whether it was from the tent hospital or from a regimental facility that those two hundred came. Despite the fact that it was believed that the wet nature of the area was bringing on fevers and diarrhea, some type of hospital seems to have remained here throughout the summer and into the fall, when it was reported that two-thirds of the sixty-five men the British killed and fourteen of those they wounded in the taking of that fort were hospital patients.[50] Whether the hospital referred to in these later documents was still a general hospital rather than a regimental facility is not apparent.

There was also a general hospital at Fort George, which was taken from the British in late May 1813 and held for several months. Although the alternating cold and heat, dryness and dampness here were blamed for the high incidence of typhus, intermittent fever, diarrhea, and dysentery among military and civilian populations alike, the water came in for its share of blame, since it was said to have "a purgative quality." A contributing factor in the high disease rate, in Mann's opinion, however, "was the effluvia from the sinks [latrines]," which filled the air with a heavy stench even when the "sinks" were covered with earth every day.[51]

In June, some of the patients at Fort George were also moved to the higher, healthier facility at Lewiston. By August, however, more than one-third of the men still there were sick and, with half the medi-

moved away from Sackett's Harbor by April because in May, the British raided the town, killing twenty-two Americans and wounding eighty-four, before being repulsed. By late June 1813, however, when a hospital surgeon was ordered to report there, a general hospital had once again been opened at Sackett's Harbor. A total of three surgeons and five mates seem to have cared for the sick and wounded here during the summer of 1813. By early September, there were 62 in the general hospital here as well as 501 in regimental ones, and conditions remained poor. It was reported that there was little good water available and that the food, particularly the bread, was bad. Great difficulty was being experienced in maintaining standards of camp sanitation because so many of the soldiers were inexperienced, and diarrhea, dysentery, and jaundice afflicted half of those who were acutely ill. The atmosphere was not considered to be healthy, and it was cal staff too ill to work, only three surgeons and four mates were available to care for six hundred to seven hundred patients. Hospital stores were running short by September when Mann decided to move the general hospital from Fort George to a site near Buffalo and to send all 100 invalids ready for discharge with a surgeon's mate from Fort George to Greenbush.[52]

It was in May 1813 that a unit Mann described as a flying hospital was opened at Lewiston in two barns and a number of hospital tents which were located about seventy feet above water level. Initially the staff there appears to have consisted of Mann and four hospital mates, who were expected to care for as many as six hundred to seven hundred patients or more, among them the wounded from the garrison hospital at Newark, near Fort George, who were moved to Lewiston in June. Later, however, two of the mates were ordered to Fort George, leaving Lewiston severely understaffed. Mann was able to obtain a sufficient number of bunks and bed sacks for this unit to assign one to each patient and located a good supply of milk for his patients.[53]

By the end of September 1813, the weather along the Niagara had become "very pleasant, and the troops generally more healthy." The convalescents at Lewiston were put on light duty and they did so well that only three experienced significant relapses. When his army left the area, General Wilkinson ordered that those not strong enough for the march be sent to Lewiston and that Mann locate winter quarters for them which would be secure from the enemy. Since, with the arrival of colder weather, the sick in the tents became uncomfortable and some developed pneumonia, Mann concluded that, although the Lewiston unit had earned an excellent reputation, it should now be abandoned. There does, however, seem to have been a hospital operating at Lewiston again in the summer of 1814.[54]

Although typhus and diarrhea had been a problem in Lewiston in 1813, Mann observed that wounds seemed to heal more quickly there than at other hospitals in the area, a fact he attributed in part to the healthy site. Of the 950 to 1,000 men cared for there, 59 died, with half of these deaths occurring within a three-week period in one sixty-man ward. Mann concluded that this tragedy had been caused by "an imprudent and injudicious administration of tartrite of antimony."[55]

When Mann broke up the Lewiston hospital, he sent approximately 100 of the strongest of his patients there to Greenbush also, but 250 others were sent to Williamsville, the site he had chosen near Buffalo. They were taken first in wagons from Lewiston to Fort Schlosser, where they boarded boats to travel to Black Rock. Before they could disembark into the wagons which took them the final forty miles to Williamsville, however, a sudden rainstorm and wind arose and some of the hospital stores and baggage were lost. Six "of the most enfeebled" patients died on the way.[56]

The hospital at Williamsville was located in an extensive barracks which had been renovated for use as a hospital. Since some of the men brought to this facility lacked adequate clothing, it was doubly fortunate that it was possible here to keep the rooms warm. Only six men were assigned to each ward, the rooms were easy to keep clean, and the patients tended to recover their health quickly. Having settled his patients in Williamsville's wholesome accommodations, Mann set out to join General Wilkinson at his winter camp at Malone, leaving surgeon's mate Joshua Whitridge, a physician whose "services . . . cannot be too highly appreciated," in charge. It seems probable that this facility, too, was closed at some time in the winter of 1813–14 or the spring of 1814.[57]

The regimental surgeons and mates of the units in the North also established their own hospitals or infirmaries. Beaumont described one aspect of the work of a regimental surgeon in his account of the attack upon Toronto in the spring of 1813, when the explosion of an ammunition dump caused American casualties in excess of 300, 109 of whom came from his regiment, including 65 deaths. "Wading in blood," he personally operated on fifty patients in a two-day period. "Their wounds were of the worst kind, compd fractures of *legs, thighs, & arms* and fractures of *Sculls*." "I cut and slashed for 48 hours, without food or sleep—My God! who can think of the shocking scene, where his fellow creatures lye mashed & mangled in evry part with a leg—an Arm—a head, or a body ground in pieces." Although Beaumont performed his operations at Toronto, some surgeons seem to have worked on board ships of the American Great Lakes squadron.[58]

The patients at Toronto were placed on a boat when it was time to evacuate them, but for several days bad weather kept the vessel in harbor. The men were not removed, however, and they spent a total of eight days on board, including the single day required for the voyage itself. They were so crowded that the surgeons could not effectively care for them. Although his wound was slight, one man died, apparently of suffocation in the close quarters. Diarrhea and dysentery also began to make inroads among his patients, but Beaumont commented that they survived in better condition than he would have expected under the circumstances. After their evacuation from Toronto, these casualties were hospitalized first at Newark and late in June were moved to Lewiston.[59]

After the unsuccessful attempt on Montreal in the fall of 1813, General Hampton was criticized for his handling of his wounded, who were reportedly "very much neglected, as far as regards comfortable quarters and transportation and . . . were strewed along the roads through which we marched, without care or attendance." General Wilkinson's wounded, however, received the benefit of organized care during the winter of 1813–14 after they arrived at winter camp. A regimental hospital was established at French Mills, in northern New York, sixteen miles from General Wilkinson's headquarters at Malone. Nevertheless, the patients here had to endure shortages of hospital stores and medicines and a poor diet, as well as the rigors of the weather, since they were for a short time sheltered in tents, the two houses taken over for their use being too small to shelter all the sick and wounded. The shortage of bedding required that some patients lie upon straw on the floor. The available blankets were of an inferior quality, and by early December, shirts for the patients had not yet been received. The port wine was reportedly not pure, the chocolate was so poor as to be inedible,[60] and the flour was "so sour and damaged, as to prove unhealthy." The bread his men ate, according to General Wilkinson, contained lime, soap, "and other extraneous and even *feculent* ingredients." The water used in making the bread seems to have been at the root of the problem, since it was "impregnated with, and contains a diffusion of excrementitious matter."[61] Sick and death rates were high in one instance; 75 men of a 160-man unit were ill, 39 with diarrhea and dysentery, 18 with pneumonia, 6 with typhus, and 12 with "paralysis of all the extremities."[62]

From June 1812, when war was declared, to June 1813, when Tilton was appointed Physician and Surgeon General of the Medical Department, the medical support of the Army continued to be, for all practical purposes, entirely in the hands of individual surgeons. The creation of the office of the Physician and Surgeon General, however, put Tilton in a position to assign and reassign surgeons, surgeon's mates, and hospital attendants on the basis of the overall need of the service and with due consideration for the skills and experience of the personnel of the Medical Department as a group. In the Northwest, slow communication and transportation made it impossible for any significant effects of the new organization to be felt in the period of scarcely a year remaining after Tilton's appointment before the end of the campaign season of 1813–14. In the Northeast, however, the benefits of centralization could be seen even in this short period of time in the sending of Mann, who had personally established an efficient hospital out of the chaos he found at Greenbush, to help his less experienced colleagues with the management of other hospitals caring for war casualties in upstate New York and New England.

9
Defeat and Final Victory, 1814 to 1815

Enemy attacks on the Baltimore-Washington area in the summer of 1814–15 made it obvious that the British posed a threat not only to the northern tier of states but also to the borders of the entire nation. Although by this time the care given the soldiers fighting in the North was beginning to show the benefits of the efforts and experience of the Medical Department's surgeons assigned to that area, the facilities available to the regulars defending Washington and New Orleans were in some degree overwhelmed by the sudden need to care for militia and volunteer casualties as well.

Campaign in the North

Although the campaign season of 1814 in the Northeast began with the failure of a northward move by Maj. Gen. James Wilkinson from the Lake Champlain area, operations to the west, along the Niagara River, reflected great credit upon the American forces, in large measure because of the training given to many of the men by Brig. Gen. Winfield Scott and the leadership of General Scott and Maj. Gen. Jacob Brown. Both the Americans and the British suffered heavy losses in these engagements; the Americans, for example, lost 227 wounded in the 5 July action along the Chippewa River and more than 850 in total casualties in the 25 July Battle of Lundy's Lane. Unfortunately, both General Brown and General Scott were wounded in the course of the summer, and in October, Maj. Gen. George Izard, who led reinforcements in from the east, ordered the Americans to withdraw from Canadian territory.[1]

Reinforcements for the Niagara area, however, had been taken from among the forces along Lake Champlain. The enemy quickly attempted to take advantage of the situation, but the success of American naval forces in the Battle of Plattsburg Bay and the resultant loss by the British land forces of their naval support led to the withdrawal of the British into Canada and the end of the threat of British invasion from the north.

The Burlington hospital continued to be one of the major Army facilities in this area during the last months of the war. In charge at Burlington were, first, Dr. James Mann, the surgeon with the greatest seniority in the 9th District and therefore presumably its medical director, and later, Dr. Henry Huntt, a hospital surgeon of junior status. Under their supervision at one time or another in the period January 1814 to April 1815 were more than 3,700 patients, fewer than 200 of whom died.[2] *(Table 9)*

If one can generalize from Mann's account, the most persistent problems confronting the surgeons staffing this hospital were those caused by regimental officers and regimental physicians. Often the required records did not accompany the patients to the hospital, an omission which at times may have been deliberate. A shortage of blankets and bedding was aggravated by the failure of regimental surgeons to send the bed sacks along with the men they sent to the general hospital. Some patients, furthermore, were sent from regimental

TABLE 9—ADMISSIONS AND DEATHS AT THE BURLINGTON GENERAL HOSPITAL, JANUARY 1814–APRIL 1815

Month	Admissions	Deaths
Total	3,707	184
1814		
January	180	7
February	671	17
March	931	29
April	630	22
May	151	17
June	59	6
July	30	1
August	33	0
September	729	31
October	105	25
November	52	11
December	13	5
1815		
January	35	6
February	56	3
March	20	2
April	12	2

SOURCES: Mann, *Sketches*, p. 144; Huntt, "Burlington," p. 179.

facilities to the general hospital only after they had reached "a moribund state." Mann was particularly angered, however, when regimental officers, often without even consulting a member of the hospital staff, informed one of his patients that if he did not return to duty at once, he would be considered a deserter. Mann believed that no officer was entitled to command a soldier to leave the hospital without a specific order to that effect from his commanding general.[3]

The strain placed upon the Burlington hospital increased in the late summer of 1814 after patients from Plattsburg were evacuated there in the face of the enemy advance. An estimated 650 to 815 patients arrived at the Vermont facility in open boats, "a great number of them ... unable to walk; and some were so reduced by disease as to be unable to tell their names." A sizable majority of the men had diarrhea and dysentery[4] and some developed what was diagnosed as typhus. It was noted at this time that the suffering of such of these men as had recently come in from the south seemed to be greater than that of others under these circumstances. Although the hospital itself could hold only 300 at a time, a barracks was taken over for the use of these new patients, and each man was washed and placed in a clean bed. In early September 1814, after the Battle of Plattsburg, seventy-nine more patients entered the Burlington hospital, fifty-five of whom were seriously wounded. Dysentery and diarrhea were now afflicting so many that physicians "could hardly enter a ward without seeing half a dozen on the close-stool," and care was taken to keep close-stools filled with limewater to reduce the odor.[5]

The men hospitalized at Plattsburg were not so fortunate as those at Burlington. In December 1813, first priority had been given here to building barracks for able-bodied soldiers and thus the hospital facilities were very disorganized when an epidemic similar to that of the previous year hit the Northern Army in the early months of 1814. As a result, some of the sick reportedly died from the cold. By the early summer of 1814, the weather and "ill-judged" troop movements were blamed for a "prodigious mortality," and by mid-August 1814, when there were 100 men in the general hospital within the Plattsburg camp, Mann was the only physician available to care for them. Another thirty patients were hospitalized in the village itself at this time under Wheaton's management and regimental surgeons were responsible for another fifty to ninety men. By 1 September, surgeons at Plattsburg were caring for more than seven hundred men.[6]

Although General Izard and his men marched for Sackett's Harbor in late August 1814, they left more than nine hundred patients and convalescents from both regimental and general hospitals behind at Plattsburg. Those still hospitalized at Plattsburg in early September were evacuated to Burlington in the face of the British advance. Initially, however, because of the lack of adequate transportation, they were moved two and a half miles to Crab Island, where for several days Mann, aided only by a surgeon's mate who was himself sick, cared for them as they lay on the wet ground, sheltered only by tents from the rainy weather. Finally, however, in the care of the surgeon's mate, they were moved in large open boats the remaining twenty-five miles to Burlington.[7]

Although he stayed with his patients while they were on Crab Island, Mann continued in overall charge of both Army and Navy wounded from the Battle of Plattsburg and reported that while the guns were firing, surgeons were exposed to danger as they moved from one protected area to another to care for the wounded. After the battle, more than thirty major operations were performed and these with such skill that Mann could write that "the medical gentlemen of our army and navy were . . . superior to the medical gentlemen of the British navy."[8]

The unit at Plattsburg appears to have been reopened once the threat to the town had passed, and by the end of the year, as the war drew to an end, 174 were patients still hospitalized in regimental units and 210 in general hospitals in the Lake Champlain area, including Burlington and Plattsburg.[9]

In the hospital at Malone, New York, the situation had deteriorated seriously by February 1814. Two hundred patients had been sent in from the camp at nearby French Mills and every house available for the purpose in the village was taken over to shelter the total of 450 patients now hospitalized in Malone. An adequate supply of blankets, bed sacks, hospital stores, and medicines, however, could not be located. The sick were suffering so intensely from the severe weather that four of them, according to Mann, died from the cold. "Humanity," Mann commented, "shudders at the appearance of these unfortunate men."

It now became necessary to send the men arriving at this hospital to other facilities, despite their "deplorable condition." Mann noted that this was not the first time the Medical Department had been overwhelmed by circumstances.[10]

On 9 February 1814, all the patients whose condition permitted it were moved away and the hospital at Malone was broken up. Under Mann's supervision, more than 450 men were sent first to Plattsburg, a journey of about seventy miles, and then on to Burlington. They were moved in sleighs in small groups to avoid overtaxing the accommodations of the sparsely settled areas through which they had to pass. Twenty of those in the poorest condition, however, were left at Malone under the care of a civilian physician and were captured by the British, while six of those who attempted the journey died on the way.[11]

Despite the crowding at Malone in the early winter of 1814 and the reappearance of the pneumonia experienced in the North the previous winter, only twenty men of the 380 admitted in the period 1 January to 9 February 1814 died at Malone. Some of the victims of this form of pneumonia died in a very short time after the first appearance of their symptoms. Among the complications attending this illness were "swelled feet and legs; some of these were accompanied with mortifications; the consequence of long confinement and inactivity in the boats, wet and cold, during the passage of the army down Lake Ontario and the river St. Lawrence."[12]

The hospital located at Sackett's Harbor, New York, remained there at least through the summer of 1814 despite dissatisfaction with the site. In the winter of 1814, the Apothecary General complained that the surgeons at this facility were wasteful, and the surgeon in charge pointed out that the 2,500 soldiers there had no regimental surgeons or mates with them and that, although hospital surgeons had taken over these responsibilities, more physicians were needed at Sackett's Harbor.[13]

For the final two years of the war there was also a general hospital at Brownville, New York, near Sackett's Harbor. It appears to have been closely linked with the Sackett's Harbor unit and from January 1814 to April 1816 was under the supervision of Dr. Hosea Blood. Unfortunately, however, Blood's report concerning deaths among the patients under his care does not break the figure down between Sackett's Harbor and Brownville. In the period 23 October 1813 to 20 January 1814 at Sackett's Harbor and 20 January 1814 to April 1816 at Brownville, 325 of his patients died. Tilton seems to have believed that the Brownville site was well chosen since the air and water there were good, but he urged that tents continue to be used during the summer of 1814 and that a large number of them be kept on hand to meet any eventuality, since huts should be used only in cold weather.[14]

A general hospital remained at Greenbush, New York, on the east bank of the Hudson, opposite Albany, as late as the earliest weeks of 1816. Little detail is available on conditions there, but the site was considered to be high enough to avoid the great danger posed by the fogs rising from the river. In the fall of 1813, a group of patients from the hospital at Lewiston, New York, had been evacuated to Greenbush, and early in 1814, two hundred to three hundred more were sent in from Buffalo. In his report of August 1814, however, Tilton listed only sixty-seven patients remaining in the Greenbush general hospital, but by 31 December 1814, the number of patients at Greenbush had again increased markedly, partly because the facility was now caring for 161 wounded British prisoners as well as 160 Americans.[15]

In 1814, the hospital at Williamsville, New York, did not occupy the same quarters it had used the previous year, and patients were sheltered in tents while awaiting the completion of buildings designed specifically for use as a hospital. Progress on the construction was extremely slow, however, and General Izard wrote that "the jealousy and quarrels between surgeons and the Quartermaster's department of General Brown's division" were to blame. In early November 1814, the new building was still "far from ready for the reception of the sick and wounded."[16] Some of the construction may have been complete by 26 November, for General Izard referred to the Williamsville facilities at that time as an "extensive hospital establishment," but in early November, because of the inadequacies of the facility, General Izard, following a suggestion from the hospital's senior surgeon, ordered that as many as could tolerate the journey be sent on to Greenbush. Nevertheless, almost two thousand patients were in such poor condition that they had to remain behind in the tents at Williamsville.[17]

There was, for a time, also a hospital set up at Buffalo in 1814 in the tents left behind when camp there was broken. The Americans wounded in July's battle at Chippewa and some of the enemy wounded, probably those from the Battle of Lundy's Lane, were sent to Buffalo. Among the British patients were some so badly burned in the explosion of a powder magazine that their "faces and hands were so crisped that the skin peeled off like a baked pig." Among a number of American wounded who were rowed up the Niagara River in a flat-bottomed boat to Buffalo was General Scott himself. Only those in the poorest condition were retained at Buffalo for any length of time, however, and although some difficulties were experienced in obtaining transportation, all but eighty to ninety men too seriously injured to be moved were sent eastward, apparently within a few weeks, to the facility at Williamsville. The Buffalo facility was closed on 23 December 1814.[18]

Because of the casual nature of some

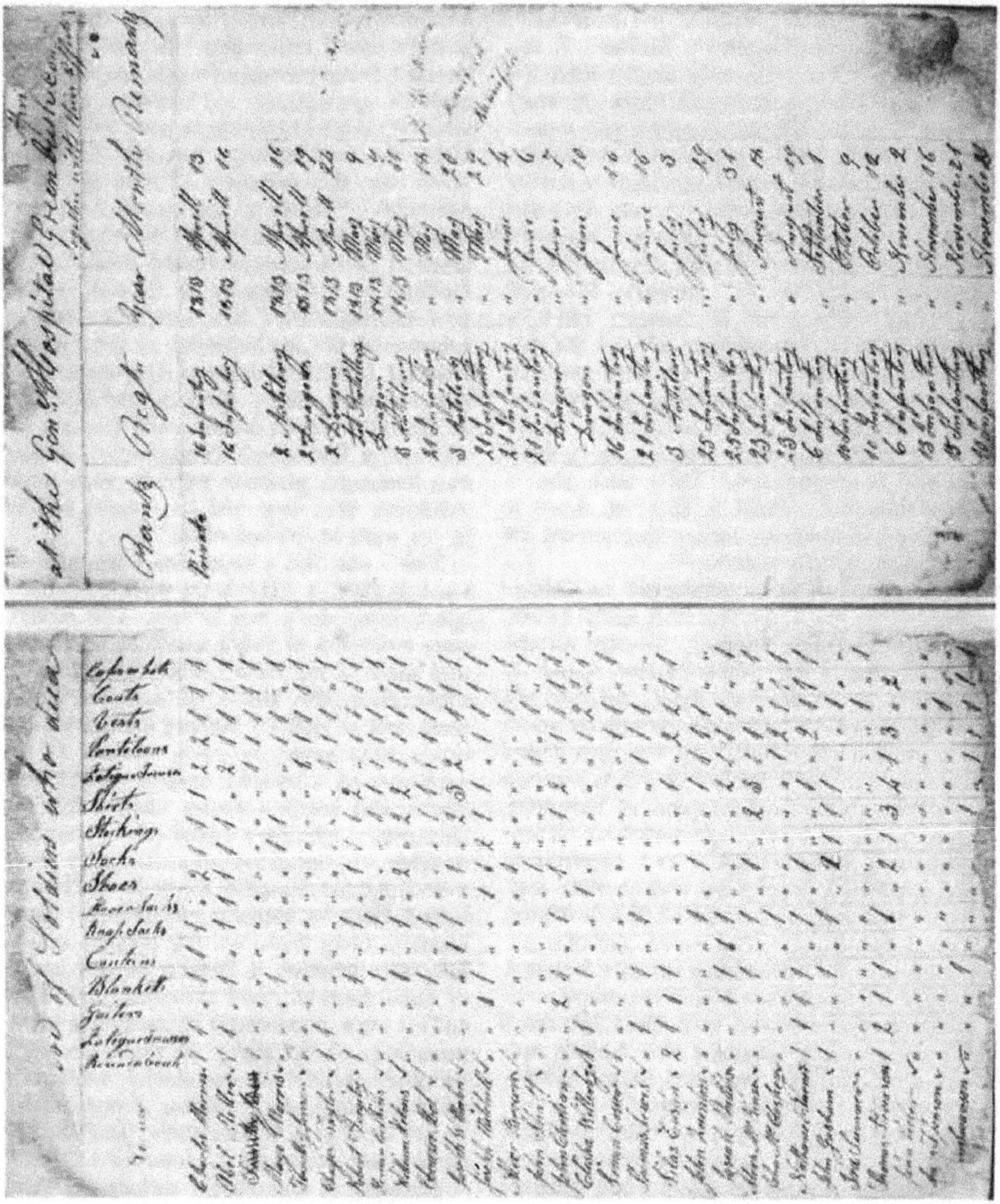

of the reports which survive from the time of the War of 1812, it is difficult to be sure of the nature of all of the hospitals serving the Army during that time. The Tilton report of 20 August 1814, for example, mentioned a return from a hospital surgeon, E. W. Bull, concerning the sick and wounded from Chippewa. It did not, however, make clear whether Bull was referring to men who became incapacitated during the battle of that name or to men hospitalized at some facility or facilities at or near Chippewa. If the former is true, however, the figures furnished Tilton by Bull (approximately 900 wounded, 300 sick) are, as Tilton commented, surprisingly high and probably included, as the Physician and Surgeon General commented, British casualties. It is difficult to believe that 300 men would fall ill as a result of one battle, and therefore it is likely that the reference was to the number of patients at a hospital. There is no record of a general hospital at Chippewa, however, but since the reporting physician was a hospital surgeon rather than a regimental surgeon, it is reasonable to assume that the Chippewa facility was a flying hospital.[19]

Patients at Fort Erie, which was taken from the British in July, were cared for by regimental surgeons who received high praise in the summer of 1814. The men there suffered from the high rate of illness which was to be expected in the area, but by early August, they were in better health than had been expected. Not long thereafter, however, the British began an unsuccessful five-week siege of Fort Erie, during which a strongpoint blew up just as the British were about to take possession of it. The wounded left behind by the British, their faces, in some cases, "so fearfully disfigured, that the sight of them was sickening," were carried to the American hospital. The care two surgeons and three mates gave the men entrusted to them at Fort Erie [20] led the commanding general to comment upon their "active, humane, and judicious treatment of the wounded, both of the enemy and of our own." [21]

The final report for the Medical Department in the 9th District in the War of 1812, covering the last months of 1814, noted that in the right wing there were 174 men remaining in regimental facilities and 210 in general hospitals, and in the Niagara area, the left wing, 365 in all facilities. In the vicinity of Sackett's Harbor, the central division, the total number of patients reported to Tilton was 581, but he questioned the accuracy of this figure.[22]

In the Northwest's 8th District, even after the departure of Maj. Gen. William Henry Harrison and approximately seven hundred regulars for the Niagara front, surgeons were unequal to the task which confronted them. The same agues and fevers which severely afflicted the civilian population in the area of Lower Sandusky, Ohio, and the country around Fort Stephenson struck at the garrisons holding the area. The physician responsible for the health of the soldiers here, Nathan Boulden, regimental surgeon for the 28th Infantry, also attempted to care for the thirty families living near the fort, even after he himself fell ill. He commented that the low-lying land was "astonishingly fruitful in the production of marsh miasmata" and that there were occasions when every member of a family was sick at the same time.[23]

Upon his arrival in the Northwest as hospital surgeon for the 8th District late in 1814, another Army surgeon, Adam Hays, commented that "there had been no kind of system in this district, but I shall endeavor to cleanse the Augean stable." He emphasized the shortage of hospital surgeons, pointing out that the Army would save money in the long run by sending out two good hospital mates and three garrison mates and thus eliminating the need to hire private physicians with wasteful habits.[24] By mid-January, however, the situation in the Northwest had deteriorated to the point where Boulden "fled for his life," after "having lost his health in the sickly region of Sandusky," and Hays was threatening to resign because of a shortage of physicians so severe that those who remained were "worn out."[25]

Although Tilton's attempt to put the Army's medical services on a systematic basis fell short of its goal and the care offered the sick and wounded in the Northwest's 8th Military was far from the ideal in the 9th Military District where the Army had concentrated both its most skilled physicians and many of its finest military leaders, by 1814 the picture was not entirely a dark one. "Intermittent fevers, dysentery, diarrhoea and jaundice" were regarded as "endemic diseases" here,[26] but because of the efforts of both physicians and military leaders, the only formidable sources of disease in 1814 appeared to be new troops, "the miserable refuse of society who never had energy to demonstrate that they lived." "The mystical power of strict discipline and rigid police" which could prevent even "the demon diarrhoea" was now recognized [27] and utilized in both camp and hospital. The recognition of the need for order and system was already leading to improvements in the care offered the sick and wounded of the Army in the North.

In the districts of the North where there was no military action, however, few patients required the attention of Medical Department physicians. In the 2d District (Rhode Island and Connecticut), for example, at the end of 1814 thirty-five patients were reported to the Physician and Surgeon General, all of them in a regimental infirmary, while in the general hospital of the 3d District (southern New York State and adjacent New Jersey), there were but fifty-eight patients remaining at this time, twenty-two of whom were from the militia.[28]

CAMPAIGN IN THE SOUTH

The demands made upon the Army Medical Department in the South, where relatively few Regular Army units saw action during the War of 1812, were quite different from those encountered in the North. Unfortunately, however, few of the surgeons on the small staff in the South left records of their work, and, as a result, only fragmentary information is available on the activities of department physicians below the Mason-Dixon line.

During the War of 1812, most of the area below the Mason-Dixon line lay in the 5th, 6th, and 7th Military Districts and, after the summer of 1814, in the newly created 10th Military District, which included the District of Columbia. *(Map 12)* At the end of 1813, there were a total of four hospital surgeons, six hospital surgeon's mates, one garrison surgeon, and six garrison surgeon's mates assigned to the first three of these districts. In the following year, a fifth hospital surgeon and five more hospital surgeon's mates were added to the staff in the South, but, even so, there were fewer physicians assigned to the hospitals and garrisons of the entire South than to the northern 9th District.[29]

In anticipation of an enemy attack upon Washington, the 10th Military District was formed on 2 July 1814, to include the area from Baltimore south through northern Virginia, and Brig. Gen. William H. Winder was placed in command. Estimates of the number of men, both militia and regulars, vary, but the latter did not exceed 500 and may have been no more than 300. More than 93,000 militia were alerted, but the entire force at General Winder's disposal at the time of the British landing near Benedict, Maryland, on the Patuxent River on 19 August probably did not exceed 1,700 men.

Although approximately five thousand to six thousand Americans, a large majority of

[Ch. 9] Defeat and Final Victory: 1814–1815   179

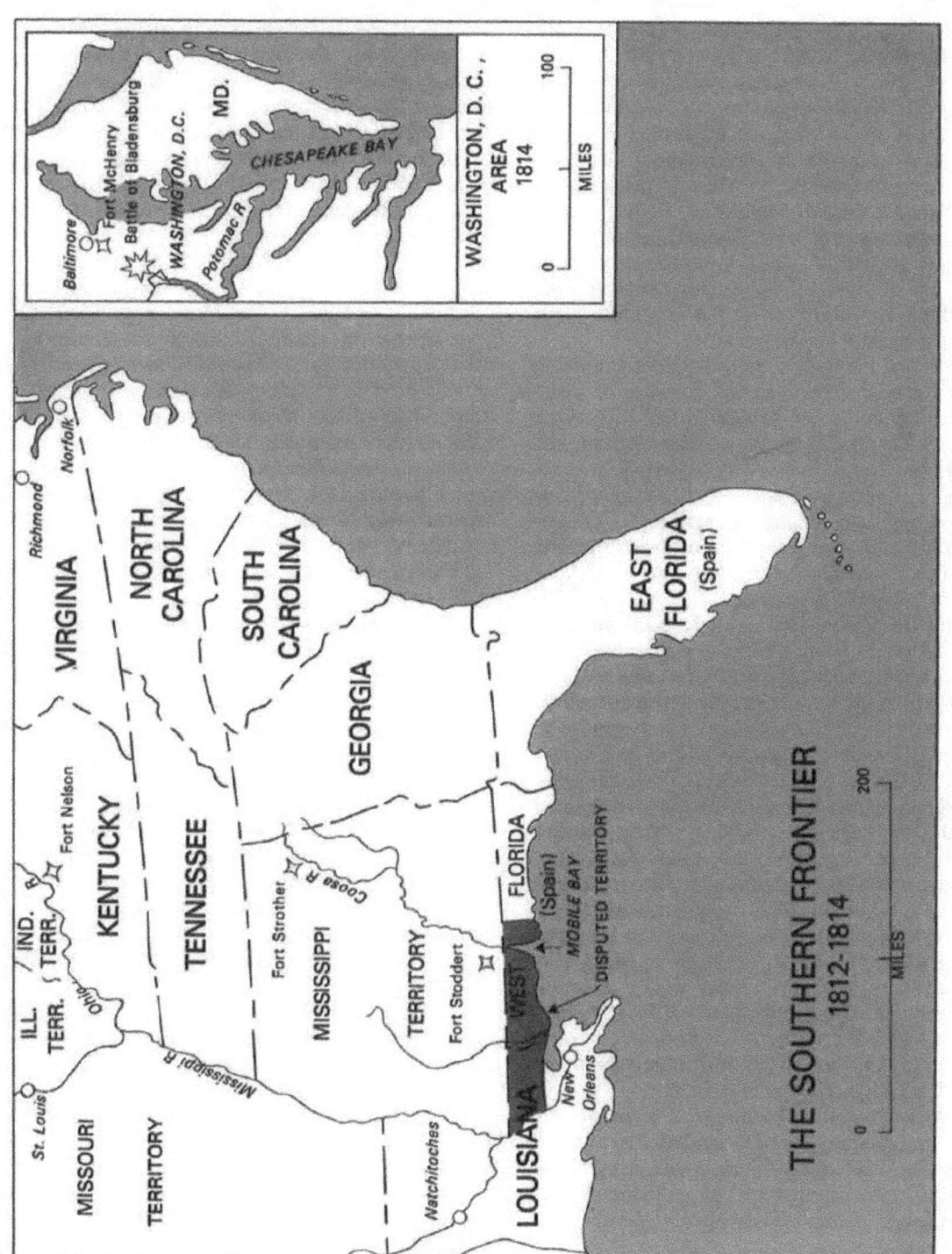

MAP 12

them untrained militia and volunteers, were in the vicinity of the capital by 24 August, the British won an easy victory in the Battle of Bladensburg and then moved on Washington to burn the Capitol, the White House, and other government buildings before withdrawing to their ships and reembarking on 30 August. A British attack on Baltimore in early September was defeated by militia and volunteers, without the aid of regulars except for those at Fort McHenry, where 24 of 600 regulars were wounded and 4 killed.[30]

Several facilities appear to have cared for the Army's patients in the summer of 1814 in the vicinity of Washington, D.C. One Army hospital, under the direction of Dr. William Jones, who was probably a hospital surgeon's mate at the time, was operating at a location described as Greenleaf's Point, now the site of Fort McNair at the junction of the Potomac and Anacostia Rivers, as early as the fall of 1813. The care offered soldiers before the summer of 1814 in what would become the 10th Military District nevertheless seems to have left much to be desired and the establishment of the new district does not appear to have markedly improved it. The day before the Battle of Bladensburg, Physician and Surgeon General James Tilton complained that the district was in great disorder largely because no one was officially in charge of medical support there. He urged the appointment of a hospital surgeon to provide leadership and proposed a personal visit to the area. Although it appears that it was not until 1 October that a hospital surgeon was moved to the 10th District, within three months he was able to bring at least some order to the management of medical support in that area.[31]

Because of the absence of a hospital surgeon in August 1814, wounded from action in the Washington area were apparently placed under the overall supervision of Dr. Hanson Catlett, who was referred to in a House of Representatives report as "the superintending surgeon." He is listed in the official records as the regimental surgeon for the 1st Infantry [32] and referred to himself as having been specifically "attached to the suite of General Winder, as staff surgeon." [33] Shortly after the Battle of Bladensburg, Catlett went through the British lines to aid in the care of injured American prisoners. Two other American physicians, at least one of whom was apparently himself also a captive, aided him here. By 2 September, the hospital Catlett had been ordered to set up on Capitol Hill was ready to take all the patients who might be sent there. When the British reembarked, they left several surgeons and their most seriously wounded behind them, and these men, too, became an American responsibility. There is no indication whether any of these prisoners were cared for in the Capitol Hill unit, which was still in operation as late as September 1814.[34]

In addition to the Greenleaf's Point and Capitol Hill facilities, there was also a third military hospital in the District of Columbia. Here some of the sick and wounded, both American and British, were cared for by a prominent civilian physician, Dr. James Ewell, who was assisted by a second civilian doctor. Ewell wrote that the Acting Secretary of War had ordered a militia facility established next door to his unit. This "militia-murdering hospital" was run by a surgeon's mate who had barely started his medical training at the time when he was appointed to care for the militia's wounded.[35]

By the end of 1814, the regular troops in the 10th District were in good condition but the health of the men of the militia was reported to be suffering because of their lack of discipline. The militia's sick were being discharged, however, and at the end of the year there were only eighty sick in regimental infirmaries and seventy in the general hospital. By January 1815, the troops still in the Washington, D.C., area were again sickly and a hospital surgeon was ordered to investigate conditions in a small barracks "near the President's Square." It was pointed out to this surgeon that the hospital at Greenleaf's Point was not filled to capacity and could accommodate more patients than it then held.[36]

Although regular units were also distributed among garrisons and forts throughout the deep South, many of the operations there during the War of 1812 were, like those in the North, conducted by militia and volunteers. The men operating against the Creek Indians in the Southeast beginning in the summer of 1813 were reinforced by regulars only in February 1814 when the 600-man 39th Infantry Regiment moved from Tennessee to Fort Strother on the Coosa River in what is now northeastern Alabama. *(See Map 12.)* On 28 May 1814, Andrew Jackson was named major general in the Regular Army to command the 7th Military District, which included Louisiana and the Mississippi Territory and, believing that the British were planning a move in the South, the Secretary of War began concentrating troops, both regular and militia, there. By 1 July, there were reportedly more than 2,000 regulars in the 7th Military District [37] and militia was being raised within Louisiana and neighboring states for the defense of that area.

General Jackson did not remain in the vicinity of New Orleans at this time but moved against West Florida with both regulars and volunteers. He did not return to New Orleans until 2 December. On 10 December, the British fleet was sighted at anchor not far from New Orleans, at a time when the only regulars there were elements of two regiments and an artillery detachment, totaling six hundred to eight hundred men or fewer.[38] Militia and volunteer units continued to pour in, however, and by 22 December, General Jackson had more than 2,000 men at New Orleans.

The first engagement with the British at New Orleans took place on 23 December 1814 and was followed by three more battles, on the 28th of December and the 1st and 8th of January 1815. The battle of 8 January resulted in a decisive victory over the British with only minor losses for the Americans. On the morning of 19 January, it was discovered that the British had slipped away from New Orleans, leaving behind eighty of their wounded.[39] Minor clashes between the British and Americans continued in the South, however, until mid-February when Congress ratified the Treaty of Ghent and brought the War of 1812 officially to a close.

Other than physicians accompanying militia and volunteer units and such of the department's regimental medical staff as may have accompanied detachments of regulars into the 7th Military District, the medical staff in this district was composed of a single hospital surgeon, who was stationed at the general hospital at New Orleans, two hospital surgeon's mates, whose precise locations cannot be determined, a garrison surgeon at New Orleans, and four garrison surgeon's mates, two of whom were at Fort Stoddert, north of Mobile Bay, and a third at Natchitoches, in west central Louisiana. The location of the fourth garrison surgeon's mate does not appear in the reports of the period.[40]

There was neither a surgeon nor a mate assigned to Fort Strother, and as late as December 1813, the 39th Infantry was without a surgeon. It is likely, therefore, that the medical care of regular units based there during two successful months of campaigning early in 1814 was provided by a regimental surgeon's mate.[41] The records of the medical care of General Jackson's men are very sparse, however, and the few details which can be pieced together concern the hospital and physicians at New Orleans.

According to Dr. Oliver Spencer, the

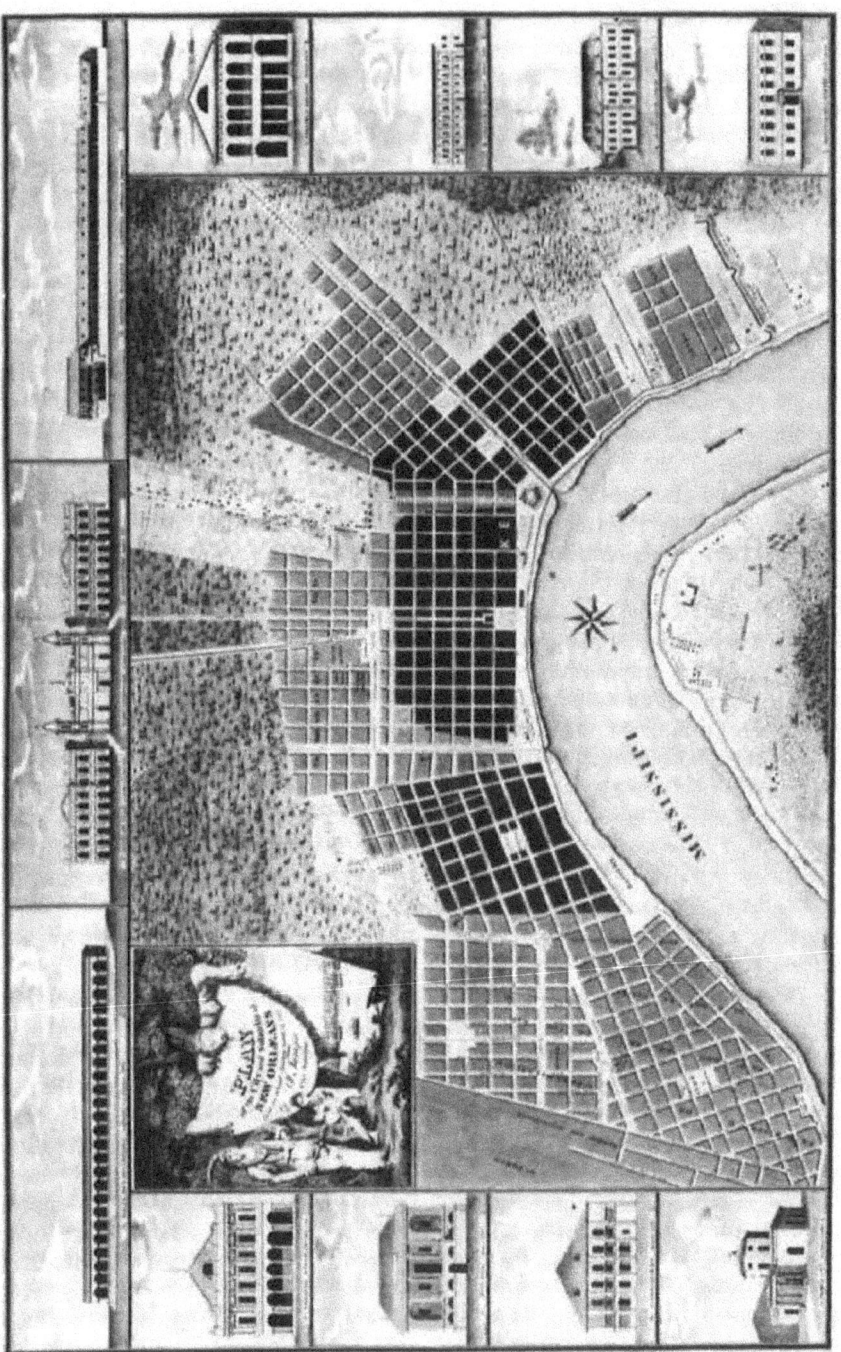

New Orleans in 1815. Military hospital at upper right corner. (Courtesy of Historic Urban Plans, Ithaca, N.Y.)

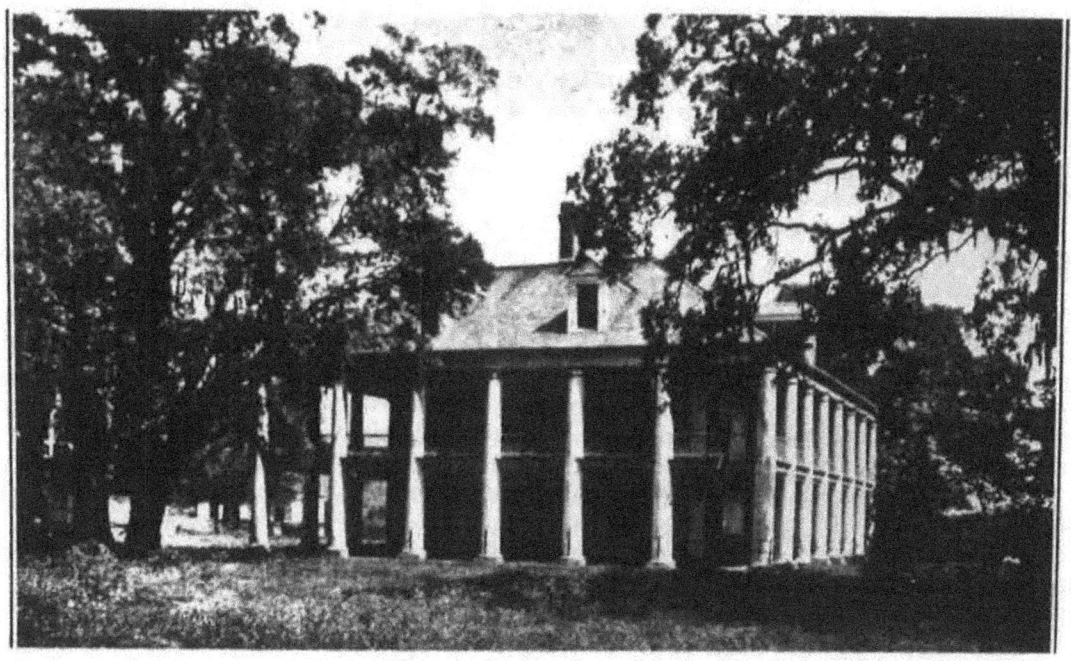

THREE OAKS MANSION. *(From Arthur, New Orleans.)*

garrison surgeon for that post, before General Wilkinson's last nine-month command in the 7th Military District, which ended in the spring of 1813, the general hospital in the New Orleans area moved with the units it served when they left the city itself. Since that time and despite the "acknowledged insalubrity" of the location, the facility had remained within the city, which was known not only for its permeation by "poisonous exhalations" from the river and marshes but also for its "extraordinary profligacy and licentiousness." [42]

Even before the War of 1812, the general hospital at New Orleans was apparently located very near an Ursuline convent, the unit's presence having been described as a "great inconvenience" for "the ladies of the convent." As early as April of 1812, it had been suggested that the hospital building and lot be given to the Ursulines in exchange for property which they owned elsewhere, but as late as mid-June of 1815, the trade had not been carried out, even though General Jackson himself was in favor of moving the facility outside the city. [43]

From time to time, other buildings were apparently also used to shelter Army patients near New Orleans. During the action around New Orleans on 8 January, hospital facilities were set up near the field of battle. It seems likely that a building was used rather than a tent, since the hospital surgeon, Dr. David Kerr, later stated that when the action was at its height, Louisiana's governor Claiborne rode his horse behind the hospital, "where he was entirely shelter'd from the balls of the enemy." This unit could have been the hospital set up in late December in a mansion house outside the city, one which was so damaged by this use that, according to its owner, $550 would be required to repair it. There was a mansion known as Three Oaks in this area which served as a hospital during the defense of New Orleans. Other patients were cared for in the schoolroom of the Ursuline convent, which had been abandoned by its pupils on 23 December. Fifty beds were reportedly set up there and it seems possible that the sisters also served as nurses elsewhere.[44]

Kerr was the director of the New Orleans general hospital during the last months of the War of 1812 and as such was apparently also responsible for collecting the required reports from the regimental and garrison surgeons and mates in the 7th District. Kerr reported to Tilton, however, that as of 30 July 1814 he had been unable to acquire reports from the other physicians in his district, although there were forty-nine patients under his own care in the general hospital.[45]

References pertaining to the medical care received by the troops defending New Orleans are not always easy to interpret because of a tendency to refer to participants in the struggle by their last names only and because there were two physicians with the last name of Kerr involved. It is, therefore, not always possible to be sure from the context to which of the doctors Kerr reference is being made. By the time of the British assault on New Orleans, Spencer had resigned as garrison surgeon, but Dr. Christopher Backus, of "the Drs. Apothecary Generals department," remained in the city. A native of Louisiana, Backus had been appointed Assistant Apothecary General in August 1814. Also aiding in the care of the wounded near New Orleans was a Dr. Flood, who appears to have owned land upon which General Jackson's line was at one time camped and who seems, like John Kerr, to have volunteered his services. Dr. Lewis Heerman was a third volunteer whose name, like that of Flood, does not appear on the rolls of the Army Medical Department.[46]

Because the climate was taking its customary toll, the burden on the hospital facilities in the New Orleans area in December 1814 and January 1815 was great, despite the low number of American casualties. Many contracted "pernicious fever and dysenteries" and in one month 500 men reportedly died from disease alone. Large numbers of wounded British prisoners were also the responsibility of the U.S. Army at this time. The captives were taken to New Orleans the evening of 8 January, but, since the facilities there were already filled with Americans, an appeal was made to the citizens of the city for help. Pillows, old linen for dressings, and 140 mattresses were brought forward, and many civilians volunteered to take British casualties into their homes and to care for them there until space could be found for them within the hospital. All civilian physicians in the city at this time were called upon to care for the enemy wounded. They appear to have responded without hesitation and some even left town and went out to meet the wounded to render more prompt care.[47] On 8 January, General Jackson assured the British Commander that "The wounded on the field shall be sought after, and every comfort administered them until they are recd." [48]

General Jackson also sent a friend who happened to be a native of New Orleans back to check on the condition of his own wounded, who were scattered about the city, but despite his concern, the death rate among the hospitalized in New Orleans in the early winter of 1815 was reported to be very high. Militia and volunteer surgeons were ordered retained in the service to care for their patients who were housed in Army hospitals. General Jackson himself was on the sick list at one time, laid low by a "serious attack of disentry . . . brought on by cold and fatigue." His cure, achieved through the efforts of "Doctor Kerr Hospital surgeon," [49] undoubtedly confirmed his earlier evaluation of the care the sick and wounded received during and after the defense of New Orleans which had led him to conclude that "The medical staff has merited well of the country."[50]

In the 5th and 6th Military Districts, unlike the 7th, there were no major military operations in the last year and a half of the War of 1812, although enemy raids occurred from to time along the eastern coast. In the 5th Military District, the headquarters of the Medical Department was at Norfolk, an area which the hospital surgeon in charge found to be healthier than he had anticipated. Assigned to Norfolk in 1814 were the district's only hospital surgeon, two hospital surgeon's mates, and a garrison surgeon's mate. There was also a garrison surgeon's mate at nearby Fort Nelson.[51]

When the hospital surgeon at Norfolk reported to Tilton in the summer of 1814, there were but forty-three patients in his general hospital and 618 in the "regimental infirmary." Elsewhere within the district, however, there seems to have been much confusion. The Deputy Quartermaster General in Richmond, Joseph Wheaton, maintained that he was forced to act as physician, superintendent, and manager of hospitals in Richmond from 1 January 1814 to 19 November 1817[52] because "there was no hospital or medical department, nor even a United States physician at Richmond" to care for the many sick who, after their discharge from the Army, went through Richmond on their way from Norfolk. He had personally taken the initiative, arranged to obtain the use of a building for a hospital, signed on a surgeon's mate, and appointed nurses. He apparently also supervised the care of patients from the militia units in the area.[53]

The troops in the Carolinas and Georgia were served by a relatively large medical staff, which as of 29 December 1813 included, on paper, three hospital surgeons, three hospital mates, and two garrison mates. Tilton appears to have had as little success in extracting reports from this district as he had in many others.[54]

The last year of the War of 1812 illustrated in the North the improvements in the care of the sick and wounded which could result from the effort and planning of experienced physicians when they were given adequate time and resources. Hospitals there were clean and efficiently managed and there is no evidence that in the North they became the hotbeds of infection which they had been in the Revolutionary War. In the South, where a high rate of disease was to be expected but where relatively few regular troops were stationed, the situation was quite different. Since casualties here were few among American regulars, any unusual strain upon the department's physicians resulted largely from the wounded militia, volunteer, and enemy troops entrusted to their care.

10

The Lessons of War: 1815 to 1818

The experiences of two wars and several expeditions against the Indians made it obvious not only that Army surgeons, like their colleagues everywhere in the late seventeenth and early eighteenth centuries, were unable to treat a large proportion of their patients successfully but also that the U.S. Army was unable to deliver the best medical care, as determined by the standards of the time, to its sick and wounded. After hostilities ended in 1815, a number of surgeons published journal articles about their professional experiences during the War of 1812, but since there was no central authority to coordinate their observations or to study their conclusions and since they had little understanding of the causes of disease and infection, the significance of their contributions was limited.

A number of the nation's political leaders were also brought by the experiences of that war to urge the creation of a permanent, professional, and quickly expandable Army. Although their concepts failed to achieve wide acceptance in the years following the war and their efforts were to a significant degree frustrated, a permanent Medical Department was nevertheless established in 1818 when, as a result of the efforts of Secretary of War John Calhoun, legislation created a number of permanent staff departments for the Army. The disciplined, co-ordinated collection and study of data systematically gathered by the department from different areas of the country and over a long period of time now became possible; as a result, as the value of statistical studies received greater recognition, the department would be in a position to make important contributions to medical science. The existence of a permanent organization, furthermore, would also guarantee that a nucleus of experienced and disciplined military surgeons would be available at all times in the future to advise concerning the prevention of disease and to care for the Army's sick and wounded.

INDECISION AND DECISION, MARCH 1815 TO APRIL 1818

The confusion and suffering caused by the fact that the Medical Department was created after the War of 1812 had begun and therefore could not prepare for the care of large numbers of sick and wounded in the War of 1812 did not prevent the breakup of its central organization within a short time after the hostilities ended. The office of Physician and Surgeon General was eliminated by the legislation of 3 March 1815, which reduced the Army in size to 10,000 men, but the positions of Apothecary General and two assistants, considered still needed because of "principles of convenience and real economy,"[1] were provisionally retained through an order of 17 May 1815. (*See Appendix K.*) The ratio of one surgeon and two mates per regiment was not altered, however, and a maximum of five hospital surgeons, fifteen hospital mates, and twelve post surgeons per division was also permitted. Many of the most experienced physicians were dropped, either temporarily or permanently, from the service, even in those instances when they had expressed a wish to be retained. By the end of the year, however, Secretary of the Army William H. Crawford was urging Congress to recognize the fact that the military should be given "in time of peace, the organization which it must have to render it efficient in a state of war." Even so, he did not suggest the creation of the post of surgeon general, but merely proposed that a permanent staff include an apothecary general, whom he would have stationed at Philadelphia.[2]

In April 1816, legislation was passed to clarify the organization of the medical support to be provided the Army and the positions of the Apothecary General and his two assistants were now made permanent. The Army was divided into a Northern Division with four geographical departments and a Southern Division with five. A ratio of four hospital surgeons and eight mates for each of the two divisions was established, and the position formerly known as garrison surgeon was officially redesignated post surgeon. Although there was now a small permanent staff to handle the supply of drugs and medicines, when John Calhoun became Secretary of War late in 1816, there was still no single superior over the entire department through whom the Apothecary General, Francis LeBaron, could work in estimating the overall needs of the Army's surgeons.[3]

Apparently some critics of the medical care available to the men of the U.S. Army at this time blamed inadequacies in large measure upon "the irregular and injudicious mode which government has pursued in the organization of a medical department." Calhoun, however, was a young man of both energy and ambition. He was convinced of the necessity of expanding the work of his predecessor in creating a peacetime staff organization which would be able to meet the challenge of war whenever it might come. By April 1818, the new Secretary of War was able to add to the permanent staff posts of the Army that of the Surgeon General of the Army Medical Department.[4]

At least twenty-two physicians who had served with the Army during the War of 1812 informed Tilton, who himself retired in the spring of 1815, that they wished to remain in the Army. It appears, however, that by January 1816, only seven of the twenty-two had actually been retained in any capacity whatever and that at least one of the seven was very unhappy with the position to which he had been assigned. One of those who was dropped from the Army commented to Tilton that "a just and honorable reward for public service is seldom bestowed on the humane and faithful physician and surgeon." Although he remained in the Army, a second physician, Dr. J. H. Sackett, who had served as a hospital surgeon's mate during the war, joined those who complained of the Army's attitude. Sackett had at first been dropped from the Army's rolls in May 1815, but after being asked to remain the following month, was assigned the position of a mere garrison surgeon's mate.[5]

Despite the fact that Dr. James Mann, in Tilton's words, "the oldest surgeon on our register," was recommended for reappointment by both Tilton and LeBaron, among others, and wished to remain in the Army, he was not initially asked to do so. He appears, however, to have remained on duty at least through mid-April. He became quite bitter over what he regarded as the Army's unfairness, since he had a family to support and had given up his private practice upon entering the Army. By the spring of 1816, however, he had apparently been reappointed and was serving as one of the four hospital surgeons in the Northern Division, along with Benjamin Waterhouse, Joseph Lovell, and Tobias Watkins.[6]

Even after hostilities ceased, large numbers of bills which Apothecary General Francis LeBaron had difficulty paying continued to come in to his office. Among the expenses he was required to handle were the costs of care for the men who were treated by private physicians after falling ill along the roadside when units of the Northern Army were on the march. Through the entire spring of 1815, LeBaron continued to press for the funds he needed to meet the department's expenses, and during the summer the Secretary of War decided that one way of meeting some of these claims against the department would be to sell off all hospital supplies no longer needed.[7]

Early in 1816, LeBaron began to urge measures to eliminate waste and extravagance. Since surgeons were accumulating unnecessarily large quantities of supplies, specific regulations should be drawn up "for the economy of supplies in this Dept." LeBaron's problems continued, however, and the spring of 1817 found him still concerned about the accountability of surgeons and others who handled supplies. He maintained that a one-quarter savings could result if surgeons were made responsible to the Apothecary General and the Apothecary General in turn to "some higher source." He reported that he had been able, even so, to save some money by having old instruments repaired, but old medicines tended to deteriorate and those of his drugs which had been long in storage were losing in value with every passing day. They should, therefore, be sold at once.[8]

Another economy suggested by LeBaron in March 1815 was a consolidation of hospitals to reduce the cost of transporting supplies. The Apothecary General urged that the men then in facilities at Burlington, Brownville, and Williamsville be sent to Greenbush, but he agreed with Waterhouse that an invalid hospital should be opened to serve the northern and western states. His suggestions, however, appear to have been to some degree ignored, since the hospital at Brownville was in operation as late as the fall of 1817 and that at Burlington was still open when the hospital surgeon who was in charge there in the winter and spring of 1815 left the Army that summer.[9]

LeBaron made a number of other suggestions for improving the efficiency of the department's supply system, but it is not always possible today to ascertain to what extent his ideas were carried out. He appears to have succeeded to some degree in limiting the frequency of supply deliveries to any given area to once a year and hoped that, as a result, he would receive fewer of those small orders which could be easily lost. He requested that estimates of need be made up by March of each year, pointing out that timely returns could have saved $10,000 of the $36,000 to $37,000 which was spent on drugs in the twelve-month period ending in the summer of 1817.[10]

The path of distribution of supplies to the regimental surgeons lay through the quartermasters at such central points as Philadelphia, Boston, and New York. In early 1815, for example, the assistant apothecary general assigned to Richmond, Virginia, was receiving all of his medicines from the deputy commissary in that city. There was at least one request that a storage depot also be established at Baltimore, but LeBaron believed that taking this step would unnecessarily complicate the handling of supplies.[11]

LeBaron hoped to take advantage of water transportation wherever he could. With this in mind, he pointed out that New York City, where he wished to make his headquarters, was an ideal location. He apparently experienced difficulty in receiving permission to make the move and in the spring of 1816 was still urging that this step be taken. He pointed out to the Secretary of War that the rivers leading to the west from Philadelphia could be used for transport from a depot there and that New Orleans could serve as a center from which the deep South could be supplied. LeBaron's work was complicated, however, not only by such occasional problems as the "uncommon scarcity of Water of the Mohawk" but also by the fact that he

STATEMENT ON HOSPITAL SUPPLIES SENT FROM NEW YORK. *(Courtesy of National Archives.)*

could not be sure what forts were in use at any given time.[12]

The Apothecary General made an inspection trip in the late summer and early fall of 1816. It was planned to take him along the northern frontier, which was in an "unsettled state" as far as the Medical Department was concerned. He hoped to visit Brownville, Sackett's Harbor, Niagara, and Detroit, and possibly Michilimackinac as well. When he learned that the men constructing a "military road" near Detroit would probably suffer a high rate of disease, LeBaron decided to take two wagonloads of items which they might need along with him when he left Albany. He seems to have set out upon this three-month voyage in the late summer of 1816, but in addition to being "sick most of the time," he was shipwrecked on Lake Ontario.[13]

Despite his efforts to improve the supply operations of the Medical Department, LeBaron's position was made insecure by continuing criticism of the quality of the supplies he sent out. In February 1817, although the exact nature of the complaint was not spelled out in the Secretary of War's letter to the Apothecary General, LeBaron was tersely informed that if there were further complaints on this score, "the government [will] . . . discontinue your services."[14]

Much of the work of Army surgeons in the period immediately after the end of the War of 1812 involved the sick and wounded still remaining in need of care or new patients from among the troops originally concentrated as a result of the war. In February 1815, for example, there were still "sundry considerable armies & cantonments" in the 9th Military District. As late as March there were also sick and wounded British prisoners in a hospital at Pittsfield, Massachusetts. Even in 1817, Army surgeons were still concerned with the veterans of the War of 1812. The certificate of an Army physician was required for some types of pensions, but apparently not all of the certificates issued were accurate. In at least one instance, a surgeon stated that a man had been wounded in action at a time when the individual had not yet joined the Army. The physicians involved, however, were not accused of fraud but rather of a lack of awareness which made them the easy victims of dishonest soldiers.[15]

Although there were still patients requiring care in the vicinity of Lake Champlain, Dr. Henry Huntt was on leave and Mann was attending the court-martial of Maj. Gen. James Wilkinson at Utica, leaving no hospital surgeon on duty in this area. By April, however, when Mann had returned to Plattsburg, the men were in excellent health, a fact he attributed to the "rigid discipline and judicious police" which prevailed among them. He also noted that the regimental units were well managed. Huntt was ordered to the general hospital at Burlington early in February 1815, but in June he was relieved of duty there and left the Army.[16]

By the end of June 1817, Dr. Joseph Lovell appears to have become, at least unofficially, the head of the Northern Division. He turned in a report of that date which was entitled "Remarks on the Sick Report of the Northern Division for the Year Ending June 30, 1817"[17] and later that fall was referred to as "Inspecting hospital Surgeon, at Head Quarters."[18] As a result of his inspections he was able to report that the health of the men in the North was very good. More than 2,100 patients had been treated in the preceding twelve months, 838 of whom were suffering from fevers "and other important complaints," 193 from wounds, and 55 from venereal diseases.[19]

THE STATE OF THE ART

Two wars and a number of campaigns against the Indians offered the physicians who served with the American Army before the spring of 1818 opportunities they would not otherwise have had to observe diseases and their treatment and the effects of climate, weather, and geography upon health. Some of these surgeons attempted to record either formally or informally for the benefit of others what they had seen while in the Army and the conclusions they had reached, but the speedy disbanding of the Medical Department made the most effective use of their professional experiences during the war impossible.

Most of the observations of the military physicians of this period seem to have been directed at the practice of medicine rather than that of surgery. Concern continued to be shown for the prevention of disease, through improved hygiene and, in the case of smallpox, through the new process of vaccination. The prevalent types of treatment were also examined with a critical and discriminating eye.

Vaccination was not used within the Army with the enthusiasm which might have been expected, despite the fact that an early supporter of the procedure, Dr. Benjamin Waterhouse, joined the Army Medical Department during the War of 1812. Since, in addition, no deliberate effort was made to study the effectiveness of the procedure, a valuable scientific opportunity was lost. LeBaron, as Apothecary General, attempted in late April of 1813 to have all nonimmune troops vaccinated and urged that the material necessary be sent out at once so that all susceptible men could be immunized before the new campaign began. Although he sent out the "vaccine virus" to various commanding officers, LeBaron did not have the authority to order the troops to undergo the procedure. He made no reference to the existence of any smallpox within the Army, but pointed out that immunization was necessary because some of the localities through which the troops would have to pass were experiencing smallpox epidemics. He emphasized that no special preparation was deemed necessary before vaccination and that after the procedure had been completed, the men could continue with their normal routines.[20]

Not long after he became head of the Medical Department in 1813, the Physician and Surgeon General appointed six young surgeon's mates to form a vaccinating team to go out to immunize the Northern Army. Like LeBaron, however, Tilton made no mention of any smallpox epidemic within the ranks of the Army. Whether the mission he assigned was actually accomplished cannot be ascertained, but the next summer Maj. Gen. George Izard, alarmed by a single case of smallpox within his camp, sent "an express" to Albany to obtain "kine pox matter" and commented that his troops should have been vaccinated earlier.[21]

Although none of these documents refers to an epidemic of smallpox within the Army in the War of 1812, the fear that there might be one was evident. Since references to devastating smallpox epidemics were common in the documents of the Revolution, and since the disease was still dreaded, it is unlikely that similar epidemics in the War of 1812 would go unmentioned.

Discipline as a key to the prevention of disease was well recognized by the War of 1812 and was emphasized by the future Surgeon General, Joseph Lovell, who pointed out that one of the reasons for retaining a "military establishment" in peacetime was the fact that military experience was necessary to an understanding of regulations and their importance. The precautions recommended for the prevention of disease included not only the obvious sanitary measures but also the locating of camps in dry areas and the starting of fires early in the evening on the windward side of camp if circumstances made the pitching of camp in a damp area unavoidable.[22]

Proper clothing was considered to be very important. No new conclusions on the subject appear to have been reached during the War of 1812, however; faith was still placed in the wearing of woolen shirts, particularly north of Philadelphia, and Lovell recommended that the advice of Benjamin Franklin on that subject be followed: woolen shirts should be worn "until mid-summer" and put on again "the *next day*." Surgeons in the War of 1812 were apparently also familiar with the damage which cold and damp could cause to the feet. Lovell emphasized the importance of proper footgear, commenting that "the most important circumstance perhaps of all is to enable the soldier to keep his feet warm and dry by a liberal allowance of woolen socks and laced shoes, reaching at least to the ankle." Lovell also believed, however, that letting the feet remain wet and cold for any length of time had "deleterious effects upon the constitution through the lungs and bowels." [23] Tilton shared Lovell's faith in flannel worn next to the skin, but he believed that wearing clothing which was too warm in the summer was also unwise. In hot weather the soldier should wear "pantelets & shoes, without stockings," but in every kind of weather, he should wear gaiters.[24]

Mann's experiences, however, had not led him to great optimism concerning what preventive medicine could accomplish with the average soldier. The Army enlisted many men who were already "habitually intemperate, with constitutions broken down by inebriation and its consequent disease; whose bloated countenances exhibited false and insidious marks of health" and these "contribute to fill our hospitals." "It has been too much an object with officers on the recruiting service, to fill up their rolls with numbers." "The surgeons of the army," Mann lamented, "are made mere scapegoats, on whom are heaped a multitude of sins." [25]

Although hospital records surviving from the War of 1812 list fevers and digestive and respiratory ills as the most prevalent diseases, some patients suffered from "nothing" or even "rascality." [26] One Army surgeon, however, recommended a cure for this kind of ailment. Blistering, he said, was "a good test, in doubtful cases, whether a man was really sick. Rather than submit to the pain of blistering a second time, unless absolutely diseased, he would prefer going to duty . . . so that, whether a man was actually sick or only feignedly ill, blistering was an excellent remedy." [27]

If there were a disease deserving of the name of "camp disease" in the War of 1812, Lovell believed it would have to be diarrhea and dysentery. The primary cause of this problem was, in his opinion, not bad food or water, but cold and damp weather. To treat diarrhea and dysentery, physicians tried inducing perspiration by warm baths, warm drinks, warm coverings, and medicines believed to increase perspiration, such as Dover's powder, a combination of opium and ipecac.[28]

Another goal of the physician treating dysentery was the emptying of the digestive tract by purges and emetics, an approach which was accepted with little or no question. There seems to have been some difference of opinion, however, on whether the purge should precede or follow the emetic. Waterhouse believed that ipecac should be administered before the purge, and that jalap, senna, aloes, rhubarb, and "perhaps calomel" should not be used for purging the sufferer from this disease because they increased "peristaltic motion." Epsom salts, manna, castor oil, and extract of butternut, on the other hand, were appropriate since they operated by "increasing the secretion of the glands of the intestines." Heustis, however, favored administering the purgative, preferably castor oil, before the dose of ipecac or tartar emetic. For severe and chronic dysentery he also recommended the raising of blisters just above the ankle and the administration of 1.5 to 2 grams of opium, to be combined in the case of heavy drinkers suffering from this disease with 2 to 3 grams of sugar of lead. Waterhouse used opium only when his "patient has been thoroughly evacuated," but admitted that the sufferer's pain alone might make the use of opium necessary.[29] Mann, however, warned that the sudden checking of chronic diarrhea could bring on dropsy, which was best relieved by "drastic purges." [30] Waterhouse also recommended the use of "decoction of wild cherry" as an "astringent in the latter stage of dysentery." [31]

Neither Waterhouse nor Heustis seems to have believed in the unrestricted use of bleeding for dysentery and diarrhea. Heustis stated that only feverish patients should be bled, while Waterhouse recommended venesection only when the sufferer was young and had "a very hard and crowded pulse," accompanied by "severe pains in his back and loins." Even in these instances, however, Waterhouse warned that patients should be bled but once.[32]

There was considerable agreement on the appropriate diet for the patient with diarrhea or dysentery. Heustis and Waterhouse agreed that meat in any form should be avoided, along with alcohol. Heustis encouraged the use of ripe fruit, especially mangoes, guavas, and pomegranates, for "scorbutic dysentery," while Waterhouse emphasized that the fruit must be truly ripe since green fruit would have a harmful effect. Heustis favored a milk and vegetable diet for these patients,[33] and Mann added that "No article prescribed proved so beneficial as milk and its preparations . . . By milk alone, it was my persuasion, that many lives were saved, which, without it, would have been lost." [34]

Physicians in the early nineteenth century continued to question whether many of the fevers so prevalent among the Army's patients were separate entities; nothing of significance had been learned about these diseases since the time of the Revolution. In 1817, for example, Heustis wrote: "Briefly, my opinion is, that the intermitting, remitting, yellow fever, and plague, are only gradations and modifications of the same disease." In 1813, Dr. John Warren, who had served with the Hospital Department in the Revolution, speculated as to whether the disease known in the tropics as yellow fever was identical with typhus, although he was confident that the yellow fever which struck Boston in 1798 and 1802 was not typhus. Warren did distinguish between inflammatory fever and typhus, but he seems to have used the terms *typhoid* and *typhus* almost interchangeably.[35] A physician thus might describe a fever as being "a typhoid type" and characterized by a "total loss of appetite, great thirst, parched brown tongue, sordes on the teeth, increased heat of the skin." [36]

By 1817, studies arising from the interest in the possible effects of weather and climate, however, seem to have somewhat lessened the prevalent enthusiasm for the idea that the origin of fevers might be in "those changes in the air that are pointed out by the thermometer, barometer, or hygrometer." Waterhouse began to believe that the origin of these "wide spreading maladies, as well as endemics, or local disorders" lay in "some secret movement, or alterations in the earth, or on its surface." He noted that while "Epidemics seem to accompany or follow a blighted state of vegetation," they also seemed "to accompany an abundant harvest, but whether in the series of cause and effect, is not fully known." He then terminated his discussion with an abrupt "As to myself, I'm weary of conjecture!" [37] Not long after the permanent organization of the department, Army surgeons would be required to begin contributing detailed and systematic reports to the study of the question Waterhouse and others had raised.

Although the physicians of the early nineteenth century may not have been sure of the identity of typhus, at least one left a particularly vivid picture of the effects upon a patient of a disease to which he gave that name. Describing a case he had encountered in the vicinity of Niagara, Lovell wrote:

In the course of the 4th week, a small circumscribed spot of inflammation shewed itself in the face, generally, near the angle of the mouth. In a few days, the side of the face swelled; this tumour was very hard and pale, resembling the colour of a white swelling of the joints. It was not in the seat of the parotid gland but anterior to the branch of the lower jaw, and was attended with a most profuse and fetid salivation . . . . In a few days more, the red spot began to assume a vivid appearance, and symptoms of incipient mortification. In a short time the mouth was literally extended from ear to ear, exposing the backmost grinders on both sides.

Lovell ruled out the use of mercury as a cause of this horrible disfigurement, pointing out that "in the majority of these cases, not a particle of mercury had been used in any form." [38]

The treatment of whatever diseases might have been included in the term "typhus" varied. Lovell noted that militia doctors in the summer of 1814 treated it by blistering "the patient almost from the crown of his head to the soles of his feet; so that the chief difficulty was to remove the irritative fever induced by this *empirical, slovenly* practice." Some physicians also placed great reliance upon mercurial medicines [39] and still others upon the use of leeches and cupping, although they might believe that venesection itself was harmful and had in some instances "destroyed patients." [40]

When treating fevers described as intermittents, Mann resorted to bleeding and also reported the use of medicines other than "bark" (by which, presumably, he meant cinchona bark), including aromatics, bitters, wine, snakeroot, and arsenic compounds; Lovell commented that he had been unsuccessful in the use of bark against a tertian form of intermittent. Mann also failed to relieve tertian intermittents with bark except when the patient was already convalescent, although he had used "an arsenical preparation" with this type of fever and it had "acted almost like a charm." Lovell, on the other hand, observed that intermittents which responded to arsenicals in 1813 had not done so in 1814.[41] The question of the best drugs and dosages to use against malaria was to be taken up by the department and thoroughly studied with the aid of data collected from surgeons in the field after the permanent organization of the department in 1818.

By mid-1817, however, intermittents were for some reason no longer being seen with any frequency in the North except in the new 5th Military Department and particularly Detroit. Lovell's report of 30 June 1817 listed 164 cases of intermittent fevers in the North, of which 141 were in the 5th Military Department, 120 in Detroit itself. In the same report, Lovell listed 266 cases of inflammatory fevers, including colds and pleurisy, "which no *ordinary* care can prevent." [42]

Among other conditions mentioned in the records of this period was epilepsy, which Mann treated at Burlington with nitrate of silver. He concluded that "By this medicine alone, the morbid action, which constituted the disease, was entirely subdued." [43] Mumps also appeared from time to time in the Army, and on one occasion Hanson Catlett maintained that it had been brought on by "exposure to severe cold weather, & storms of snow & rain, which we have had for some days past" at Fredericksburg, Virginia. Catlett maintained that mumps might prove fatal on this occasion unless the men were moved to drier quarters.[44]

On some occasions, Army surgeons used autopsies to further their understanding of the diseases they were encountering. Waterhouse recorded that postmortems on patients who died of dysentery showed him small ulcers all along the lining of the victim's intestines. He concluded, as a result, that dysentery *"is to the intestines what smallpox is to the skin."*[45] Mann described many autopsies done in late 1812, in 1813, and in early 1814 upon patients who died from the prevalent "pneumonia notha."[46]

By the end of the War of 1812, some surgeons who had cared for troops in that period were beginning to have reservations about a number of the remedies used. Opium, of course, was suspect because of its potential for causing "an interruption of the natural actions of the small intestines." Since it "corrects nothing, expels nothing; and only assuages and benumbs," opium was apparently not highly regarded.[47] Sugar of lead, however, "was, at one time, a fashionable remedy among the surgeons of the army for chronic diarrhea." Surgeon Henry Huntt was familiar with a patient who used this remedy extensively for the better part of a year. Over that period the victim slowly developed constipation, loss of appetite, "profuse perspirations," an abscess on one leg, an ulcer on the other, and ever more violent pain. Before death brought release, he had become completely paralyzed. Although Mann noted that sugar of lead, like opium, could also lead to dropsy, Huntt placed the blame for its adverse effects not so much upon the medicine itself as upon its use in a fickle climate.[48]

The need for care in the use of mercurial compounds was now also recognized by at least some Army surgeons, since misuse could lead to the "destruction of not only the muscles, but the bones of the face." Mann recorded "Four cases, under these formidable effects of mercurial ptyalism" who were admitted to the Lewiston general hospital. Of these, three died with their jaws and faces dreadfully mutilated.

The fourth recovered, but with the loss of the inferior maxilla on one side and the teeth on the other. "He lived a most wretched life . . . incapable of taking food, except through a small aperture in place of his mouth." Mann doubted, furthermore, that calomel administered during a campaign ever completely cured syphilis. He suggested that it should be used only after the troops had entered winter camp, since, if carelessly used in the field, it was "frequently injurious to the bowels." It should never be given to patients "when exposed to cold and moisture," since if the skin could not be kept warm, "either the bowels or the glands of the mouth suffered."[49]

Reservations concerning such time-honored remedies as the antimonials and venesection were also now being expressed. Mann urged that the former not be used when the men were being sheltered from changeable weather in tents, and Waterhouse pointed out that although "If a thick muscular part is inflamed, we can, at once, remove that inflammation, by taking off its tension, by bleedings," "if the mucous membrane, lining any internal cavity, more especially of the intestine, be inflamed, we cannot take off its tension by bleeding, without hazarding life."[50]

The Army's physicians of the early nineteenth century did not often comment on their experiences in the field of surgery. Apparently little surgery was performed outside the areas of major military activity; in the 3d Military District during the entire war only two amputations and one operation for the correction of hydrocele were recorded. When surgery, such as the setting of broken bones, became necessary at posts where there was no surgeon, the procedure might well be done by someone without any training whatever. Mann was very much concerned about the quality of the surgery which Army surgeons were performing and urged that his colleagues pay particularly close attention to the work of the famous

French military surgeon, Dominique Larrey.[51]

One surgeon, W. E. Horner, in the 9th Military District where most of the action of the War of 1812 took place, wrote a series of articles on the surgical cases he had encountered and the conclusions he had drawn from them. He noticed, for example, that buckshot wounds rarely proved dangerous unless a vital organ was hit and that bullet injuries which hit neither bones nor the "great cavities" also did not usually pose a great problem. He believed that the large size of English musket balls made amputation necessary when one of the "large cylindrical bones" was hit.[52]

Major amputations posed a number of further problems. The onset of hot weather greatly decreased the patient's chances for survival; mortification quickly set in, muscles retracted to an unusual degree, and many patients died. There was still considerable debate over the advisability of postponing amputations. Horner believed that if a patient did not have to be moved, it might be wise not to inflict the shock of amputation upon a man still suffering from the shock resulting from his wounding. Indeed, if a limb had been torn off, something could be said, he maintained, in favor of letting nature take care of the situation, since "by her law if a bone protrudes beyond the limit of its covering by muscles and skin, she in a few weeks, reduces its length to the proper mark by the process of exfoliation."[53]

Horner was familiar, however, with Larrey's preference for immediate amputation and credited the French surgeon as well as his English colleagues with the preference Americans showed in favor of early operation, even when they were familiar with instances during the War of 1812 when the survival rate among those whose amputations were temporarily postponed was higher than that among those whose surgery was performed at the first possible moment.[54]

Among those undergoing amputation who were discussed by Horner was one patient who greatly puzzled him. This soldier underwent the excruciating procedure with complete serenity, "smoking tranquilly during the whole operation; his ease not seeming to be an affectation," while his leg was removed.[55]

Several physicians with experience gained in the War of 1812 criticized the plan developed for a military hospital by Tilton during the Revolution. *(See Chapter 5.)* Surgeon William Barton was vigorously opposed to Tilton's design and, in a "treatise on various types of military hospitals," ridiculed Tilton's notion that earth floors and a center fireplace without a chimney would reduce the spread of disease. He maintained that wooden floors were entirely safe if kept clean and thickly covered with sand and added that he did "not think any plan was ever conceived, so fraught with mischief as this; and which certainly does not reflect either credit upon the inventor's ingenuity or discernment." Barton was apparently unaware of the existence of Tilton-type huts at Brownville, New York, where the surgeon in charge was quite pleased with the design, and at least one other site, for he claimed that "not withstanding the elevated rank of Dr. Tilton during the war, his plan was never adopted by a single surgeon."[56] There is no evidence, however, that Tilton ever attempted during the War of 1812 to have such a hut constructed.

Mann's experiences in the War of 1812 led to criticism of the Tilton plan which was milder than that of his outspoken colleague. He agreed that it was desirable that a hospital, particularly a temporary one, be only one story high, making proper sanitation easier and eliminating possible disturbance from footsteps overhead, but he disagreed with his superior on many other aspects of hospital design. Wood floors were warmer than those of earth, he noted, and in hot weather tents were better than huts. The smoke which filled Tilton-style units aggravated coughs and chest problems, and unless the required lumber were standing in the immediate vicinity, obtaining logs needed for the Tilton units could be very expensive.[57]

As Mann envisioned it, a military hospital should have windows on the east and west and, "On the west, a closed passage should extend the length of the hospital 12 feet wide, into which the doors of the several wards open." This passage would shield the western windows from the summer heat. Within the building, each separate ward should be thirty feet by twenty-four feet in size and thus large enough to hold twenty patients, with ceilings at least eleven feet high. Since ventilation without drafts was of great importance, hospital windows should be double-sashed. Each ward would require the attention of two nurses, unless more were required to handle the cooking. Wards for patients with contagious diseases should contain fewer patients than other wards, surgical patients should be kept separate from those with fevers, and men with either venereal disease or scabies should be kept away from all others. There should also be a separate room where patients about to be admitted could be washed with tepid water and dressed in clean linen.[58]

Mann pointed out that while the medical staff of each army on the move should be prepared to set up a field hospital and to provide transportation to this facility for its patients, each permanent hospital should have its own separate staff. In the temporary hospital, instead of the customary bunks, Mann suggested the use of "canvas bed-bottoms, constructed with loops on the side, through which pass poles for their support. The bed-bottoms are supported by stakes drove into the earth with a fork on the top to support the poles, to which the bottoms are attached. These beds may be put up in a few minutes."[59]

Mann urged also the keeping of systematic hospital records concerning patients and prescriptions, but he pointed out that, except for the Burlington hospital in the winter of 1813–14, this was not generally done. Lovell, in his report of June 1817, went even further than Mann and urged that hospital surgeons and mates also keep careful records of weather and local climate;[60] he would later, as head of the department, require this of them.

In his *Medical Sketches* which appeared in 1816, Mann discussed not only the problems of the individual military hospital but also those of the Army Medical Department as a whole. Since his opinions were generally well received by his colleagues, it is likely that they agreed with the emphasis he placed upon the need for preparing for the medical care of the nation's soldiers before the outbreak of war and also with his plea for increased stature for the Army's surgeons.[61]

Throughout the period from 1775 to 1818, the inability to plan ahead on a long-range basis to meet the needs of the Army's sick and wounded had forced the Medical Department to function in an inefficient and, too often, ineffectual manner, handicapped by a lack of supplies and housing and by surgeons who were to varying degrees unresponsive to discipline. In addition, innumerable opportunities to evaluate the effectiveness of various forms of treatment on a wholesale basis and thus to advance the state of the art of medicine were lost because of the lack of a permanent organization to plan and conduct such studies.

The lessons so painfully learned in two wars and a host of Indian skirmishes finally became too obvious to ignore. As the new nation expanded with great rapidity and Army units took up their duties increasingly far from Washington, an ever greater need arose to attract into the Army and train physicians qualified and willing to work in isolated areas on a permanent basis. To attract and supervise such a staff and to plan and coordinate not only the care of military patients but also the highly valuable studies Army surgeons would in the future conduct, a permanent central organization was necessary. The establishment of the Army Medical Department on a permanent basis in April 1818 was, therefore, a vital step toward making the best care possible available to all the sick and wounded of the United States Army.

Appendixes

APPENDIX A
SOME INFLUENTIAL DOCTORS IN THE CONTINENTAL HOSPITAL DEPARTMENT, 1775 TO 1783

Name	Highest Responsibility	Education/Experience
Benjamin Church	Director General	Studied medicine in London
John Morgan	Director General	M.D. from Edinburgh, further medical studies in England and Europe, surgeon in French and Indian War
William Shippen, Jr.	Director General	M.D. from Edinburgh, further medical studies in England
John Cochran	Director General	Apprentice-trained in England, surgeon's mate in French and Indian War
Benjamin Rush	Physician General	M.D. from Edinburgh
Malachi Treat	Physician General, Chief Hospital Physician	Professor of Medicine at King's College
Ammi R. Cutter	Physician General	Served with British at Louisburg and in Indian frontier wars with rangers
William Brown	Physician General	M.D. from Edinburgh
Walter Jones	Physician General	M.D. from Edinburgh
Charles McKnight	Surgeon General, Chief Hospital Physician	Private student of William Shippen, Jr.
Philip Turner	Surgeon General	Assistant surgeon to provincial regiment under General Amherst at Ticonderoga
Jonathan Potts	Deputy Director General	Studied medicine at Edinburgh, M.D. from Philadelphia
Samuel Stringer	Director of Hospital in North	Served in British Army
James Craik	Chief Physician and Surgeon General of the Army	Trained at Edinburgh, served in French and Indian War
Peter Dott Fayssoux	Chief Physician and Surgeon General of Southern Department	Medical education at Edinburgh
Hugh Williamson	Surgeon to the North Carolina militia	Medical education at Edinburgh and London, M.D. from Utrecht
Bodo Otto	In charge of Yellow Springs hospital	Medical education in Europe
James Tilton	In charge of various hospitals, including that at Trenton	Graduate of Philadelphia

SOURCES: Gordon, *Aesculapius*, pp. 42, 47, 95, 127, 216, 304, 369, 374, 417, 476; Major, *History of Medicine*, 2: 718, 721–22; Butterfield, *Letters of Rush*, 1: 108n, 163n, 177n; Sydney H. Carney, Jr., "Some Medical Men in the Revolution," *Magazine of History* 21 (1915): 185; Duncan, *Medical Men*, p. 84; Brown, *Medical Department*, pp. 40, 41, 42, 43, 44, 47, 60.

Appendix B
Law of 27 July 1775

The Congress took into consideration the report of the committee on establishing an hospital, and the same being debated, was agreed to as follows:

That for the establishment of an hospital for an army consisting of 20,000 men the following officers and other attendants be appointed, with the following allowance or pay, viz.

1 Director general and chief physician, his pay per day	4 dollars
4 Surgeons, per diem, each	1 1/3 do.
1 Apothecary	1 1/3 do.
20 Mates, each	2/3 do.
1 Clerk	2/3 do.
2 Storekeepers, each	4 dollars per month

1 Nurse to every 10 sick, 1/15 of a dollar per day, or 2 dollars per month

Labourers occasionally.

The duty of the above officers: viz.

Director to furnish medicines, Bedding and all other necessaries, to pay for the same, superintend the whole, and make his report to, and receive orders from the commander in chief.

Surgeons, apothecary and mates: To visit and attend the sick and the mates to obey the orders of the physicians, surgeons and apothecary.

Matron: To superintend the nurses, bedding, etc.

Nurses: To attend the sick, and obey the matron's orders.

Clerk: To keep accounts for the director and storekeepers.

Storekeeper: To receive and deliver the bedding and other necessaries by order of the director . . . .

The Congress then proceeded to the choice of officers for the Hospital, when

Benjamin Church was unanimously elected as director of, and chief physician in, the hospital.

Resolved, That the appointment of the four Surgeons and the Apothecary be left to Doctr. Church.

That the Mates be appointed by the Surgeons; that the number do not exceed twenty; that the number be not kept in constant pay, unless the sick and wounded should be so numerous as to require the attendance of twenty, and to be diminished as circumstances will admit; for wch. purpose, the pay is fixed by the day, that they may only receive pay for actual service.

That one Clerk and two storekeepers and one nurse to every 10 sick be appointed by the Director.

SOURCE: Ford, *Journals of the Continental Congress,* 2: 209–10, 211.

Appendix C
Law of 17 July 1776

The Congress took into consideration the report of the Committee on the memorial of the director general of the American hospital; Whereupon,

Resolved, That the number of hospital surgeons and mates be increased, in proportion to the augmentation of the army, not exceeding one surgeon and five mates to every five thousand men, to be reduced when the army is reduced, or when there is no further occasion for such a number:

That as many persons be employed in the several hospitals, in the quality of store keepers, stewards, managers, and nurses, as are necessary for the good of the service, for the time being, to be appointed by the directors of the respective hospitals:

That the regimental chests of medicines, and chirurgical instruments, which are now, or hereafter shall be, in the possession of the regimental surgeons, be subject to the inspection and inquiry of the respective directors of hospitals, and the director general; and that the said regimental surgeons shall, from time to time, when thereto required, render account of the said medicines and instruments to the said directors, or if there be no director in any particular department, to the director general; the said accounts to be transmitted to the director general, and by him to this Congress; and the medicines and instruments not used by any regimental surgeon to be returned when the regiment is reduced, to the respective directors, and an account thereof rendered to the director general and by him to this Congress:

That the several directors of hospitals, in

the several departments, and the regimental surgeons, where there is no director, shall transmit to the director general regular returns of the number of surgeons' mates and other officers employed under them, their name and pay; also an account of the expenses and furniture of the hospital under their direction; and that the director general make a report of the same, from time to time, to the commander in chief and to this Congress.

That the several regimental and hospital surgeons, in the several departments, make weekly returns of the sick to the respective directors in their departments:

That no regimental surgeon be allowed to draw upon the hospital of his department, for any stores except medicines and instruments: and that, when any sick person shall require other stores, they shall be received into said hospital, and the rations of the said sick persons be stopped, so long as they are in said hospitals, and that the directors of the several hospitals report to the commissary the names of the sick, when received into, and when discharged from the hospitals, and make a like return to the Board of Treasury:

That all extra expences for bandages, old linen, and other articles necessary for the service, incurred by any regimental surgeon, be paid by the director of that department, with the approbation of the commander thereof:

That no more medicines belonging to the continent be disposed of, till further order of Congress:

That the pay of the hospital surgeons be increased to one dollar and two thirds of a dollar by the day; the pay of the hospital mates to one dollar by the day; and the pay of the hospital apothecary to one dollar and two-thirds of a dollar by the day; and that the hospital surgeons and mates take rank of regimental surgeons and mates:

That the director general, and the several directors of hospitals, be empowered to purchase, with the approbation of the commanders of the respective departments, medicines and instruments for the use of their respective hospitals, and draw upon the paymaster for the same, and make the report of such purchases to Congress.

SOURCE: Ford, *Journals of the Continental Congress*, 5: 568–71.

APPENDIX D
LAW OF 7–8 APRIL 1777

Resolved, That there be one director general of all the military hospitals which shall be erected for the continental army in the United States, who shall particularly superintend all the hospitals between Hudson and Potowmack rivers:

That there be one deputy director general, who, in the absence of the director general, shall superintend the hospitals to the eastward of Hudson's river:

That there be one deputy director general, who, in the absence of the director general, shall superintend the hospitals in the northern department:

That when the circumstances of the war shall require it, there be one deputy director general, who in the absence of the director general, shall superintend the hospitals in the southern department:

That the director general, or, in his absence, the deputy director general in each respective department, be empowered and required, with the advice and consent of the commander in chief therein, to establish and regulate a sufficient number of hospitals, at proper places, for the reception of the sick and wounded of the army, to provide medicines, instruments, dressings, bedding, and other necessary furniture, proper diet, and every thing requisite for the sick and wounded soldiers, and the officers of the hospitals; to pay the salaries and all other expences of the same:

That there be assistant deputy directors, to superintend the hospitals committed to their care, and assist in providing the articles before specified, under the orders and controul of the director or deputy director general of the respective districts:

That there be one apothecary general for each district, whose duty it shall be, to receive, prepare, and deliver medicines, and other articles of his department to the hospitals and army, as shall be ordered by the director general, or deputy directors general, respectively:

That the apothecaries [general] be allowed as many mates as the director general, or respective deputy director generals, shall think necessary:

That there be a commissary of the hospitals in each of the aforesaid districts, whose duty it shall be, to procure, store, and deliver provisions, forage, and such other articles as the director, or deputy director general shall judge necessary for the use of the hospitals; in the purchase of which, he shall frequently consult with the commissary and quarter master general, and be regulated by the prices which they give:

That the commissary be allowed such assistants and store keepers, as the director general, or deputy director general of the district, shall judge necessary:

That a steward be allowed for every hundred sick or wounded, who shall receive provisions from the commissary, and distribute them agreeable to the orders of the director general, or in his absence, of the deputy director general, or physician, or surgeon general, and be accountable to the commissary for the same:

That a matron be allowed to every hundred sick or wounded, who shall take care that the provisions are properly prepared; that the wards, beds, and utensils be kept in neat order, and that the most exact oeconomy be observed in her department:

That a nurse be allowed for every ten sick or wounded, who shall be under the direction of the matron:

That an hostler or stabler be allowed to each hospital, to receive the horses from the commissary, and to take care of the waggon, and other horses belonging to the hospital, pursuant to orders from the director general, or, in his absence, the deputy director general, or such other officer as he shall appoint:

That there be a clerk in each district, whose business it shall be, to keep the accounts of the hospitals, and to receive and deliver the monies agreeable to the orders of the director or deputy director general:

That a sufficient number of assistant clerks be allowed:

That such officers and soldiers as the general shall order to guard the hospitals and to conduct such as shall be weekly discharged the hospitals, to their respective regiments, shall, while on this duty, obey the director or deputy director general, or the physicians and surgeons general;

That the director and deputy directors general be respectively empowered to appoint and discharge their assistant deputy directors, and other said officers and attendants of the hospitals, in such numbers as the necessities of the army may require, and the commander in chief of the department shall, in writing, approve; report of which to be immediately made to Congress, as hereafter directed:

That there be also one physician and one surgeon general in each district, to be appointed by Congress, whose duty it shall be, respectively, to superintend the practice of physic and surgery in all the hospitals of the district to which they shall be appointed, and, in the absence of the director or deputy director general, they shall have power to order the physicians, surgeons, and other officers of the several hospitals, to such duty as they shall think proper, and shall report weekly to the director general, or, in his absence, to the deputy director general, or, in his absence, to the assistant deputy director, the state and number of the sick and wounded in the hospitals, and the delinquent officers of the same, and see that such, as may be fit, shall be delivered every week to the officer of the guard, to be conducted to the army:

That there be allowed, also, senior physicians and surgeons, who shall attend, prescribe for, and operate upon, and see properly treated, such sick and wounded, as shall be allotted them by the director general, deputy director general, or assistant director, or physician, or surgeon general; the number for the district to be determined by the director or deputy director general, and appointed by the surgeon and physician general:

That there be also such a number of second surgeons as the director or deputy director general for the district shall judge necessary, to assist the senior surgeons, and be under the same direction, and to be appointed by the physician and surgeon general as aforesaid:

That there be also such a number of mates as the director general or deputy director general of the district shall direct, who shall assist the surgeons in the care of the wounded, and see that the medicines are properly and regularly administered, and appointed in the manner before directed for senior and second surgeons:

That a suitable number of covered and other waggons, litters and other necessaries for removing the sick and wounded, shall be supplied by the quarter master or deputy quarter master general, and in cases of their deficiency, by the director or deputy director general:

That there be one physician and surgeon general for each separate army, who shall be subject to the orders and controul of the director general and deputy director general of the district wherein he acts: That his duty shall be, to superintend the regimental surgeons and their mates, and to see that they do their duty, to hear all complaints against the said regimental surgeons and mates, and make report of them to the director general, or, in his absence, to the deputy director, or, in their absence, from the said army, to the commanding officer thereof, that they may be brought to trial by court martial for misbehavior; to receive from the director general or deputy director general, a suitable number of large strong tents, beds, bedding, medicines, and hospital stores, for such sick and wounded persons as cannot be removed to the general hospital with safety, or may be rendered fit for duty in a few days; and shall also see that the sick and wounded, while under his care, are properly attended, and dressed and conveyed, when able, to the general hospital, for which last purpose he shall be supplied by the director general, or deputy director, with a proper number of convenient waggons and drivers:

That each physician and surgeon general of the armies shall appoint such a number of surgeons, nurses, and orderly men, as the director general or deputy director general shall judge necessary for the more effectual care and relief of the sick and wounded, under the care of such physician and surgeon general as provided in the last foregoing section; and the said physician and surgeons general shall have under them, in each army, a steward to receive, and properly dispense such articles of diet as the director general, or deputy director general shall give, or order to be given him by the commissary of the army or hospital:

That whenever any regimental surgeon or mate shall be absent from his regiment without leave from the said surgeon general, or the commander in chief of the army where his duty lies, the said surgeon general shall have power to remove such surgeon or mate, and forthwith to appoint another in his stead:

That the director, deputy directors, physicians, and surgeons general, and all other officers before enumerated, shall be tried by a court martial for any misbehaviour, or neglect of duty, as the commander in chief of the several armies shall direct:

That the physician and surgeon general of each army, shall cause daily returns to be made to him, of all the sick and wounded, which have been removed to the hospitals, all that remain in the hospital tents, all that are become fit for duty, all that are convalescent, and all who may have died, specifying the particular maladies under which the sick and wounded labour:

That the said physicians and surgeons general shall cause weekly returns of the same to be made to the director or deputy director general respectively:

That the physicians and surgeons general of the hospitals, cause like daily returns to be made in every hospital, and the like weekly returns to their respective directors, *mutatis mutandis;*

That the deputy directors general cause the like returns to be made, once every month, to the director general, together with the names and denominations of all the officers in the respective hospitals.

And that the director general make a like return for all the hospitals and armies of these United States, once every month, to the Medical Committee:

That the Medical Committee have power to appoint any of their members to visit and inspect all or any of the medical departments, as often as they shall think proper, to enquire into the conduct of such general officers of the hospital as shall be delinquent in this or any parts of their duty, and to report their names to Congress, with the evidence of the charges, which shall be brought against them. . . .

Resolved, That in time of action and on any other emergency, when the regimental surgeons are not sufficient in number to attend properly to the sick and wounded, that cannot be removed to the hospitals, the director, or deputy director general of the district, be empowered and required, upon the request of the physician and surgeon general of the army, to send, from the hospitals under his care, to the assistance of such sick and wounded, as many physicians and surgeons as can possibly be spared from the necessary business of the hospitals.

That the director, deputy directors general, assistant deputy directors, physicians and surgeons general, be, and they are hereby required and directed to employ such parts of their time, as may conveniently be spared from the duties before pointed out to them, in visiting and prescribing for the sick and wounded of the hospitals under their care.

That the establishment of the medical department be as follows:

1 director general,	6 dollars a day and 9 rations	
3 deputy directors general,	5 do.	6 do.
Indeterminate assistant deputy director,	3 do.	6 do.
4 physicians general and 4 surgeons general each,	5 do.	6 do.
1 to each army, physician and surgeon general of the army,	5 do.	6 do.
Senior Surgeons,	4 do.	6 do.
Second Surgeons,	2 do.	4 do.
Surgeons' mates,	1 1/3 do.	2 do.
Apothecaries general,	3 do.	6 do.
Mates,	1 1/3 do.	2 do.
Commissary,	2 do.	4 do.
Clerk, who is to be pay master,	2 do.	4 do.
Assistant clerks,	2/3 do.	1 do.
Stewards,	1 do.	2 do.
Matron,	1/2 do.	1 do.
Nurses,	24–90	1 do.
Stabler,	1 do.	1 do.
Regimental surgeons,	2 do.	4 do.
Ditto, mates	1 1/3 do.	2 do.

Ordered, That the regulations respecting hospitals be published.

SOURCE: Ford, *Journals of the Continental Congress,* 7: 231–37, 244–46.

APPENDIX E
LAW OF 6 FEBRUARY 1778

Congress took into consideration the report of the committee to whom the letters from Dr. Shippen, Dr. Rush, and others were committed; and thereupon came to the following resolutions:

For the better regulating the hospitals of the United States,

Resolved, That there be a deputy director general for the hospitals between Hudson and Potomack rivers; and that the superintending care of the director general be extended equally over the hospitals in every district, and that he be excused from the duty of providing supplies, when the deputy director general shall be ready to enter upon the office:

That the several officers of the hospitals shall cease to exercise such of their former powers as are herein assigned to other officers thereof:

That in the absence of the director general from any district, the physician general and surgeon general shall hereafter determine the number of hospitals to be provided by the deputy director general for the sick and wounded, and shall superintend and control the affairs of such hospitals:

That the director general shall consult with the physician general and surgeon general in each district, about the supplies necessary for the hospitals, and shall give orders in writing to the deputy director general thereof to provide the same; and, in the absence of the director general, the physician general and surgeon general shall issue such orders:

That each deputy director general shall appoint one or more of the assistant deputy directors, under him, to the sole business of providing beds, furniture, utensils, hospital cloathing, and such like articles; and shall appoint one or more to provide medicines, instruments, dressings, herbs, and necessaries of a similar kind:

That the director general shall frequently visit the hospitals in each district, and see that the regulations are carried into effect; shall examine into the number and qualifications of the hospital officers, report to Congress any abuses that may have taken place, and discharge the supernumerary officers, if there be any, that all unnecessary expence may be saved to the public; and when the director general is in any particular district, the physician general and surgeon general in that district shall not appoint any officers without his consent:

That, on the settlement of hospital accounts, the officers entrusted with public money shall produce vouchers to prove the expenditure, and receipts from the proper officers of the hospitals, specifying the delivery of the stores and other articles purchased; and the apothecaries, mates, stewards, matrons, and other officers, receiving such stores and other articles, shall be accountable for the same, and shall produce vouchers for the delivery thereof from such officers, and according to such forms as the physicians general and surgeons general have directed, or shall, from time to time, direct; which forms and directions the physicians and surgeons general shall report to the Board of Treasury:

That the director general, or, in his absence from the district, the physician general, and surgeon general, shall appoint a ward master for each hospital, to receive the arms, accoutrements and cloathing of each soldier admitted therein, keeping entries of, and giving receipts for such articles, which, on the recovery of the soldier, shall be returned to him, or, in case of his death, the arms and accoutrements shall be delivered to the commissary or deputy commissary of military stores, and receipts be taken for the same; and the ward master shall receive and be accountable for the hospital cloathing; and perform such other services as the physician general or the surgeon general shall direct:

That the physicians general and surgeons general shall hereafter make no returns to the deputy directors general, but the returns shall be made by the said officers respectively to the director general, who shall carefully transmit copies of each with his monthly return to Congress, and suspend such of the officers aforesaid as neglect this or any other part of their duty, and shall report their names to Congress:

That the director and deputy directors general forthwith prepare their accounts, and adjust them with the commissioners of claims, at the Board of Treasury.

That four dollars a day, and the former allowance of rations, be hereafter allowed to each assistant deputy director and the commissary of the hospitals in each district; and one dollar a day, and two rations, to each ward master:

Resolved, That Dr. Potts be called from the northern district, and appointed to act as deputy director general in the middle district.

Resolved, That the eldest assistant deputy director in the northern district shall execute the office of the deputy director general in the said district, until the further orders of Congress:

That the salaries of the hospital officers and debts contracted for the hospitals of the middle district to the time of Dr. Potts's entering upon the office of deputy director general therein, shall be adjusted and paid by the director general, who shall deliver all the public stores in his possession to the deputy director general or his order, taking duplicate receipts for the same, and transmitting one of each to the Board of Treasury; and the same rule shall be observed by Dr. Potts with respect to the salaries and debts of the hospitals of the northern district, and the public stores thereof, which are to be delivered to his successor in office in that district.

SOURCE: Ford, *Journals of the Continental Congress,* 10: 128–31.

APPENDIX F
LAW OF 30 SEPTEMBER 1780

Whereas, the late regulations for conducting the affairs of the general hospital are in many respects defective; and it is necessary that the same be revised and amended, in order that the sick and wounded may be properly provided for and attended, and the business of the hospitals conducted with regularity and oeconomy; therefore,

Resolved, That there be one director of the military hospitals, who shall have the general direction and superintendance of all the hospitals to the northward of North Carolina; that, within the aforesaid limits, there be three chief hospital physicians, who shall also be surgeons; one chief physician, who shall also be a surgeon, to each seperate army; fifteen hospital physicians, who shall also be surgeons; twenty surgeons mates for the hospitals; one purveyor, with one assistant; one apothecary; one assistant apothecary; and to each hospital a steward, matron, orderly men and nurses, as heretofore:

That the director, or, in his absence, one of the chief hospital physicians, be empowered and required, with the advice and consent of the Commander in Chief, or commander of a seperate army, to establish and regulate such a number of hospitals, at proper places, for the reception of the sick and wounded of the army, as may be found necessary:

That the director be authorised and instructed to enjoin the several chief hospital physicians, and other officers of the hospitals under his superintendance, to attend at such posts or stations as he may judge proper, and also to attend and perform such duties, at any post or place, as a change of the position of the army, or other circumstances, may from time to time make necessary, and shall be required by the Commander in Chief; and that, in case of any dispute concerning their seniority or precedence, the director shall determine the same in the first instance, the party supposing himself aggrieved being at liberty to appeal for redress to the Medical Committee.

That in time of action, and on any other emergency, when the regimental surgeons are not sufficient in number to attend properly to the sick and wounded that cannot be removed to the hospitals, the director, or, in his absence, the nearest chief hospital physician, be empowered and required, upon request of the chief physician and surgeon of the army, to send from the hospitals under his care, to the assistance of such sick and wounded, as many surgeons as can possibly be spared from the necessary business of the hospitals:

That the director, or, in his absence, two of the chief hospital physicians, shall make out and deliver, from time to time, to the purveyor, proper estimates of hospital stores, medicines, instruments, dressings, and such other articles as may be judged necessary for the use of the hospitals; also direct the apothecary or his assistant, to prepare and deliver medicines, instruments, dressings, and other articles in his possession to the hospitals and surgeons of the army and navy, as he or they may judge necessary:

That the director authorise and instruct the purveyor and apothecary to supply, for the use of the regimental surgeons, such medicines and refreshments as may be proper for the relief of the sick and wounded, before their removal to a general hospital, and to be dispensed under the care, and at the direction of the chief physician of the army:

That the director, or, in his absence, the chief hospital physicians, respectively, be empowered occasionally to employ second mates, when the number of the sick shall increase so as to make it necessary, and to discharge them as soon as the circumstances of the sick will admit:

That the director, or, in his absence, the chief hospital physicians, respectively, shall appoint a ward master for each hospital, to receive the spare regimental cloathing, arms, and accoutrements of each soldier admitted therein, keeping entries of and giving receipts for every article received, which, when the soldier shall be discharged, shall be accounted for by the said ward master with the commanding officer of the regiment to which such soldier belonged, or the officer directed to take charge of the convalescents from the said hospital; or, in case of the death of the soldier, shall be accounted for with, and delivered to the quartermaster of the regiment to which the said soldier belonged; and the ward master shall receive and be accountable for the hospital cloathing, and perform such other services as the chief hospital physician shall direct.

That the director shall make returns of all the sick and wounded in the hospitals, once every month, to the medical committee, together with the names and ranks of all the officers and others employed in the several hospitals:

That the director be required to employ such part of his time as may be spared from the duties before pointed out to him, in visiting and prescribing for the sick and wounded of the hospitals; and that he pay particular attention to the conduct of the several officers in the hospital department, and arrest, suspend and bring to trial, all delinquents within the same:

That the duty of the chief hospital physicians shall be, to do and perform all the duties herein before enjoined them to do in the absence of the director; to receive and obey the orders of the director, made and delivered to them in writing, to superintend the practice of physick and surgery in the hospitals put under their particular care by the director, or which, by the order of the commander in chief or the commander of a seperate army, may be by them established; to see that the hospital physicians and other officers attending the same, do their duty; and make monthly returns to the director, of the state and number of the sick and wounded in the hospitals under their care; and also make returns to the director, and to the medical committee, of all delinquent officers, in order that they may be speedily removed or punished; and to take measures that all such sick and wounded as are recovered and fit for duty be delivered weekly to the officer of the guard, to be conducted to the army: when present at any hospital, to issue orders to the proper officers for supplying them with necessaries; and generally, in the absence of the director, to superintend and controul the business of such hospitals, suspend delinquent and remove unnecessary non-commissioned officers, making report to the director; and, when in their power, to attend and perform or direct all capital operations:

That the hospital physicians shall take charge of such particular hospitals as may be assigned them by the director: They shall obey the orders of the director, or in his absence, of the chief hospital physician: They shall have power to suspend officers under them, and to confine other persons serving in the hospitals under their charge, for negligence or ill-behaviour, until the matter be regularly inquired into: They shall diligently attend to the cases of the sick and wounded of the hospitals under their care, administering at all times proper relief, as far as may be in their power: They shall respectively give orders, under their hands, to the assistant purveyor or steward at the hospital, for the issuing provisions and stores, as well as for the procuring any other small articles that the exigencies of the hospital may require, and which the store is not provided with, having always a strict regard to oeconomy, as well as the welfare of the sick then to be provided for: They shall make weekly returns to the nearest chief hospital physician, of the state of the hospitals under their respective care.

The mates shall each take charge of and attend the patients assigned them and perform such other duties as shall be directed by the director, chief or other physicians and surgeons.

The chief physician and surgeon of the army shall be subject to the orders and controul of the director: His duty shall be to superintend the regimental surgeons and their mates, and to see that they do their duty: To hear all complaints against the said regimental surgeons and mates, and make report of them to the director, or, in his absence, to the Commander in Chief or commanding officer of a seperate army, that they may be brought to trial by court-martial for misbehaviour: To draw for and receive from the purveyor a suitable number of large strong tents, beds, bedding and hospital stores, and from the apothecary, or his assistant, proper medicines, for such sick and wounded persons as cannot be removed to the general hospital with safety, or may be rendered fit for duty in a short time. He shall also see that the sick and wounded, while under his care, are properly attended and provided for, and conveyed, when fit to be removed, to the general hospital; for which last purpose, he shall be supplied by the quartermaster general, with a proper number of convenient waggons and drivers; he shall have a steward, which he is to appoint, to receive and properly dispense such articles of diet and refreshment as shall be procured for the sick; and also shall appoint such a number of nurses and orderly men as may be necessary for the attendance of the sick and wounded under his care. He shall cause daily returns to be made to him of all the sick and wounded which have been removed to the hospitals, all that remain in the hospital tents, all that are become fit for duty, all that are convalescent, and all who may have died, specifying the particular maladies under which the sick and wounded labour, and shall make a monthly return thereof to the director, who shall add it to his general hospital returns, to be transmitted monthly to the Medical Committee.

That whenever any regimental surgeon or mate shall be absent from his regiment, without leave from the chief physician and surgeon or commander of the army where his duty lies, the said chief physician and surgeon shall have power to remove such surgeon or mate and forthwith appoint another in his stead.

That the purveyor provide, or cause to be provided, all hospital stores, medicines, instruments, dressings, utensils, and such other articles as shall be prescribed by the written order of the director, or two of the chief hospital physicians, and deliver, or cause the same to be delivered, upon written orders, under the hands of the director, or chief hospital physician, or one of the hospital physicians, having the charge of a particular hospital, or of a chief physician and surgeon of the army, which, with receipts thereon for delivery of the same, shall be his sufficient vouchers. He shall be allowed a clerk, and as many store keepers as occasion may require, and the director shall approve of. He shall also pay the salaries of the officers, and all other expences of the hospitals. He shall render his accounts every three months to the Board of Treasury for settlement, and make application for money to the Medical Committee, before whom he shall lay estimates of articles necessary, which shall previously have been approved and signed by the director or two of the chief hospital physicians; at the same time he shall render to them an account of the expenditure of the last sum of money advanced to him; and the said Medical Committee shall lay such estimates before Congress, with their opinion thereon:

That the assistant purveyor shall procure such supplies, and do and perform such parts of the purveyor's duty, as by him shall be particularly assigned to him.

That the apothecary and his assistant receive, prepare and deliver medicines, instruments and dressings, and such other articles of his department, to the hospitals and army, on orders in writing from the director or either of the chief hospital physicians, or chief physician and surgeon of the army; and that he be allowed as many mates as occasion may require, and the director shall approve of:

That the director, or in his absence, the chief hospital physician, shall appoint a steward for each hospital, whose duty it shall be to purchase vegetables and other small articles, under the direction of the purveyor, and to receive hospital stores from the purveyor, and provisions from the commissary general, and issue the same for the use of the sick and wounded, agreeably to the order of the physician and surgeon attending such hospital; the steward to account with the purveyor for all such issues:

That the director, or, in his absence, the chief hospital physician, appoint a proper number of matrons, nurses, and others, necessary for the regular management of the hospitals, and fix and ascertain their pay, not exceeding the sums heretofore allowed; and point out and prescribe their particular duties and employments, in writing, which they are enjoined to observe and obey:

That the director, with two chief hospital physicians, be empowered to fix the pay of second mates, and of such clerks, store keepers, and other persons, as may occasionally be employed; and also make such regulations, and point out and enjoin, in writing, such further particular duties for the several officers in the hospital department, as they may judge necessary for the regular management of the same; which duties shall always be consistent with, and in no wise contradictory to any of the duties herein before particularly enumerated, and which being reported to, and approved of by the Medical Committee, shall thereupon become obligatory to all those concerned:

That the quartermaster general furnish the hospital department, from time to time, as occasion may require, with such a number of horses and wagons as may be necessary for removing the sick and wounded, and for transporting the hospital stores; but that no other horses than those belonging to the officers of the department, for which forage may be herein allowed, be kept seperately and at the expence of the department.

That no person concerned in trade, on his own account, shall be suffered to act as an officer in the hospital or medical department of the army:

That no officer or other person in the hospital department, except the sick and wounded, be permitted to use any of the stores provided for the sick:

That the director, chief hospital physicians,

and the chief physicians and surgeons of the army, physicians and surgeons, purveyor, apothecary, assistant purveyor, and assistant apothecary, be appointed and commissioned by Congress; the regimental surgeons and mates to be appointed as heretofore:

That the director, with the advice and concurrence of two of the chief hospital physicians, appoint all hospital mates, which appointments shall be certified by warrants under the hand of the director; in which appointments no person shall be admitted under the age of twenty-one years:

That all the officers in the hospital or medical departments, shall be subjected to trial by courts-martial for all offences, in the same manner as officers of the line of the army.

Resolved, That the pay and establishment of the officers of the hospital department, and medical staff, be as follows:

Director, one hundred and fifty dollars per month, two rations for himself, and one for his servant, per day, and forage for two horses:

Chief physicians and surgeons of the army and hospitals, each, one hundred and forty dollars per month, two rations per day, and forage for two horses:

Purveyor and apothecary, each, one hundred and thirty dollars per month:

Physicians and surgeons of the hospitals, each, one hundred and twenty dollars per month, one ration per day, and forage for one horse:

Assistant purveyors and apothecaries, each, seventy-five dollars per month:

Regimental surgeons, each, sixty-five dollars per month, one ration per day, and forage for one horse:

Surgeons' mates in the hospitals, fifty dollars per month, one ration per day:

Surgeons' mates in the army, forty-five dollars per month, one ration per day:

Steward for each hospital, thirty-five dollars per month, one ration per day:

Ward master for each hospital, twenty-five dollars per month, one ration per day.

Resolved, That none of the aforesaid officers, or other persons employed in any of the hospitals, be entitled to rations of provisions or forage when on furlough.

Resolved, That the chief physician of the army be allowed a two horse covered waggon for transporting his baggage:

That the several officers abovementioned shall receive their pay in the new currency, emitted pursuant to a resolution of Congress of the 18th day of March last; and that they be allowed and paid at the rate of five dollars of said currency per month for every retained ration; and shall each be entitled annually to draw cloathing from the stores of the cloathier general, in the same manner and under the same regulations as are established for officers of the line, by a resolution of Congress of the 25th November, 1779:

That the returns for cloathing for officers in the medical staff (regimental surgeons and their mates, who are to draw with the regimental staff, excepted) be signed by the directors, or one of the chief hospital physicians; and such cloathing shall be delivered either by the cloathier general or any sub-cloathier in the state in which the officer to receive cloathing shall reside, in the same manner as is provided in the cases of other staff officers not taken from the line:

That the several officers whose pay is established as above (except the stewards and ward masters) shall at the end of the war be entitled to a certain provision of land, in the proportion following, viz.

The director to have the same quantity as a brigadier-general;

Chief physicians and purveyor, the same as a colonel;

Physicians and surgeons and apothecary, the same as a lieutenant colonel;

Regimental surgeons and assistants to the purveyor and apothecary, the same as a major;

Hospital and regimental surgeons' mates, the same as a captain;

That the former arrangements of the hospital department, and all resolutions heretofore passed touching the same, so far as they are inconsistent with the foregoing, be repealed, excepting that the hospitals in the southern department, from North Carolina to Georgia, inclusive, be continued under the same regulations as heretofore, until the further order of Congress.

SOURCE: Ford, *Journals of the Continental Congress,* 18: 878–88.

Appendix G
Hospitals Serving Washington's Army

In the period covered by Chapter 4, a large number of hospitals served General Washington's army. Among those not discussed in the text are the following: [1]

Buckingham Meeting House, Pennsylvania. On 15 November 1777, General Washington ordered the sick of his army to be sent here, but on 18 November the government of the state of Pennsylvania apparently ordered that no more sick be sent to that town. As of 24 November, the Buckingham unit contained 259 patients, 10 of these being wounded and another 10 convalescent. This unit was among those closed after the British occupation of Philadelphia.

French Creek, Pennsylvania. The hospital here was established in the winter of 1777–78 in the Lutheran Zion and German Reformed churches as well as in the parsonage they shared a few miles north of Yellow Springs. Ill will was stirred up by the arbitrary manner in which the buildings were requisitioned, but when he arrived at nearby Yellow Springs, Dr. Bodo Otto was able to smooth the matter over. The facility was still in operation in the spring of 1778, and the various components, one of which held more than 60 patients and another almost 100, were described at that time as "clean" and "airy." [2]

Lancaster, Pennsylvania. This facility seems to have been established sometime in the fall of 1777 and was the final destination of Brig. Gen. Anthony Wayne's wounded after the Paoli engagement. On 11 October 1777, the unit held 59 patients. It was apparently suffering the effects of overcrowding in late January and by early February was said to be caring for as many as 400 to 500 patients. On 26 April 1778, Brig. Gen. Lachlan McIntosh reported that 203 patients were in the hospital there, 98 had died or deserted, and 340 had been discharged since 1 January 1778. He added to his report the fact that among the latter there may have been some of the patients sent to Lancaster from Lititz.[3]

Limerick, Pennsylvania. A letter of Dr. Benjamin Rush to John Adams of 13 October 1777 mentions a hospital located here, 26 miles from Philadelphia, on the road to Reading.[4]

Manheim, Pennsylvania. A Manheim church was apparently used as a hospital and at least some medical supplies were stored in the town until March, when Shippen ordered them to be moved to Yellow Springs. Shippen reported 62 patients in this hospital on 24 November 1777, of whom 17 were sick, 5 wounded, and 40 convalescent.[5]

North Wales, Pennsylvania. Mention is made in at least one contemporary account of a hospital established in a Quaker meetinghouse on the North Wales road. Shippen reported on 24 November 1777 that there were in this unit 100 sick and 59 convalescents.[6]

Phoenixville, Pennsylvania. William Shainline Middleton, in his article "Medicine at Valley Forge," mentions a hospital located in a German Reformed church near Phoenixville in the spring of 1778.[7]

Plumstead (Plumsteadville), Pennsylvania. A report dated 10 December 1777 lists a hospital here which admitted 40 patients at the end of November, of whom by 10 December 2 had died and 10 had been discharged, leaving 28 remaining. On 19 December 1777, the patients remaining here were removed by General Washington's orders, escorted by a surgeon, to Lititz.[8]

Red Lion (Red Lyon, Lionville), Pennsylvania. The Uwchlan Quaker Meeting House here was taken over by force to be used as a hospital in the winter of 1778. A hospital was still in existence at Red Lion in June 1778 and was sheltering 127 patients as of 14 June 1778.[9]

Reamstown (Rheimstown), Pennsylvania. This unit was opened in December 1777 and closed on 17 March 1778. From 21 January to 17 March, 19 Reamstown patients either died or deserted.[10]

Schaefferstown, Pennsylvania. This unit must have been established at essentially the same time as those at Ephrata and the other towns in the same general area. General McIntosh's report on Schaefferstown covers the period 1 January 1778 to 19 April 1778 and lists 76 patients remaining as of the latter date, 7 having died or deserted in the period and 103 returned to duty.[11]

Warwick (Warrick), Pennsylvania. At least

some of the patients at this hospital were located in a Lutheran church, but General McIntosh's report of 26 April speaks of "Three Churches, Warwick." The unit was closed 7 April 1778 and its remaining two patients went to Manheim. Of the men cared for here, 41 were reported dead or deserted, 142 returned to camp.[12]

York(town), Pennsylvania. Although in late March the hospital here was reported as sheltering few patients, General McIntosh reported 23 still in this facility as of 27 April 1778 and the journal of the Rev. Dr. James Sproat implies that this facility was still open on 9 June 1778.[13]

Black River, New Jersey. A hospital existed here for at least part of the spring and summer of 1777. In June, General Washington urged the replacement of the male nurses here by women, although there is no record of whether this was actually done.[14]

Mendham, New Jersey. A hospital existed here in a barn and a church near General Washington's army at Morristown for at least several months of the winter and spring of 1778. As in the case of Black River, New Jersey, General Washington wished the male nurses here to be replaced by women.[15]

Red Bank, New Jersey. Dr. Benjamin Rush was assigned the task of opening a hospital here to care for the wounded of the Delaware River forts in November 1777. It is unlikely, however, that he was able to progress far with his task, because Fort Mifflin, across the river from Fort Mercer, was abandoned by the Americans the night of 15-16 November and Fort Mercer five days later.[16]

APPENDIX H
AN ACT TO REGULATE THE MEDICAL ESTABLISHMENT, 2 MARCH 1799

Sec. 1. Be it enacted by the Senate and House of Representatives of the United States of America in Congress assembled. That in the medical establishment of the United States there shall be the following officers: A physician-general, who shall be charged with the superintendence and direction of all military hospitals, and, generally, of all medical and chirurgical practice or service concerning the army and navy of the United States, and of all persons who shall be employed in and about the same, in camps, garrisons, and hospitals. An apothecary-general, and one or more deputies, who shall be charged with the safe keeping and delivery of all medicines, instruments, dressings, and other articles, for the use of the hospital and army. A purveyor, who shall be charged with providing medicines, stores, and whatsoever else may be necessary in relation to the said practice or service. A competent number of hospital surgeons, who shall be liable to serve in the field, and who shall have the immediate charge and direction of such military hospitals as may be committed to their care, respectively. A suitable number of hospital mates, who are to observe the directions of the hospital surgeons, and shall diligently perform all reasonable duties required of them for the recovery of the sick and wounded.

Sec. 2. And be it further enacted, That each military hospital shall have a steward, with a competent number of nurses, and other attendants; which steward shall be charged with the procuring of such supplies as may not otherwise be furnished, and with the safe keeping and issuing of all supplies.

Sec. 3. And be it further enacted, That the said physician-general, hospital-surgeons, purveyor, and apothecary or apothecaries, deputy or deputies, shall be appointed as other officers of the United States; and the said mates and stewards shall be appointed by the authority, and at the direction, of the said physician-general, subject to the eventual approbation and control of the President of the United States, and shall be removable by the authority of the said physician-general; and that the surgeon of each hospital shall appoint, employ and fix the compensations of, the nurses and other attendants of such hospital, subject to the control of the said physician-general, or the hospital surgeon, of senior appointment, with a separate army, or in a separate district.

Sec. 4. And be it further enacted, That as often as the regimental sick will not suffer by the employing of regimental surgeons or mates in the temporary or other hospitals of the United States, the physician-general, or the hospital surgeon, of senior appointment, with a separate army, or in a separate district, with the consent of the general and commander-in-chief, or the officer commanding a separate army, may require the attendance of such surgeons, or surgeon's mates, as in his opinion, can be with safety so withdrawn from their regiments.

Sec. 5. And be it further enacted, That it shall be the duty of the physician-general, with two or more hospital surgeons, to frame a system of directions relative to the description of patients to be admitted into the hospitals; to the means of promoting cleanliness in the hospitals; to the prevention of idleness, skulking, and gambling, in the hospitals; to the prevention of the spread of infectious distempers in the camps and hospitals, and the government of nurses, and all others charged with the care of the sick in camps or hospitals, subject, in the first instance, to the approbation and revision of the commander-in-chief, the commander of a separate army, or in a separate district, as the case may be, and, eventually, to the approbation and control of the President of the United States: Provided always, That the said directions, having received the sanction of the commander-in-chief, or the commander of a separate army, shall be operative, and remain in full force, unless altered or annulled by the President of the United States.

Sec. 6. And be it further enacted, That the compensations of the said several officers shall be as follows: of the physician-general, one hundred dollars pay per month, and fifty dollars per month, which shall be in full compensation for forage, rations, and travelling expenses: of the purveyor, one hundred dollars pay per month, in full compensation for his services, and all expenses: of the apothecary general, eighty dollars pay per month, and thirty dollars per month, in full compensation for forage, rations, and all expenses: of each of his deputies, fifty dollars pay per month, and sixteen dollars per month, in full compensation for forage, rations and all expenses: of each hospital surgeon, eighty dollars pay per month, and forty dollars per month, in full compensation for forage, rations, and all expenses: of each mate, thirty dollars pay per month, and twenty dollars per month, in full compensation for forage, rations, and all expenses: of each steward, twenty-five dollars pay per month, and eight dollars per month, in full compensation for forage, rations, and all expenses: Provided, That none of the officers aforesaid shall be entitled to any part of the pay or emoluments aforesaid, until they shall respectively, be called into actual service.

Sec. 7. And be it further enacted, That, for the accommodation of the sick of the army and navy of the United States, the physician-general, and hospital surgeon of senior appointment, with the approbation of the general commanding the army within the district where he shall be, shall have power to provide temporary hospitals; and the physician-general, with the approbation of the President of the United States, shall have power to provide and establish permanent hospitals.

Sec. 8. And be it further enacted, That all the said officers, and others, shall, as touching their several offices and duties, be liable to the rules and regulations for the government and discipline of the army and shall be bound to obey, in conformity with law and the usages and customs of armies, the orders and directions of the chief military officers of the respective armies, and within the respective districts in which they shall respectively serve and be.

Sec. 9. And be it further enacted. That the physician-general or, in his absence, the senior medical officer, with the approbation of the commander-in-chief, or commanding officer of a separate army, be, and hereby is, authorized and empowered, as often as may be judged necessary, to call a medical board, which shall consist of the three senior medical officers, then present, whose duty it shall be to examine all candidates for employment or promotion in the hospital department, and certify to the secretary of war the qualifications of each.

(Approved, March 2, 1799.)

SOURCE: Trueman Cross, *Military Laws of the United States; to Which is Prefixed the Constitution of the United States* (Washington: Edward de Krafft, 1825), pp. 96–99.

APPENDIX I
LEGISLATION CONCERNING THE U.S. ARMY MEDICAL DEPARTMENT

March 1813: That, for the better superintendence and management of the hospital and medical establishment of the army of the United States, there shall be a physician and surgeon-general, with an annual salary of $2500, and an apothecary-general, with an annual salary of $1800; whose respective duties and powers shall be prescribed by the President of the United States.

[*January-March 1814:* legislation reaffirming ratio of one surgeon and two mates per regiment.]

March 1814: That, from and after the first day of June next, the officers of the army shall be entitled to waiters, agreeable to grade, as follows: . . . the physician and surgeon general, two; . . . hospital surgeon, each, one. . . .

That the President of the United States be authorized to appoint so many assistant apothecaries as the service may, in his judgment, require; each of whom shall receive the same pay and emoluments as a regimental surgeon's mate.

That the physician and the surgeon general of the army be entitled to two rations per day, and forage for two horses; and that in addition to their pay, as at present established by law, the regimental surgeons and regimental surgeons' mates be entitled to $15 per month each.

SOURCES: Callan, *Military Laws,* pp. 246, 253–55; William O. Owen, ed., *A Chronological Arrangement of Congressional Legislation Relating to the Medical Corps of the United States Army From 1785 to 1917* (Chicago: American Medical Association, 1918), pp. 10–11.

APPENDIX J
DUTIES OF MEMBERS OF THE MEDICAL DEPARTMENT, 1814

Physician and Surgeon General:
1) establish rules for management of Army hospitals and see that they are enforced;
2) appoint stewards and nurses;
3) request and receive returns of medicines, surgical instruments, hospital stores;
4) authorize, regulate supply of regimental medicine chests;
5) report twice a year on regimental medicine chests, sick in hospitals to War Department;
6) report yearly to War Department on estimated supply needs.

Apothecary General:
1) assist Physician and Surgeon General in his duties;
2) obey orders of Physician and Surgeon General.

Apothecary General and his assistants:
1) receive and manage all hospital stores, medicines, surgical instruments, dressings, bought by commissary general of purchases or his deputies;
2) account to superintendant general of military supplies for all disbursement of items under 1) above;
3) pay monthly wages of stewards, ward masters, nurses of hospital;
4) compound, prepare, and issue medicines under direction of Physician and Surgeon General or on estimates and requisitions of senior hospital surgeons and regimental surgeons;
5) regulate, under supervision of superintendant general of military supplies, forms of returns made quarterly to apothecary general's office by deputy apothecaries, surgeons, mates, or those having charge of instruments, medicine, hospital stores, hospital equipment of any kind.

Senior hospital surgeons:
1) direct medical staff in army or district to which he is attached;
2) live at or near headquarters;
3) countersign all requisitions of regimental surgeons or mates made on apothecary general or his assistants;
4) inspect hospitals under him, correcting abuses and reporting delinquencies;
5) make quarterly reports to Physician and Surgeon General on sick and wounded in his hospital and on medicines, instruments, hospital stores received, expended, on hand, and wanted;

6) keep diary of weather, medical topography of country where he is serving;

7) report to commanding officer concerning anything concerning the health of the troops.

Hospital surgeons:

1) superintend everything relating to hospital;
2) order steward to furnish whatever is needed by the sick;
3) visit sick and wounded in hospital every morning;
4) require from resident mate report on all changes since morning;
5) instruct mate in writing on care of patients;
6) have police rules of hospital displayed in each ward;
7) assign appropriate wards to patients;
8) keep register of all patients admitted;
9) keep case book of every important or interesting case of disease and report on it monthly.

Mates:

1) visit patients with surgeon, take note of his prescriptions;
2) keep case book;
3) attend to carrying out of surgeon's prescriptions;
4) dress all wounds;
5) enforce discipline;
6) one mate, at least, to remain on call;
7) responsible for medicines and instruments.

Steward:

1) receive and take charge of all hospital stores, furniture, utensils, under surgeon's direction;
2) keep accurate account of all issues;
3) responsible to Apothecary General or his assistant.

Ward master: under steward's direction:

1) receive arms, accoutrements, clothing of every patient admitted;
2) have clothes immediately washed, numbered, labeled with name, regiment, company of patient and properly stored;
3) responsible for cleanliness of wards and patients;
4) call roll every morning and evening;
5) supervise handling of closestools, seeing that they are cleaned at least three times a day and always have proper quantity of water or charcoal in them;
6) see that beds and bedding are properly aired and exposed to sun, weather permitting;
7) see that straw in each bed sack changed at least once a month;
8) see that each patient washed and has hair combed every morning;
9) see that bed and bedding of patient who has been discharged or has died is cleaned and straw burned;
10) see that nurses and attendants are kind and attentive to patients;
11) supervise all attendants.

SOURCE: Paraphrased from Palmer, *Historical Register*, 3: 7–9.

APPENDIX K
LEGISLATION AFFECTING THE ARMY MEDICAL DEPARTMENT, MARCH 1815 TO APRIL 1818

March 1815: That there shall be . . . such number of hospital surgeons and surgeon's mates as the service may require, not exceeding five surgeons and fifteen mates, with one steward and one ward-master to each hospital. [This act also reaffirmed the ratio of one surgeon and two mates for each regiment.]

April 1816: . . . and that the apothecary-general, as heretofore authorized, be allowed two assistant apothecaries.

That the medical staff shall be so extended that there shall be four hospital surgeons and eight hospital surgeon's mates, to each division, with as many post surgeons as the service may require, not exceeding twelve to each division; who shall receive the same pay and emoluments as hospital surgeon's mates. . . .

. . . and that the garrison surgeons and mates be hereafter considered as post surgeons.

April 1818: That so much of the act "fixing the military peace establishment of the United States," passed the 3d of March 1815, as relates to hospital stewards and ward-masters, and so much of the "Act for organizing the general staff, and making further provision for the army of the United States," passed April 24, 1816, as relates to hospital surgeons, hospital surgeon's mates, . . . be and the same is hereby repealed.

That there shall be one surgeon-general, with a salary of two thousand five hundred dollars per annum, one assistant surgeon-general with the emoluments of a hospital surgeon, . . . to each division . . . and that the number of post-surgeons be increased, not to exceed eight to each division.

SOURCES: Owen, *Legislation*, pp. 10–11; Callan, *Military Laws*, pp. 266, 273–76, 285.

Notes

CHAPTER 1

1. Unless otherwise indicated, this chapter is based on these secondary sources: Erwin Heinz Ackerknecht, *A Short History of Medicine* (New York: Ronald Press Co., 1955); Stanhope Bayne-Jones, *The Evolution of Preventive Medicine in the United States Army, 1607–1939* (Washington: Government Printing Office, 1968); John B. Beck, *Medicine in the American Colonies: An Historical Sketch of the State of Medicine in the American Colonies, From Their First Settlement to the Period of the Revolution* (orig. printed Albany, N.Y., 1850; Albuquerque, N. Mex.: Horn & Wallace Publishers, 1966); Whitfield Jenks Bell, Jr., "Medical Practice in Colonial America," *Bulletin of the History of Medicine* 31 (1957): 442–53; Fielding H. Garrison, *History of Medicine* (Philadelphia: W. B. Saunders Co., 1914); Maurice B. Gordon, *Aesculapius Comes to the Colonies* (Ventor, N.J.: Ventor Publishers, 1949); L. S. King, *The Medical World of the Eighteenth Century* (Chicago: University of Chicago Press, 1958); R. H. Major, *A History of Medicine* (Springfield, Ill.: Charles C Thomas, 1954); Richard Harrison Shryock, *The Development of Modern Medicine: An Interpretation of the Social and Scientific Factors Involved* (New York: Alfred A. Knopf, 1947); Richard Harrison Shryock, *Eighteenth Century Medicine in America* (Worcester, Mass.: American Antiquarian Society, 1950); Richard Harrison Shryock, *Medicine and Society in America, 1660–1860* (Ithaca, N.Y.: Cornell University Press, 1960); Richard Harrison Shryock, "Public Relations of the Medical Profession in Great Britain and the United States: 1600–1870," *Annals of Medical History*, n.s. 2 (1930): 308–39; Allen O. Whipple, *The Evolution of Surgery in the United States* (Springfield, Ill.: Charles C Thomas, 1963).

Also consulted for the preceding paragraph were: Michael Kraus, "American and European Medicine in the Eighteenth Century," *Bulletin of the History of Medicine* 8 (1940): 683–84; Lyman H. Butterfield, "Benjamin Rush: A Physician As Seen in His Letters," *Bulletin of the History of Medicine* 20 (1946): 150; George W. Corner, ed., *The Autobiography of Benjamin Rush: His "Travels Through Life" Together With His "Commonplace Book" for 1789–1813* (Princeton, N.J.: Princeton University Press, 1948), p. 362.

2. Quoted in Joseph Carson, *A History of the Medical Department of the University of Pennsylvania, From Its Foundation in 1765* (Philadelphia: Lindsay and Blakiston, 1869), p. 85; Corner, *Rush*, pp. 81–82, 362–64; Benjamin Waterhouse, *The Rise, Progress, and Present State of Medicine* (Boston: Thomas and John Fleet, 1792), pp. 15–16, 17; Samuel Miller, *A Brief Retrospect of the Eighteenth Century*, 2 vols. (New York: T. and J. Swords, 1803), 1:264–66.

3. Quoted in Shryock, *Eighteenth Century Medicine*, p. 17; O. H. Perry Pepper, "Benjamin Rush's Theories on Blood Letting After One Hundred and Fifty Years," *Transactions of the College of Physicians of Philadelphia*, 4th ser. 14 (1946): 122, 123; Nathan Smith Davis, *History of Medical Education and Institutions in the United States From the First Settlement of the British Colonies to the Year 1850* (Chicago: S. C. Griggs & Co., 1851), p. 70; Corner, *Rush*, pp. 364–65.

4. Many authors, including Bayne-Jones, erroneously refer to Pringle as Surgeon-General. John Pringle, *Observations on the Diseases in the Army, in Camp and Garrison* (London: A. Millar, D. Wilson, and T. Payne, 1752), pp. 96–98, 101–2, quote from pp. 101–2; Robert Thomas, *The Modern Practice of Physic*, 3d American ed. (New York: Collin & Co., 1815), p. 275; Charles-Edward Amory Winslow, "The Colonial Era and the First Years of the Republic (1607–1799)—The Pestilence That Walketh in Darkness," in

C.-E. A. Winslow, Wilson G. Smillie, James A. Doull, and John E. Gordon, *The History of American Epidemiology*, ed. Franklin H. Top (St. Louis: C. V. Mosby Co., 1952), pp. 21–23; David Hosack, *Observations on the Laws Governing the Communication of Contagious Diseases and the Means of Arresting Their Progress* (New York: Van Winkle and Wiley, 1815), pp. 2, 31, 34, 41; Wilson G. Smillie, *Public Health: Its Promise for the Future: A Chronicle of the Development of Public Health in the United States, 1607–1914* (New York: Macmillan Co., 1955), p. 37; Miller, *Brief Retrospect*, p. 273; John Pringle, *Six Discourses, Delivered by Sir John Pringle, Bart. . . . , To Which Is Prefixed the Life of the Author by Andrew Kippis, D. D. F. R. S. and S. A.* (London: W. Strahan and T. Cadell, 1783), p. xii.

5. D'Arcy Power, *Selected Writings: 1877–1930* (Oxford: Clarendon Press, 1931), pp. 4–5; Silas Weir Mitchell, *The Early History of Instrumental Precision in Medicine* (New Haven: Tuttle, Morehouse & Taylor, 1892), pp. 15–16, 21–23; Logan Clendening, ed., *Source Book of Medical History* (New York: Dover Publications, 1942), p. 306; Erwin Heinz Ackerknecht, *Malaria in the Upper Mississippi Valley, 1760–1900* (Baltimore: Johns Hopkins Press, 1945), pp. 7, 54; Smillie, *Public Health*, pp. 50–51; Richard Brocklesby, *Oeconomical and Medical Observations, in Two Parts, From the Year 1758 to the Year 1763, Inclusive . . .* (London: T. Becket and P. A. De Hondt, 1764), p. 212; Donald Monro, *An Account of the Diseases Which Were Most Frequent in the British Military Hospitals in Germany, From January 1761 to the Return of the Troops to England in March 1763 . . .* (London: A Millar, D. Wilson, T. Durham, and T. Payne, 1764), p. 8.

6. Pringle, *Observations*, p. 95; James Lind, *An Essay on Diseases Incidental in Europeans in Hot Climates . . .* (London: T. Becket & P. A. De Hondt, 1768), pp. 36–38; Gerhard van Swieten, *The Diseases Incident to Armies, With the Method of Cure . . . To Which Are Added: The Nature and Treatment of Gunshot Wounds, By John Ranby, Esquire, Surgeon General to the British Army . . .* (Philadelphia: R. Bell, 1776), p. 5; John Ballard Blake, "Diseases and Medical Practice in Colonial America," in "Symposium on the History of American Medicine," *International Record of Medicine* 171 (1958): 351–53; Smillie, *Public Health*, p. 43; Monro, *An Account*, pp. 265–67; Reuben Friedman, "Scabies in Colonial America," *Annals of Medical History*, 3d ser. 2 (1940): 401–2; Alfred Hess, *Scurvy, Past and Present* (Philadelphia: J. B. Lippincott Co., 1920), p. 3.

7. Blake, "Diseases," p. 356; Smillie, *Public Health*, pp. 35, 67; Mark F. Boyd, "An Historical Sketch of the Prevalence of Malaria in North America," *American Journal of Tropical Medicine and Hygiene* 21 (1941): 229; Richard Harrison Shryock, "Medical Practice in the Old South," *South Atlantic Quarterly* 29 (1930): 160–61; A. W. Ratcliffe, "The Historical Background of Malaria—a Reconsideration," *Journal of the Indiana State Medical Association* 39 (1946): 339; Robert Hamilton, *Observations on the Marsh Remittent Fever . . .* (London: T. Gillet, 1801), p. 23; Thomas, *Modern Practice*, pp. 4–6.

8. Such authors as John Duffy, Philip Cash, and Wyndham B. Blanton maintain that physicians at the time of the American Revolution could not distinguish between the two diseases, but Fielding H. Garrison and John B. Blake have noted that the disease described as "putrid, malignant" fever may have been typhus and "slow, nervous" fevers typhoid. Neil Cantlie maintains that typhus was at this time already beginning to be recognized "as a specific entity," but Lester S. King explains that although Pringle described jail or hospital fever so well that we can recognize it today as typhus, the great British military physician did not consider this illness to be a specific entity but rather believed that any putrid disease could lead to what he called jail or hospital fever. John Duffy, *Epidemics in Colonial America* (Baton Rouge: Louisiana State University Press, 1953), p. 232; Philip Cash, *Medical Men at the Siege of Boston, April 1775–April 1776 . . .* (Philadelphia: American Philosophical Society, 1973), p. 53; Wyndham Bolling Blanton, *Medicine in Virginia in the Eighteenth Century* (Richmond: Garrett & Massie, 1931), p. 258; Garrison, *History of*

Notes to Chapter 1

Medicine, pp. 292–93; Blake, "Diseases," p. 353; Neil Cantlie, *A History of the Army Medical Department*, 2 vols. (Edinburgh: Churchill Livingstone, 1974), 1: 57; King, *Medical World*, pp. 136–37.

9. Quoted in Duffy, *Epidemics*, p. 232; Brocklesby, *Observations*, p. 212; Medical Department, United States Army, *Infectious Diseases*, Internal Medicine in World War II, vol. 2 (Washington: Government Printing Office, 1963), p. 217; Monro, *An Account*, p. 8; Van Swieten, *Diseases*, p. 86.

10. Monro, *An Account*, pp. 57–58.

11. Van Swieten, *Diseases*, p. 68.

12. Monro, *An Account*, p. 57.

13. Van Swieten, *Diseases*, pp. 67–73, quotes from p. 69; John Hunter, *Observations on the Diseases of the Army in Jamaica . . .*, 3d ed. (London: T. Payne, 1808), p. 176; Thomas, *Modern Practice*, pp. 278–80; Smillie, *Public Health*, p. 43.

14. John Hunter, *A Treatise on the Venereal Disease*, abridged by William Currie (Philadelphia: Charles Cist, 1787), p. 59, quote from p. 5; Howard Lewis Applegate, "Remedial Medicine in the American Revolutionary Army," *Military Medicine* 126 (1961): 450; Smillie, *Public Health*, pp. 48–49.

15. Quoted in Brocklesby, *Observations*, pp. 286–97; Van Swieten, *Diseases*, p. 95; Thomas, *Modern Practice*, p. 502.

16. Monro, *An Account*, p. 265.

17. Quoted in van Swieten, *Diseases*, p. 100; Monro, *An Account*, pp. 266–67; Brocklesby, *Observations*, pp. 285–86; Van Swieten, *Diseases*, pp. 100–1; Ltr, Col Robert J. T. Joy, MC, to author, 25 Mar 76.

18. Van Swieten, *Diseases*, pp. 14, 19–31, quote from p. 28.

19. David Ramsay, *A Review of the Improvements, Progress and State of Medicine in the XVIIIth Century* (Charleston: W. P. Young, 1801), pp. 18–19; Lind, *An Essay*, p. 233; John Hunter, *Hunterian Reminiscences; Being the Substance of a Course of Lectures on the Principles and Practice of Surgery, Delivered by the Late Mr. John Hunter, in the Year 1785*, ed. by J. W. K. Parkinson (London: Sherwood, Gilbert, and Pepir, 1833), p. 66; Corner, *Rush*, pp. 364–65; David Harris, "Medicine in Colonial America," *California and Western Medicine* 51 (1939): 38.

20. Quoted in Beck, *Medicine*, p. 30; Francis R. Packard, "How London and Edinburgh Influenced Medicine in Philadelphia in the Eighteenth Century," *Annals of Medical History*, n.s. 4 (1932): 227–28; Theodore Diller, *Franklin's Contribution to Medicine* (Brooklyn, N.Y.: Albert T. Huntington, 1912), pp. 9–10, 20, 25, 52, 56–57; William Pepper, *The Medical Side of Benjamin Franklin* (Philadelphia: William J. Campbell, 1911), pp. 9–10, 12, 63, 72; William Buchan, *Observations Concerning the Prevention and Cure of the Venereal Disease . . .* (Dublin: P. Wogan, J. Millikin, W. Sleater, J. Rice, P. Moore, 1796), pp. 71–72; James Thacher, *American Medical Biography . . .* (Boston: Richardson & Lord and Cottons & Barnard, 1828), pp. 27–28; John Warren, *A View of the Mercurial Practice in Febrile Diseases* (Boston: T. B. Wait and Co., 1813), pp. vi–viii, 1, 4; Ramsay, *Review*, pp. 16, 19; Miller, *Brief Retrospect*, pp. 31–34.

21. Ramsay, *Review*, p. 19.

22. John Hunter, *Treatise on the Blood, Inflammation, and Gunshot Wounds* (London: John Richardson, 1794), p. 3.

23. Warren, *Mercurial Practice*, pp. 12–16.

24. Warren, *Mercurial Practice*, pp. 5, 7–8, quote from p. 42; Thacher, *Biography*, pp. 27–28; Buchan, *Venereal Disease*, pp. 68, 70.

25. Salvatore P. Lucia, *A History of Wine as Therapy* (Philadelphia: J. B. Lippincott Co., 1963), pp. 155–56; Brocklesby, *Observations*, pp. 195, 196, 223–24; Monro, *An Account*, pp. 16, 17n; Thomas, *Modern Practice*, p. 47.

26. Ramsay, *Review*, pp. 18–19.

27. Hugues Ravaton, *Chirurgie d'armée ou traité des plaies d'armées à feu* (Paris: Didot le jeune, 1768), pp. 635–36.

28. Pringle, *Observations*, pp. 128, 131–32; Monro, *An Account*, pp. 357–60; Albert A. Gore, *The Story of Our Services Under the Crown. A Historical Sketch of the Army Medical Staff* (London: Baillière, Tindall, and Cox, 1879), p. 107; Cantlie, *History*, 1: 45, 145; Van Swieten, *Diseases*, p. 13.

29. Monro, *An Account*, pp. 357–59, 361–64, 382–85, 403–6, quote from p. 395;

Brocklesby, *Observations,* pp. 27–28, 52–53; Lind, *An Essay,* p. 165; Pringle, *Observations,* pp. 131–32.

30. Ramsay, *Review,* p. 22, quote from p. 23; Pringle, *Observations,* pp. 128–32, 133–35; Lind, *An Essay,* p. 165; John Aiken, *Thoughts on Hospitals* (London: Joseph Johnson, 1771), p. 20; Stephen Hales, *A Treatise on Ventilators* (London: Manby, 1758), pp. 1–3, 14; Thomas, *Modern Practice,* pp. 283–84; Edward Cutbush, *Observations on the Means of Preserving the Health of Soldiers and Sailors . . .* (Philadelphia: Fry and Kammerer, 1808), pp. 182–84, 190–91; Robert P. Multhauf, *A Catalogue of Instruments and Models in the Possession of the American Philosophical Society* (Philadelphia: American Philosophical Society, 1961), p. 32; Monro, *An Account,* pp. 359–65, 368–69.

31. Monro, *An Account,* pp. 365–401, quote from p. 400; Peter Middleton, *A Medical Discourse, or an Historical Inquiry into the Ancient and Present State of Medicine . . .* (New York: Hugh Gaine, 1769), p. 219.

32. John Jones, *The Surgical Works of the Late John Jones, M.D.,* 3d ed., edited by James Mease (Philadelphia: Wrigley and Berriman, 1795), pp. 161–63, first quote from p. 157; Monro, *An Account,* pp. 338–39, 344–45; Cutbush, *Observations,* pp. 3–4, 55–57, 62–64; Van Swieten, *Diseases,* pp. 7, 9, second quote from p. 9; General Committee of Defense, *Observations Relative to the Means of Preserving Health in Armies,* 7 Sep 1814; Howard Lewis Applegate, "Preventive Medicine in the American Revolutionary Army," *Military Medicine* 126 (1961): 379, 381.

33. Cutbush, *Observations,* pp. 12, 14–16; Monro, *An Account,* pp. 317–18; Jones, *Works,* pp. 158, 159; Pringle, *Observations,* pp. 116–18; Applegate, "Preventive Medicine," p. 379.

34. Quoted in Jones, *Works,* p. 163; Applegate, "Preventive Medicine," pp. 380–81; Van Swieten, *Diseases,* pp. 10–11; Pringle, *Observations,* p. 113; Ramsay, *Review,* p. 33; Cutbush, *Observations,* pp. 8–11.

35. Pringle, *Observations,* p. 112; Jones, *Works,* pp. 157, 170–71.

36. Cutbush became better known after he joined the U.S. Navy as a surgeon in 1799. Jones, *Works,* pp. 168–69; Monro, *An Account,* p. 319; Cutbush, *Observations,* pp. 22–23, 24–25, 26–27, 29, 32; Van Swieten, *Diseases,* p. 8; Pringle, *Observations,* pp. 137–38.

37. Jones, *Works,* pp. 157, 167; Pringle, *Observations,* pp. 105–9; William Buchan, *Observations Concerning the Diet of the Common People . . .* (London: A. Steahan, T. Cadell, Jr., and W. Davies, J. Balfour and W. Creich, 1797), p. 7; Applegate, "Preventive Medicine," pp. 379–80; Ramsay, *Review,* pp. 31–33; Middleton, *Medical Discourse,* pp. 9–13; Monro, *An Account,* pp. 377–79; Cutbush, *Observations,* p. 38.

38. James Lind, *A Treatise of the Scurvy . . .* (Edinburgh: Sands, Murray, and Cochran for A. Kincaid & A. Donaldson, 1753), pp. 192–95, 197–202, quotes from pp. 180, 181; Blake, "Diseases," pp. 351–53; Hess, *Scurvy,* p. 3; Van Swieten, *Diseases,* p. 7.

39. Van Swieten, *Diseases,* p. 90; William Buchan, *Domestic Medicine; or, the Family Physician . . . ,* 2d American ed. (Philadelphia: Joseph Crukshank, 1774), p. 299; Miller, *Brief Retrospect,* p. 289; Ramsay, *Review,* pp. 28–30.

40. Lind, *Scurvy,* p. 182; Cutbush, *Observations,* pp. 30–31; Blanton, *Medicine,* p. 260.

41. John Morgan, *A Recommendation of Inoculation, According to Baron Dimsdale's Method* (Boston: J. Gill, 1776), pp. 3, 7, 11–12, quote from p. 11; Cantlie, *History,* 1: 140, 281; Arnold C. Klebs, "The Historic Evolution of Variolation," *Bulletin of the Johns Hopkins Hospital* 24 (1913): 71–72; Reginald H. Fitz, "Zabdiel Boylston, Inoculator, and the Epidemic of Smallpox in Boston in 1721," *Bulletin of the Johns Hopkins Hospital* 22 (1911): 316–20; Winslow, "Colonial Era," pp. 19–20; John Ballard Blake, *Public Health in the Town of Boston, 1630–1822* (Cambridge: Harvard University Press, 1959), pp. 112, 114; Thacher, *Biography,* p. 27; Lyman H. Butterfield, ed., *Letters of Benjamin Rush: Memoirs of the American Philosophical Society,* 30, parts 1 and 2, 2 vols. (Princeton: Princeton University Press, 1951), 1: 66–67; Morris C. Leikind, "Vaccination in Europe," *Ciba Symposia* 3 (1942): 1101; Maurice B. Gordon, "Medicine in Colonial New Jersey

and Adjacent Areas," *Bulletin of the History of Medicine* 17 (1945): 45–47; Benjamin Gale, "Historical Memoirs, Relating to the Practice of Inoculation for the Smallpox, in the British American Provinces, Particularly in New England," *Royal Society of London, Philosophical Transactions* 55 (1765): 194–95.

42. John Warren, A. Dexter, James Jackson, and John C. Warren, *Report on Vaccination*, n.p., 1 Jun 1808, pp. 136–38; U.S. War Department, *Subject Index, 1809–1860, General Orders, Adjutant General's Department, Subject Index of the General Orders of the War Department From 1 Jan. 1809 to 31 Dec. 1860*, comp. under direction of Brig Gen Richard C. Drum, by Jeremiah C. Allen (Washington: Government Printing Office, 1886), p. 177; Bayne-Jones, *Preventive Medicine*, p. 75; John B. Blake, *Benjamin Waterhouse and the Introduction of Vaccination, a Reappraisal* (Philadelphia: University of Pennsylvania Press, 1957), p. 62; Anthony Wayne, "General Wayne's Orderly Book," *Michigan Pioneer and Historical Society* 34 (1904): 350; Howard Dittrick, "Medical Agents and Equipment Used in the Northwest Territory," in Jonathan Forman, comp., *Physicians and the Indian Wars* (Columbus, Ohio: Ohio State Medical Association, 1953).

43. Quoted in Owsei Temkin, "The Role of Surgery in the Rise of Modern Medical Thought," *Bulletin of the History of Medicine* 25 (1951): 259.

44. Jones, *Works*, pp. 7–8, 111–13, quote from p. 11; Power, *Writings*, p. 270; Harvey Graham, *The Story of Surgery* (Garden City, N.Y.: Doubleday, Doran & Co., 1939), p. 214; Josiah Bartlett, *A Dissertation on the Progress of Medical Science in the Commonwealth of Massachusetts* (Boston: T. B. Wait and Co., 1810), p. 15.

45. Ramsay, *Review*, pp. 10–11; Allen O. Whipple, *The Story of Wound Healing and Wound Repair* (Springfield, Ill.: Charles C Thomas, 1963), p. 68; Jones, *Works*, pp. 10–11, 33–34, 40–41; Benjamin Gooch, *A Practical Treatise on Wounds and Other Chirurgical Subjects . . .* , 2 vols. (Norwich: W. Chase, 1767), 1: 193; Henri François Le Dran, *The Operations in Surgery of Mons. Le Dran*, trans. Thomas Gataker (London: C. Hitch and R. Dodsby, 1749), p. 79; "The Medical History of Louis XIV (Editorial)," *Annals of Medical History*, 1st ser. 8 (1926): 203.

46. Hunter, *Treatise on the Blood*, pp. 207–8; Jones, *Works*, pp. 36–38, 40–41; Hunter, *Reminiscences*, p. 131; Lloyd Allan Wells, "Aneurysm and Physiologic Surgery," *Bulletin of the History of Medicine* 44 (1970): 411–24; Gooch, *Treatise*, 1: 102–3.

47. Jones, *Works*, p. 33.

48. Quote from John Ranby, "The Nature and Treatment of Gunshot Wounds," in van Swieten, *Diseases*, p. 121; Hunter, *Reminiscences*, p. 65.

49. Ranby, "Gunshot Wounds," in van Swieten, *Diseases*, pp. 125, 126; Jones, *Works*, p. 140.

50. Jones, *Works*, pp. 141, 142; Van Swieten, *Diseases*, p. 94.

51. Jones, *Works*, pp. 16–17, quote from p. 30; John S. Billings, "The History and Literature of Surgery," in Frederic Shepard Dennis, ed., *System of Surgery* (Philadelphia: Lea Brothers & Co., 1895), 1: 72. Billings has termed the Petit tourniquet "an appliance of almost as much importance as the ligature"; Owen H. Wangensteen, Jacqueline Smith, and Sarah D. Wangensteen, "Some Highlights in the History of Amputation Reflecting Lessons in Wound Healing," *Bulletin of the History of Medicine* 41 (1967): 101–2, 103; Miller, *Brief Retrospect*, pp. 299–300; Samuel Clark Harvey, *The History of Hemostasis* (New York: Paul B. Hoeber, 1929), pp. 63–64; Cantlie, *History*, 1: 59; Theodor Billroth, "Historical Studies on the Nature and Treatment of Gunshot Wounds From the Fifteenth Century to the Present Time," trans. C. P. Rhoads, *Yale Journal of Biology and Medicine* 4 (1931–1932): 235; Hunter, *Treatise on the Blood*, pp. 209–10, 211; Gooch, *Treatise*, 1: 150–51, 154; Ramsay, *Review*, p. 11; Graham, *Surgery*, p. 213. When the edges of a wound have been brought together and held in this position before the healing process has begun, the wound is said to be healing by the first intention.

52. Hunter, *Treatise on the Blood*, pp. 204, 211, quote from p. 204.

53. Wangensteen, "Amputation," pp. 103,

105; Hunter, *Reminiscences,* pp. 79, 132; Jones, *Works,* pp. 21-22.

54. Jones, *Works,* pp. 19-20, quote from p. 20; Hunter, *Reminiscences,* p. 69.

55. Hunter, *Treatise on the Blood,* pp. 496-97, 499.

56. Quote from Gooch, *Treatise,* 1: 71; Wangensteen, "Amputation," p. 106.

57. Thomas, *Modern Practice,* pp. 332-33; Benjamin Rush, *Observations on the Cause and Cure of the Tetanus* (Philadelphia, 1787), pp. 461-62.

58. Jones, *Works,* pp. 67, 134, 135-37; Hunter, *Treatise on the Blood,* pp. 530, 532, 535-36; Hunter, *Reminiscences,* p. 104; Ramsay, *Review,* p. 11; Ravaton, *Chirurgie,* pp. 86-87.

59. Wangensteen, "Amputation," pp. 105-6; Louis C. Duncan, *Medical Men in the American Revolution, 1775-1783,* Army Medical Bulletin No. 25 (Carlisle Barracks, Pa.: Medical Field Service School, 1931), p. 11; C. M. B. Gilman, "Military Surgery in the American Revolution," *Journal of the Medical Society of New Jersey* 57 (1960): 493-94; Temkin, "Surgery," pp. 252-53; Buchan, *Domestic Medicine,* p. 439; Miller, *Brief Retrospect,* p. 301; Hunter, *Reminiscences,* p. 84; Jones, *Works,* pp. 43-54, 59-60, 63-66, 70, 151, 154-55; Aiken, *Thoughts,* pp. 24-25.

60. Gooch, *Treatise,* 1: 78-79, 98-118; Jones, *Works,* pp. 35, 63-66.

61. Temkin, "Surgery," p. 251; Richard Harrison Shryock, *Medical Licensing in America, 1650-1965* (Baltimore: Johns Hopkins Press, 1967), pp. 4-5, 8-9; Henry Woodhouse, "Colonial Medical Practice," *Ciba Symposia* 1 (1940): 383; Shryock, "Public Relations," pp. 310, 312; William Shainline Middleton, "John Morgan, Father of Medical Education in North America," *Annals of Medical History,* 1st ser. 9 (1927): 18; Claude Edwin Heaton, "Medicine in New York During the English Colonial Period, 1664-1775," *Bulletin of the History of Medicine* 17 (1945): 36-37; Duncan, *Medical Men,* p. 38; Henry R. Viets, *A Brief History of Medicine in Massachusetts* (New York: Houghton Mifflin Co., 1930), p. 81.

62. William Frederick Norwood, *Medical Education in the United States Before the Civil War* (Philadelphia: University of Pennsylvania Press, 1944), pp. 9, 58; R. H. Dalton, "A Glance at the American Medical Profession Since the Beginning of the Present Century," *Journal of the American Medical Association* 21 (1893): 953; Winslow, "Colonial Era," pp. 18-19.

63. Whitfield Jenks Bell, Jr., "Philadelphia Medical Students in Europe, 1750-1800," *Pennsylvania Magazine of History and Biography* 67 (1943): 4; Norwood, *Medical Education,* pp. 32-35.

64. Bell, "Students," pp. 3, 13, 14, 18, 19; Ramsay, *Review,* pp. 8, 9-10; Kraus, "Medicine," pp. 680-81; Edgar M. Bick, "French Influences on Early American Medicine and Surgery," *Journal of the Mount Sinai Hospital* 24 (1957): 500, 502, 503; James Joseph Walsh, *History of Medicine in New York . . . ,* 5 vols. (New York: National Americana Society, 1919), 1: 40-41, 44; William Frederick Norwood, "Medicine in the Era of the American Revolution," *International Record of Medicine* 171 (1958): 395; Packard, "London and Edinburgh," p. 222; William Henry Welch, "Influence of English Medicine Upon American Medicine in Its Formative Period," in *Papers and Addresses,* ed. Walter C. Burket (Baltimore: Johns Hopkins Press, 1920), 3: 445, 446, 447; Genevieve Miller, "Medical Schools in the Colonies," *Ciba Symposia* 8 (1947): 524; William Shainline Middleton, "William Shippen, Junior," *Annals of Medical History,* n.s. 4 (1932): 442; Jones, *Works,* pp. 4-8; James Gregory Mumford, *A Narrative of Medicine in America* (Philadelphia: J. B. Lippincott Co., 1903), p. 96.

65. Richard Harrison Shryock, *American Medical Research: Past and Present* (New York: Commonwealth Fund, 1947), p. 20; Jules Calvin Ladenheim, "The Doctors' Mob of 1788," *Journal of the History of Medicine* 5 (1950): 23, 24-25, 29-35; William Dosite Postell, "Medical Education and Medical Schools in Colonial America," *International Record of Medicine* 171 (1958): 366-67; Norwood, *Medical Education,* pp. 6, 37, 38, 39, 42, 46; Walsh, *Medicine in New York,* p. 47; D. J. D'Elia, "Dr. Benjamin Rush and the American Medical Revolution," *Proceedings of the American Philosophical Society*

110 (1966): 227; Nathan Smith Davis, *Contributions to the History of Medical Education and Medical Institutions in the United States of America 1776–1876* (Washington: Government Printing Office, 1877), p. 12; Richard Hingston Fox, *Dr. John Fothergill and His Friends, Chapters in Eighteenth Century Life* (London: Macmillan and Co., 1919), pp. 367–68.

66. John Morgan, "A Discourse Upon the Institution of Medical Schools in America," in *Publications of the Institute of the History of Medicine* (orig. printed in Philadelphia by William Bradford, 1765, reprinted facsimile from first ed. with introduction by Abraham Flexner; Baltimore: Johns Hopkins Press, 1937), 2: 16–17, 30–32; Norwood, *Medical Education*, pp. 43–44, 67, 69–70.

67. Middleton, *Medical Discourse*, p. 68; Butterfield, *Letters of Rush*, 1: 31n; Brooke Hindle, *The Pursuit of Science in Revolutionary America, 1735–1789* (Chapel Hill: University of North Carolina Press, 1956), pp. 61, 111–12; Stephen Wickes, *History of Medicine in New Jersey, and of Its Medical Men From the Settlement of the Province to A.D. 1800* (Newark: Dennis, 1879), p. 53; John D. Comrie, *History of Scottish Medicine*, 2d ed., 2 vols. (London: Baillière, Tindall, & Cox, 1932), 2: 441; Bick, "French Influence," pp. 508–9.

68. Davis, *History of Medical Education*, pp. 20–21; Norwood, *Medical Education*, pp. 57, 58; Miller, "Medical Schools," p. 523; Duncan, *Medical Men*, pp. 17–18; Middleton, "Morgan," p. 14; James E. Gibson, *Dr. Bodo Otto and the Medical Background of the American Revolution* (Baltimore: Charles C Thomas, 1937), pp. 48–49; Jones, *Works*, pp. 11–12; Hindle, *Science*, p. 110; Corner, *Rush*, p. 131.

69. Duncan, *Medical Men*, pp. 18–19; Courtney Robert Hall, "The Beginnings of American Military Medicine," *Annals of Medical History*, 3d ser. 4 (1942): 122–23; Cantlie, *History*, 1: 102, 145, 147; Gore, *Story*, pp. 94–95, 104, 105; Pringle, *Observations*, pp. 131–32; Monro, *An Account*, pp. 361–64; Lind, *An Essay*, p. 165; Nicholas Senn, "The Evolution of the Military Surgeon," *Surgery, Gynecology and Obstetrics* 8 (1909): 394; Whitfield Jenks Bell, Jr., *John Morgan, Continental Doctor* (Philadelphia: University of Pennsylvania Press, 1965), pp. 31–32, 42; Billroth, "Gunshot Wounds," pp. 239–40.

CHAPTER 2

1. Unless otherwise indicated, this chapter is based on these secondary sources: P. M. Ashburn, *A History of the Medical Department of the United States Army* (Boston: Houghton Mifflin Co., 1929); Harvey E. Brown, *The Medical Department of the United States Army From 1775 to 1873* (Washington: The Surgeon General's Office, 1873); Duncan, *Medical Men;* Fielding H. Garrison, "Notes on the History of Military Medicine," reprinted from *Military Surgeon*, vols. 49–51, 1921–22 (Washington: Association of Military Surgeons, 1922); Gibson, *Otto;* Louis Clinton Hatch, *The Administration of the American Revolutionary Army*, Harvard Historical Studies, vol. 10 (New York: Lenox Hill Publ. & Dist. Co., 1904); Edgar Erskine Hume, *Victories of Army Medicine: Scientific Accomplishments of the Medical Department of the United States Army* (Philadelphia: J. B. Lippincott Co., 1943); James M. Phalen, *Chiefs of the Medical Department, United States Army, 1775–1940*, Army Medical Bulletin No. 52 (Carlisle Barracks, Pa.: Medical Field Service School, April 1940); Erna Risch, *Quartermaster Support of the Army: A History of the Corps, 1775–1939* (Washington: Government Printing Office, 1962); Charles Smart, "Medical Department, U.S. Army," *Journal of Military Service Institute* 14 (May 1893): 692–708; Oliver Lyman Spaulding, *The United States Army in War and Peace* (New York: G. P. Putnam's Sons, 1937); Russell F. Weigley, *History of the United States Army* (New York: Macmillan Co., 1967).

2. Washington to the President of Congress, 20 Jul 1775, in John C. Fitzpatrick, ed., *The Writings of George Washington From the Original Manuscript Sources, 1745–1799*, 39 vols. (Washington: Government Printing Office, 1931–44), 3: 350.

3. Worthington Chauncey Ford, Gaillard Hunt, and others, eds., *Journals of the Conti-*

nental Congress, 34 vols. (Washington: U.S. Government Printing Office, 1904–37), 2: 209.

4. Ford, *Journals of the Continental Congress,* 2: 191, quote from p. 250; 4: 344; 5: 636, 673; 6: 1006, 1065; 7: 13, 44; Medical Committee to George Washington, 13 Feb 1777, in Edmund Cody Burnett, ed., *Letters of Members of the Continental Congress,* 8 vols. (Washington: Carnegie Institution of Washington, 1921–36), 2: 249; Gibson, *Otto,* p. 109; Jennings Bryan Sanders, *Evolution of Executive Departments of the Continental Congress* (Gloucester, Mass.: Peter Smith, 1971 reprint of 1935 edition), p. 7.

5. Ford, *Journals of the Continental Congress,* 7: 193. A number of other committees of the Continental Congress became directly or indirectly involved in the affairs of the Hospital Department. Among them were the so-called Secret Committee and two appointed at different times to hear John Morgan's defense of his own conduct as the second director and his charges against his successor, William Shippen, and another formed in February 1778 after Rush attacked Shippen. Ford, *Journals of the Continental Congress,* 7: 206, 219, 225; 8: 626; Bell, *Morgan,* pp. 211–12, 219; Corner, *Rush,* p. 136.

6. George B. Griffenhagen, *Drug Supplies in the American Revolution,* U.S. National Museum Bulletin 225 (Washington: Smithsonian Institution, 1961), pp. 121–22; Ford, *Journals of the Continental Congress,* 3: 261; 5: 528; 6: 990; 17: 708; Claude Halstead Van Tyne, *The War of Independence,* 2 vols. (Boston: Houghton Mifflin Co., 1929), 2: 284.

7. Ford, *Journals of the Continental Congress,* 2: 211.

8. William Frederick Norwood, "The Enigma of Dr. Benjamin Church, A High-Level Scandal in the American Colonial Army Medical Service," *Medical Arts and Sciences* 10 (1956): 82; Church to Samuel Adams, 23 Aug 1775 in Allen French, *General Gage's Informers* (Ann Arbor: University of Michigan Press, 1932), pp. 173–75; John Sullivan to John Langdon and Josiah Bartlett, 4 Sep 1775, in John Sullivan, *Letters and Papers of Major General John Sullivan, 1771–1777,* 3 vols., Collections of New Hampshire Historical Society (Concord: New Hampshire Historical Society, 1930), 1: 82–83.

9. Norwood, "Church," p. 82; Howard Lewis Applegate, "The American Revolutionary War Hospital Department," *Military Medicine* 126 (1961): 296; Robert Jackson, *A System of Arrangement and Discipline for the Medical Department of Armies* (London: John Murray, 1805), p. 59; Edwin P. Wolfe, "The Genesis of the Medical Department of the United States Army," *Bulletin of the New York Academy of Medicine,* 2d ser. 5 (1929): 829–30.

10. General Orders, 7 Sep 1775, Fitzpatrick, *Washington,* 3: 480–81, quote from p. 481; Church to Samuel Adams, 23 Aug 1775, French, *Gage,* pp. 174–75.

11. General Orders, 7 Sep 1775, Fitzpatrick, *Washington,* 3: 481.

12. Quote from Sullivan to John Langdon and Josiah Bartlett, Sullivan, *Letters,* 1: 82; Petition to Sullivan, 1775, Sullivan, *Letters,* 1: 84.

13. Ford, *Journals of the Continental Congress,* 2: 249–50, quote from p. 249.

14. Washington's Orders, 14 and 18 Sep 1775, and Horatio Gates to Church, 24 Sep 1775, in Peter Force, ed., *American Archives: Fourth and Fifth Series, Containing a Documentary History of the United States of America From March 7, 1774, to the Definitive Treaty of Peace With Great Britain, September 3, 1783,* 9 vols. (Washington: M. St. Clair Clarke and Peter Force, 1848–53), 3: 769, 770, quote from Washington's Orders, 30 Sep 1775, pp. 857–58; General Orders, 28 Sep 1775, Fitzpatrick, *Washington,* 3: 524.

15. Quote from James Warren to John Adams, 1 Oct 1775, in *Warren-Adams Letters, Being Chiefly a Correspondence Among John Adams, Samuel Adams, and James Warren,* 2 vols., Massachusetts Historical Society Collections, 5th ser. 72 (1917), 73 (1925), vol. 1, p. 121; Henry Ward to Gen Nathanael Greene, 26 Sep 1775, Force, *American Archives,* 4th ser. 3: 809; Washington to the President of Congress, 5 Oct 1775, Fitzpatrick, *Washington,* 4: 9–11; Norwood, "Church," pp. 83–84.

16. Quote from John Adams to James Warren, 18 Oct 1775, Burnett, *Letters,* 1: 234;

Carl Van Doren, *Secret History of the American Revolution* ... (New York: Viking Press, 1941), pp. 19, 21; John Adams to Abigail Adams, 13 Oct 1775, in John Adams, *Letters of John Adams Addressed to His Wife*, ed. by Charles Francis Adams, 2 vols. (Boston: Charles C. Little and James Brown, 1841), 1: 65–66; Council of War, Cambridge, 4 Oct 1775, and Massachusetts House of Representatives, 28 Oct 1775, Force, *American Archives*, 4th ser. 3: 958, 1479n–83n, 1485–86; Samuel Adams to James Warren, 13 Oct 1775, and James Warren to Samuel Adams, 26 Oct 1775, *Warren-Adams Letters*, 1: 141–42; 2: 424.

17. Quote from Council of War, 4 Oct 1775, Force, *American Archives*, 4th ser. 3: 958, 1159–60; General Orders, 3 Oct 1775, and Washington to the President of Congress, 5 Oct 1775, Fitzpatrick, *Washington*, 4: 2, 9–11; Norwood, "Church," pp. 85–86, 87.

18. Quote from John Adams to Benjamin Kent, 22 Jun 1776, Burnett, *Letters*, 1: 502; Norwood, "Church," pp. 85–86, 88–89; Edward Alfred Jones, *The Loyalists of Massachusetts: Their Memorials, Petitions, and Claims* (Baltimore: Genealogical Publ. Co., 1969), p. 87; Washington to Jonathan Trumbull, 15 Nov 1775, Fitzpatrick, *Washington*, 4: 91; Ford, *Journals of the Continental Congress*, 3: 294–95, 4: 352; Massachusetts House of Representatives, 16 Oct 1775, 26 Oct 1775, and 11 Nov 1775, and Connecticut Committee of Safety, 22 Nov 1775, Force, *American Archives*, 4th ser. 3: 1464, 1477, 1517–18, 1636–37; John Hancock to Massachusetts Council, 3 Oct 1777, Burnett, *Letters*, 2: 506; James Warren to John Adams, 5 Jun 1776, *Warren-Adams Letters*, 1: 254–55.

19. Washington to Richard Henry Lee, 8 Nov 1775, Fitzpatrick, *Washington*, 4: 76; John C. Fitzpatrick, ed., *The Diaries of George Washington, 1748–1799*, 4 vols. (Boston: Houghton Mifflin Co., 1925), 2: 195; John Adams to James Warren, 18 Oct 1775, Burnett, *Letters*, 1: 234.

20. John Adams to James Warren, 25 Oct 1775, *Warren-Adams Letters*, 1: 165.

21. Bell, *Morgan*, p. 77.

22. Barnabas Binney to Solomon Drowne, quoted in Gibson, *Otto*, p. 261.

23. Bell, *Morgan*, pp. 143, 179.

24. Quote from Washington to Joseph Reed, 20 Nov 1775, Fitzpatrick, *Washington*, 4: 104–5; James E. Gibson, "The Role of Disease in the 70,000 Casualties in the American Revolutionary Army," *Transactions and Studies of the College of Physicians of Philadelphia*, 4th ser. 17 (1949): 122; Bell, *Morgan*, pp. 180–81, 214; Solomon Drowne, "Original Letters," *Pennsylvania Magazine of History and Biography* 5 (1881): 112.

25. John Morgan to Washington, quoted in Gibson, *Otto*, pp. 117–18; Francis R. Packard, "Editorial: Washington and the Medical Affairs of the Revolution," *Annals of Medical History*, n.s. 4 (1932): 307–8; Frederick E. Brasch, "The Royal Society of London and Its Influence Upon Scientific Thought in the American Colonies," *Scientific Monthly* 33 (1931): 459.

26. Griffenhagen, *Drug Supplies*, p. 113; Washington to the President of Congress, 31 Dec 1775, Fitzpatrick, *Washington*, 4: 199; Bell, *Morgan*, pp. 183, 214–15; Packard, "Editorial," p. 310.

27. Quote from Force, *American Archives*, 4th ser. 6: 1714n–15n; Packard, "Editorial," pp. 307–8; Bell, *Morgan*, pp. 184–85, 192.

28. General Orders, 3 Jul 1776, Regulations Agreed Upon Betwixt the Director-General of the American Hospital and the Regimental Surgeons and Mates at New-York, and Morgan to Washington, 18 Jul 1776, Force, *American Archives*, 4th ser. 6: 1271; 5th ser. 1: 108–9, 416; Bell, *Morgan*, pp. 192, 194; Ford, *Journals of the Continental Congress*, 4: 188, 243, 332; 5: 568, 569; Griffenhagen, *Drug Supplies*, pp. 112–13.

29. Ford, *Journals of the Continental Congress*, 5: 568, 569, 570; Bell, *Morgan*, p. 199.

30. Quote from Col W. Smallwood to Maryland Council of Safety, Oct 1776, Force, *American Archives*, 5th ser. 2: 1100; Ford, *Journals of the Continental Congress*, 5: 857, 858; Bell, *Morgan*, p. 185.

31. General Orders, 2 Aug 1776, Fitzpatrick, *Washington*, 5: 366, quote from Washington to the President of Congress, 24 Sep 1776, 6: 113; John Morgan, *A Vindication of His Public Character* ... (Boston: Powars and Willis, 1777), xviii; Gen Na-

thanael Greene to John Hancock, 10 Oct 1776, Force, *American Archives*, 5th ser. 2: 974.

32. Ford, *Journals of the Continental Congress*, 4: 242–43; 5: 837.

33. Washington to the President of Congress, 26 Apr 1776, Fitzpatrick, *Washington*, 4: 521; Stringer to Washington, 10 May 1776, and Washington to Congress, 15 May 1776, Force, *American Archives*, 4th ser. 4: 418; 6: 469.

34. Morgan to Samuel Adams, 25 Jun 1776, Force, *American Archives*, 4th ser. 6: 1069–70, quote from 1069; Force, *American Archives*, 4th ser. 6: 1714n.

35. Horatio Gates to Egbert Benson, 22 Aug 1776, with copy to Morgan, and General Orders, General Gates, 31 Aug 1776, Force, *American Archives*, 5th ser. 1: 1114, 1271, quote from Morgan to the President of Congress, 12 Aug 1776, 1: 921; Bell, *Morgan*, p. 193; Ford, *Journals of the Continental Congress*, 5: 673, 843.

36. Virginia Convention, 21 May 1776, Virginia Convention, 15 Jun 1776, and Continental Congress, 18 May 1776, Force, *American Archives*, 4th ser. 6: 1533, 1572–73, 1673.

37. Thomas Heyward, Jr., to Morgan, 4 Sep 1776, Burnett, *Letters*, 2: 69, quote from Oliver Wolcott to Matthew Griswold, 18 Nov 1776, 2: 158.

38. Quote from Congress to Shippen, 16 Jul 1776, quoted in Gibson, *Otto*, p. 195; Bell, *Morgan*, p. 220; Caspar Wistar, *Eulogium on Dr. William Shippen* (Philadelphia: Thomas Dobson and Son, 1818), pp. 9–12, 15–16; Bell, "Students," p. 3; Ford, *Journals of the Continental Congress*, 5: 562; Middleton, "Shippen," p. 539.

39. Ford, *Journals of the Continental Congress*, 6: 857–58, 989, quote from 857–58; Shippen to Washington, 20 Oct 1776, and Shippen to the President of Congress, 9 Nov 1776, Force, *American Archives*, 5th ser. 2: 1280; 3: 618; Washington to Shippen, 3 Nov 1776, Fitzpatrick, *Washington*, 6: 239.

40. Washington to John Morgan, 6 Jan 1779, Fitzpatrick, *Washington*, 13: 482; Morgan, *Vindication*, xvii–xviii; Ford, *Journals of the Continental Congress*, 6: 991; Gen Nathanael Greene to the President of Congress, 16 Dec 1776, Shippen to Lee, 17 Dec 1776, and Council of Safety to the President of Congress, 22 Dec 1776, Force, *American Archives*, 5th ser. 3: 1246, 1259, 1358.

41. Ford, *Journals of the Continental Congress*, 7: 24.

42. Washington to Morgan, 6 Jan 1779, Fitzpatrick, *Washington*, 13: 481, quotes from Washington to Morgan, 18 Jan 1777, and to President of Congress, 26 Jan 1777, 7: 28, 64.

43. Samuel Adams to John Adams, 9 Jan 1777, Burnett, *Letters*, 2: 211, 212.

44. Morgan, *Vindication*, pp. v, xviii, quote from pp. xxv–xxvi; Bell, *Morgan*, pp. 207, 214–15, 216, 217–18; *Pennsylvania Packet*, 1 Jul 1779.

45. Ford, *Journals of the Continental Congress*, 14: 724, quote from 8: 626; Statement of Henry Laurens, 3 Jun 1779, Burnett, *Letters*, 4: 247–48; Bell, *Morgan*, pp. 213–14, 219.

46. Rush to Lee, 14 Jan 1777, Butterfield, *Letters of Rush*, 1: 129; Corner, *Rush*, p. 131.

47. Washington to Cochran, 20 Jan 1777, to the President of Congress, 14 Feb 1777 and 14 Mar 1777, Fitzpatrick, *Washington*, 7: 45, 149–50, 287–88, Washington to Shippen, 27 Jan 1777, quoted in Gibson, *Otto*, p. 134; Ford, *Journals of the Continental Congress*, 7: 162.

48. Ford, *Journals of the Continental Congress*, 7: 178, 193, 199–200, 206, 219, 225; Washington to John Warren, 23 Feb 1777, quoted in Gibson, *Otto*, p. 139.

49. See Appendix D for the complete text of the law of 7–8 April and also Corner, *Rush*, p. 131; Ford, *Journals of the Continental Congress*, 7: 162, 198–99.

50. Adams, *Letters to His Wife*, 1: 209; Roger Sherman to Jonathan Trumbull, 17 Apr 1777, Burnett, *Letters*, 2: 329; Ford, *Journals of the Continental Congress*, 7: 178; Matthew Thornton to Jonathan Potts, 12 Apr 1777, Burnett, *Letters*, 2: 320n–21n; John Hancock to Washington, 9 Apr 1777, in Jared Sparks, ed., *Correspondence of the American Revolution: Being Letters of Eminent Men to George Washington, From the Time of His Taking Command of the Army to the End of His Presidency*, 4 vols. (Boston: Little, Brown and Co., 1853), 1: 364.

51. Ford, *Journals of the Continental Congress*, 7: 162, 257; 18: 878; William Shippen, "Text of William Shippen's First Draft of a Plan for the Organization of the Military Hospital During the Revolution," *Annals of Medical History* 1 (1917–18): 176.

52. Ford, *Journals of the Continental Congress*, 7: 289–90.

53. Quoted in Gibson, *Otto*, p. 138; Letter of 13 Apr 1777, Adams, *Letters to His Wife*, 1: 213; Ford, *Journals of the Continental Congress*, 7: 253–54; Washington to the President of Congress, 14 Feb 1777, Fitzpatrick, *Washington*, 7: 149; Butterfield, *Letters of Rush*, 1: 121n.

54. Wistar, *Shippen*, pp. 9–13, 28, 31, quotes from pp. 15–16, 36; Bell, *Morgan*, p. 220; Whipple, *Evolution*, p. 11; Bell, "Students," p. 3; Betsy Copping Corner, *William Shippen, Jr.: Pioneer in American Medical Education* (Philadelphia: American Philosophical Society, 1951), pp. 117–18, 122, 123.

55. Bell, *Morgan*, p. 220; Benedict Arnold, *The Present State of the American Rebel Army, Navy and Finances, Transmitted to the British Government, October 1780*, ed. by Paul Leicester Ford (Brooklyn: Historical Printing Club, 1891), p. 10; Corner, *Shippen*, p. 112; Wistar, *Shippen*, p. 29.

56. Washington to John Augustine Washington, 10 Jun 1778, Fitzpatrick, *Washington*, 12: 43.

57. Quote from letter of 13 Apr 1777, Adams, *Letters to His Wife*, 1: 212–13.

58. Griffenhagen, *Drug Supplies*, pp. 121–22.

59. Washington to the President of Congress, 17 Nov 1777, and Washington to Gov William Livingston, 31 Dec 1777, Fitzpatrick, *Washington*, 10: 76, 233; Ford, *Journals of the Continental Congress*, 8: 608–9; 10: 941; John W. Jordan, "The Military Hospitals at Bethlehem and Lititz During the Revolution," *Pennsylvania Magazine of History and Biography* 20 (1896): 147.

60. Washington to Gov William Livingston, 31 Dec 1777, Fitzpatrick, *Washington*, 10: 233.

61. Corner, *Rush*, p. 133, quote from p. 135; Ford, *Journals of the Continental Congress*, 10: 23.

62. John Witherspoon to William Churchill Houston, 27 Jan 1778, James Lovell to John Langdon, 8 Feb 1778, and Henry Laurens to the Governor of Rhode Island, 3 Jan 1778, Burnett, *Letters* 3: 59, 97; 13: 11; Rush to John Adams, 21 Oct 1777, Rush to John Adams, 31 Oct 1777, and Rush to William Duer, 8 Dec 1777, Butterfield, *Letters of Rush*, 1: 159–62, 165, 171, 172–73; Ford, *Journals of the Continental Congress*, 10: 9, 23, 93, 128, 129; Applegate, "Hospital Department," pp. 301–2; Van Tyne, *War*, 2: 284; Potts to Medical Committee, 10 Apr 1779, in Washington, Library of Congress, Manuscript Division, Papers of Jonathan Potts.

63. Burnett, *Letters*, 5: 287–88, quote from Committee at Headquarters to President of Congress, 10 May 1780, 5: 134.

64. Cochran to Jonathan Potts, 18 Mar 1780, in Thornton Chard, "Excerpts From the Private Journal of Doctor John Cochran," *New York History* 42 (1944): 375.

65. General Orders of 2 Jan, 20 Aug 1778, 26 Mar, 6 May, 16 Jun, 23 Dec 1780, Washington to Committee of Conference, 8 Jan 1779, Fitzpatrick, *Washington*, 10: 248; 12: 338; 13: 490; 18: 160, 337–38; 19: 17–18; 21: 9, quote from Washington to Committee of Congress, 29 Jan 1778, 10: 394.

66. Ford, *Journals of the Continental Congress*, 8: 626. It is difficult to be precise about the position of Rickman in the years 1776–80. He functioned independently of the Director of the Hospital Department and his principal "territory" during this period was Virginia. It appears that he was never officially designated Deputy Director General for the Southern Department. Nevertheless, in July 1780, Gen. Horatio Gates referred to Rickman as the "Director of the Hospitals in the Southern Department" (Gates to Director of the Hospitals in the Southern Department, 19 Jul 1780, in Horatio Gates, "Letters of General Gates on the Southern Campaign," *Magazine of American History* 5 [1880]: 284) and as "Director to the General Hospital of the Southern Army," (Gates to President of the Board of War, Gates, "Letters," p. 288), which suggests that General Gates considered Rickman's authority to extend beyond Virginia. In February 1781, furthermore, in a

communication from the Continental Congress to Thomas Bond, Rickman was referred to as the "late deputy director" (Ford, *Journals of the Continental Congress,* 19: 118). One can only conclude that in this instance, as in others, titles were used casually and the limits of the authority of the individual officer not always clearly marked.

67. The terms used in the legislation and other documents of the period are often confusing to the modern reader. It should be borne in mind that although Army physicians were repeatedly referred to as "medical officers" in legislation concerning the Hospital Department, they had no rank in the period 1775–1818.

68. Washington to Maj Gen Alexander McDougall, 5 Apr 1779, and Washington to Dr. Isaac Foster, 28 Mar 1780, Fitzpatrick, *Washington,* 14: 339; 18: 174; Ford, *Journals of the Continental Congress,* 15: 1214, 1216, 1294–96; 18: 887.

69. Burnett, *Letters,* 5: 112n, also Nathaniel Scudder to Nathaniel Peabody, 6 Dec 1779, and Committee at Headquarters to President of Congress, 18 Jul 1780, 4: 533; 5: 275; Ford, *Journals of the Continental Congress,* 16: 10–12; 19: 68–69; Washington to John Cochran, 6 Nov 1780, Fitzpatrick, *Washington,* 20: 307; William T. R. Saffell, *Records of the Revolutionary War . . .* (New York: Pudney & Russell, 1859), pp. 402–3.

70. Ford, *Journals of the Continental Congress,* 10: 101; 14: 1, 733; Washington to Morgan, 5 Jan 1779, to Committee of Conference, 8 Jan 1779, and to Council of General Officers, 26 Jul 1779, Fitzpatrick, *Washington,* 13: 479, 489; 15: 488–89; James Lovell to John Langdon, 8 Feb 1777, Richard Henry Lee to Shippen, 18 Apr 1779, and John Fell Diary, entry for 16 Apr 1779, Burnett, *Letters,* 3: 77; 4: 159, 163; Rush to John Adams, 8 Feb 1778, Rush to Daniel Roberdeau, 9 Mar 1778, and Rush to John Adams, 12 Feb 1812, Butterfield, *Letters,* 1: 199–200, 204–7; 2: 1122.

71. Shippen to Lee, 16 Apr 1780, and Cochran to Jonathan Potts, 18 Mar 1780, quoted in Gibson, *Otto,* pp. 253–54, 256.

72. Quoted in Gibson, *Otto,* p. 275; Bell, *Morgan,* p. 227.

73. Quoted in Bell, "Students," p. 7; Rush to John Adams, 8 Aug 1777, and Richard Peters to Secretary of State Pickering, 7 Oct 1797, Butterfield, *Letters,* 1: 153; 2: 1210.

74. *Pennsylvania Packet,* 9 Dec 1780.

75. Bell, *Morgan,* pp. 229, 230, 233.

76. Quotes from Verdict of Court-Martial, 27 Jun 1780, quoted in Gibson, *Otto,* pp. 263–64; Ford, *Journals of the Continental Congress,* 17: 744–45.

77. *Pennsylvania Packet,* 26 Jun 1779, 18 Nov 1780, 25 Nov 1780, 6 Dec 1780, 9 Dec 1780; Rush to John Adams, 8 Aug 1777, Rush to William Duer, 8 Dec 1777, Rush to Morgan, Jan 1778, and Rush to John Adams, 12 Feb 1812, Butterfield, *Letters,* 1: 153, 173, 226; 2: 1121.

78. Quoted in Ford, *Journals of the Continental Congress,* 17: 638; Washington to President of Congress, 15 Jul 1780, quoted in Gibson, *Otto,* p. 264.

79. Corner, *Rush,* p. 137.

80. John Mathews to Washington, 15 Sep 1780, Burnett, *Letters,* 5: 372–73; Ford, *Journals of the Continental Congress,* 16: 708; 17: 879–88, 908.

81. John Mathews to Washington, 15 Sep 1780, Burnett, *Letters,* 5: 372–73; Joseph Jones to Washington, 2 Oct 1780, in Joseph Jones, *Letters of Joseph Jones of Virginia, 1777–1787,* ed. by Worthington Chauncey Ford (New York: New York Times, 1971 reprint of 1889 edition, 1971), pp. 32–33; Ford, *Journals of the Continental Congress,* 18: 878, 885, 887–88.

82. Ford, *Journals of the Continental Congress,* 18: 908–10; Washington to Joseph Jones, 9 Sep 1780, and General Orders, 19 Oct 1780, Fitzpatrick, *Washington,* 20: 18–19, 218; Jones to Washington, 2 Oct 1780, and to Madison, 17 Oct 1780, Jones, *Letters,* pp. 32–33, 36.

83. Ford, *Journals of the Continental Congress,* 19: 15, quote from 18: 1126; William Shippen to General Washington, 4 Jan 1781, in Washington, Library of Congress, Manuscript Division, Papers of George Washington.

84. Quoted in James Thacher, *A Military Journal During the American Revolutionary War, From 1775 to 1783 . . . ,* 2d ed. (Boston: Cottons & Barnard, 1827), p. 252; Ford,

Journals of the Continental Congress, 19: 48, 56, 65; John Cochrane, "Medical Department of the Revolutionary Army," *Magazine of American History* 12 (1884): 258.

85. Quote from Cochran to Dr. Peter Turner, 25 Mar 1781, and Cochran to James Craik, 26 Mar 1781, Cochrane, "Medical Department," pp. 245, 246.

86. Ford, *Journals of the Continental Congress*, 19: 68–69.

87. Ford, *Journals of the Continental Congress*, 19: 292–94; 20: 506.

88. Proceedings of the Board of War, Burnett, *Letters*, 6: 146–47; Ford, *Journals of the Continental Congress*, 20: 570.

89. Ford, *Journals of the Continental Congress*, 21: 1093; 22: 4–6.

90. Ford, *Journals of the Continental Congress*, 23: 408–12, 645; General Orders of 6 Aug 1782, Fitzpatrick, *Washington*, 24: 479.

91. Cochrane, "Medical Department," p. 252, quote from Cochran to the President of Congress, 24 May 1781, p. 248; John Cochran to Thomas Bond, 1781, in Morristown, N.J., Morristown Historical Park, John Cochran Letter Book, microfilm 5168; Ford, *Journals of the Continental Congress*, 21: 103; Cochran to Abraham Clark, 28 Feb 1781 and Apr 1781, Chard, "Cochran," pp. 366–67, 369; Washington to Cochran, 12 Feb 1781, and to James and Horace Hooker, 25 Feb 1781, Fitzpatrick, *Washington*, 21: 217, 292–93.

92. Fitzpatrick, *Washington*, 24: 489n; Washington to President of Congress, 15 Dec 1781, 23: 392, quote from Washington to Gov John Hancock, 14 Jul 1781, 22: 380; Cochran to John Warren, 30 Jun 1781, Chard, "Cochran," p. 370; Victor Leroy Johnson, "Robert Morris and the Provisioning of the American Army During the Campaign of 1781," *Pennsylvania History* 5 (1939): 11; *Pennsylvania Packet*, 14 Nov 1780, p. 2.

93. Ltrs, Robert Morris to Thomas Bond, 19 Feb 1782 and 19 Jun 1783, Xeroxes of letters held by Library of Congress, obtained from Miss Elizabeth Thomson.

94. Cochrane, "Medical Department," p. 251.

95. Cochran to George Campbell and to Abraham Clark, 2 and 30 Apr, 8 May 1781, quote from Cochran to Robert Morris, 26 Jul 1781, Chard, "Cochran," pp. 368–69, 372; Cochrane, "Medical Department," p. 252; Ford, *Journals of the Continental Congress*, 21: 1072–73; John Cochran to Peter Turner, 25 Mar 1781, Cochran Letter Book.

96. Cochrane, "Medical Department," p. 254; Ford, *Journals of the Continental Congress*, 21: 81–82; John Cochran to Samuel Huntington, 24 May 1782, Cochran Letter Book.

97. Ford, *Journals of the Continental Congress*, 29: 208; Saffell, *Records*, pp. 406–7.

98. Quote from Cochran to Hagen, 8 May 1781, Chard, "Cochran," p. 370.

99. Quote from Cochran to Hagen, 8 May 1781, Chard, "Cochran," p. 370; John Cochran to Board of War, 4 Jul 1781, and to Robert Morris, 26 Jul 1781, Cochran Letter Book; Washington to Maj Gen William Heath, 1 Aug 1781, and Washington to the Board of War, 5 Aug 1781, Fitzpatrick, *Washington*, 22: 441, 463; Ford, *Journals of the Continental Congress*, 20: 625; 21: 979.

100. Ford, *Journals of the Continental Congress*, 21: 980.

101. Ford, *Journals of the Continental Congress*, 22: 7; The President of Congress to Cochran, 25 Sep 1781, Burnett, *Letters*, 6: 225.

102. Washington's letters to Secretary of War, 16 Aug 1782, to Sir Guy Carleton, 18 Aug 1782, to Heath and Knox, 23 Sep 1782, Fitzpatrick, *Washington*, 25: 26, 38, 196.

103. Richard Peters, by order to John Cochran, 10 Oct 1781, Cochran Letter Book, with quote from Cochran to Binney, 22 Oct 1781; Cochran to President of Congress, 10 Oct 1781, to James Craik, 10 Oct 1781, and Cochran to John Warren, 10 Oct 1781, Chard, "Cochran," pp. 363–64, 365, 372; Cochran to Barnabas Binney, 22 Oct 1781, *Pennsylvania Magazine of History and Biography* 5 (1881): 230.

104. John Cochran to Barnabas Binney, 22 Oct 1781, and Cochran to John Warren, 22 Feb 1781, Cochran Letter Book; Cochran to Warren, 10 Oct 1781, Chard, "Cochran," p. 372.

105. Report of Nov 1782, Cochran to Binney, 22 Oct 1781, and Cochran to Richard

Peters, 20 Oct 1781, Cochran Letter Book; Cochran to Warren, 10 Oct 1781, Chard, "Cochran," p. 372.

106. Quoted in Ford, *Journals of the Continental Congress*, 25: 740; John C. Fitzpatrick, *The Spirit of the Revolution* (Boston: Houghton Mifflin Co., 1924), p. 211.

107. Jones, *Works*, pp. 152–54.

Chapter 3

1. For the location of towns in the vicinity of Boston mentioned in the text, see Map 1. Unless otherwise indicated, the account of the Boston area is based upon these sources: Bell, *Morgan*; Brown, *Medical Department*; Cash, *Medical Men*; and Duncan, *Medical Men*. Except where otherwise indicated, statistics throughout this and subsequent chapters are based on Charles H. Lesser, ed., *The Sinews of Independence: Monthly Strength Reports of the Continental Army* (Chicago: University of Chicago Press, 1976). It should be noted, however, that, as Lesser himself points out, there are many serious difficulties involved in any attempt to rely upon statistics concerning the rate of sickness in the Continental Army during the Revolution. Despite Washington's concern for the keeping of accurate records, care and precision with statistics were not generally characteristic of those submitting returns in this period, particularly before the winter of 1778–79, and the gathering of accurate figures was often impossible. Statistics obtained from different reports apparently covering the same units for the same period of time may, therefore, vary. A return of 29 June 1776 in Lesser, for example, lists strength and sickness statistics at variance with those cited in a strength report for the preceding day by Washington, as published in Fitzpatrick, *Washington*, 5: 194n, but the Fitzpatrick citation may not include all of the units included in the Lesser return. Attempts to use the returns published in Lesser in analyzing the work of the Hospital Department are complicated by the fact that the pertinent column headings appear somewhat ambiguous to the modern researcher; "sick present," used in the official army monthly reports, may or may not include the figures for regimental and flying hospitals, while "sick absent" may include those in general hospitals, those sick or convalescent at home or in the care of civilians outside camp, and those who deserted after their discharge from these facilities but before returning to their units (see Fitzpatrick, *Washington*, 10: 526–27, for example). Hospital Department returns, on the other hand, often use another ambiguous category, "sick in camp," or a similar term which, because of the manner in which it is used, clearly includes regimental and flying hospitals but may or may not include the sick of units stationed at some distance from the main body of the army. Figures given by the department's report are, with some exceptions, significantly smaller than those cited by Lesser, a situation which may reflect those inaccuracies in regimental returns sent directly to the Adjutant General which moved General Washington to angry comment in May 1778 (Fitzpatrick, *Washington*, 11: 454–55). The number of officers sick, when available, is listed separately in Lesser, but even when given, the figure is often partial, limited in many instances to the officers of the artillery. Percentages in this and following chapters concerning the Revolution have, therefore, been calculated from figures for the rank and file alone to establish a uniform basis for comparisons.

Also consulted for the preceding paragraph were: Gibson, "Role of Disease"; and James Stevens, "Revolutionary Journal," *Essex Institute Historical Collections* 48 (1912): 53.

2. Church to Samuel Adams, 23 Aug 1775, French, *Gage*, pp. 175–76.

3. Quote from Morgan to Washington, 12 Dec 1775, Force, *American Archives*, 4th ser. 4: 263; Church to Samuel Adams, 23 Aug 1775, French, *Gage*, pp. 175–76. Most of the papers of the Board of War from the period of the American Revolution were destroyed in a fire on 8 November 1800 and the surviving records sustained further serious losses when the British looted the fireproof room which contained them in 1814. Washington, National Archives, *Preliminary Inventories: War Department Collection of Revolutionary War Records* (Washington:

National Archives and Records Service, General Services Administration, 1970), p. 1.

4. Church to Samuel Adams, 23 Aug 1775, French, *Gage*, pp. 176–77; Norwood, "Church," p. 82; John Warren to John Hancock, Oct 1775, Duncan, *Medical Men*, p. 67; Return of the Sick & Wounded in the General Hospital at Cambridge & Roxbury, 25 Nov–2 Dec 1775, in Washington, National Archives, War Department Collection of Revolutionary War Records, Record Group 93, Revolutionary War Rolls 1775–83, Microfilm Publication M246, Miscellaneous, Hospital Department, roll 135, folder 3–1, item 15.

5. Quote from General Orders, 29 Aug 1775, in Washington, National Archives, War Department Collection of Revolutionary War Records, Record Group 93, Miscellaneous Numbered Records, 1775–84, series 6, Microfilm Publication M859, roll 2, frame 154; Fitzpatrick, *Washington*, 3: 439–40.

6. Gordon, *Aesculapius*, p. 241; Returns of 26 Nov–2 Dec 1775, RG 93, M246, folder 3–1, item 15.

7. Morgan to Washington, 12 Dec 1775, Duncan, *Medical Men*, p. 80.

8. Morgan to Washington, 12 Dec 1775, Duncan, *Medical Men*, p. 80; Returns of 16 Dec 1775–30 Mar 1776, RG 93, M246, roll 135, folder 3–1, items 17–27.

9. Returns of 16 Dec 1775–30 Mar 1776, RG 93, M246, roll 135, folder 3–1, items 17–27.

10. Quote from Morgan to Washington, 12 Dec 1775, Force, *American Archives*, 4th ser. 4: 263; Washington's letters during the period, Fitzpatrick, *Washington*, 4: 118, 145–62; Robert H. Harrison to Council of Massachusetts, 3 Dec 1775, Force, *American Archives*, 4th ser. 6: 168; Massachusetts Provincial Congress, quoted in Duncan, *Medical Men*, p. 53.

11. Thacher, *Journal*, p. 35; Morgan, *Vindication*, p. 3; Returns of 13 Jan, 30 Mar 1776, RG 93, M246, roll 135, folder 3–1, items 20–27.

12. Thacher, *Journal*, pp. 45–46; Gibson, *Otto*, pp. 90, 93; General Orders, 25 Mar 1776, Fitzpatrick, *Washington*, 4: 430; Morgan, *Recommendation*.

13. Morgan to a Committee of the Massachusetts Assembly, 11 Apr 1776, Force, *American Archives*, 4th ser. 5: 859; 6: 176n; Ephraim Eliot, "Account of the Physicians of Boston," *Proceedings of the Massachusetts Historical Society* 6 (1863–64): 178; Morgan to Washington, 22 Apr 1776, Force, *American Archives*, 4th ser. 5: 1025; Griffenhagen, *Drug Supplies*, pp. 114, 115, 121–22; Deposition of Dr. John Warren, 9 Apr 1776, in Henry Barton Dawson, *Battles of the United States*, 2 vols. (New York: Johnson, Fry and Co., 1858), 2: 97.

14. Griffenhagen, *Drug Supplies*, pp. 112–13, 115; Washington to Morgan, 3 Apr 1776, Duncan, *Medical Men*, p. 114; Morgan to Washington, 22 Apr 1776, Force, *American Archives*, 4th ser. 5: 1024; Gibson, *Otto*, p. 93; Morgan, *Vindication*, p. 4.

15. General Orders, 4 Mar 1776, Fitzpatrick, *Washington*, 4: 368–69; Gibson, "Role of Disease," p. 122.

16. Morgan, *Vindication*, pp. 3–4; Charles Lee to President of Congress, 9 Feb 1776, Force, *American Archives*, 4th ser. 4: 965; Washington to Morgan, 3 Apr 1776, and Morgan to Washington, 22 Apr 1776, Force, *American Archives*, 4th ser. 5: 783–84, 1024.

17. Unless otherwise indicated, the section on the Northern Department is based on the following sources: Brown, *Medical Department*; Duncan, *Medical Men*; Gibson, *Otto*; and Henry B. Carrington, *Battles of the American Revolution, 1775–1781: Historical and Military Criticism With Topographical Illustration*, 6th ed., revised (New York: A. S. Barnes & Co., 1968). The preceding paragraph is also based on Gibson, "Role of Disease," p. 122; and Schuyler to Samuel Stringer, 27 Aug 1775, Force, *American Archives*, 4th ser. 3: 443.

18. Ford, *Journals of the Continental Congress*, 2: 249–50; Schuyler to Stringer, 27 Aug 1775, Force, *American Archives*, 4th ser. 3: 443.

19. Arnold to Washington, 27 Feb 1776, Force, *American Archives*, 4th ser. 4: 1513; Lewis Beebe, *Journal of Dr. Lewis Beebe* (New York Times & Arno Press, 1971), pp. 325–27; Kenneth Lewis Roberts, ed., *March to Quebec: Journals of the Members of Arnold's Expedition* (New York: Doubleday,

Doran & Co., 1938), pp. 121, 195; John Codman, *Arnold's Expedition to Quebec* (New York: Macmillan Co., 1902), pp. 163, 186.
20. Arnold to Schuyler, 10 May 1776, and Washington's General Orders, 20 May 1776, Force, *American Archives*, 4th ser. 6: 452, 525; Gibson, "Role of Disease," p. 123; Beebe, *Journal*, p. 328; Arnold to Washington, 8 May 1776, Maj Gen John Thomas to Washington, 8 May 1776, and Arnold to commissioners in Canada, 15 May 1776, Sparks, *Correspondence*, 1: 194, 197–99, 516; Timothy Bedel to Brig Gen Arnold, 10 May 1776, RG 93, M859, roll 101, frame 168.
21. Stringer to Washington, 10 May 1776, Force, *American Archives*, 4th ser. 6: 417–18; Washington to Congress, 15 May 1776, Fitzpatrick, *Washington*, 5: 46; Ford, *Journals of the Continental Congress*, 4: 378.
22. Quote from Beebe, *Journal*, p. 330; Ford, *Journals of the Continental Congress*, 4: 344; Potts to Continental Congress, 29 Apr 1776, Gibson, *Otto*, p. 105; Washington to President of Congress, 26 Apr 1776, Fitzpatrick, *Washington*, 4: 520–21.
23. Schuyler to Washington, 22 May 1776, Force, *American Archives*, 4th ser. 6: 586.
24. Arnold to Schuyler, 13 Jun 1776, Morgan to Samuel Adams, 25 Jun 1776, Force, *American Archives*, 4th ser. 6: 1039, 1069, quote from extract of letter from John Adams, 26 Jun 1776, 6: 1083; Gates to John Adams, 24 Jun 1776, in Bernard Knollenberg, ed., "The Correspondence of John Adams and Horatio Gates," *Proceedings of the Massachusetts Historical Society* 67 (1941–44): 145; Arnold to Washington, 25 Jun 1776, and Arnold to Schuyler, 6 Jun 1776, Sparks, *Correspondence*, 1: 237–38, 526; Bell, *Morgan*, p. 189.
25. Quotes from Beebe, *Journal*, pp. 333, 334, 335–36.
26. Stringer to Potts, 7 Jul 1776, in Philadelphia, Historical Society of Pennsylvania, Manuscript Department, Papers of Jonathan Potts, 1766–80, 1: 70; Morgan to Samuel Adams, 26 Jun 1776, and Gates to Moses Morse, 12 Jul 1776, Force, *American Archives*, 4th ser. 6: 1069–70; 5th ser. 1: 238; Beebe, *Journal*, p. 343; John Trumbull, *Autobiography, Reminiscenses and Letters of John Trumbull, From 1756 to 1841* (New Haven: B. L. Hamlen, 1841), p. 28; Ltr, Dr. Meyrich, 1835, and John Trumbull to Governor of Connecticut, Trumbull, *Autobiography*, pp. 300, 304; Morgan, *Vindication*, pp. 50, 52; Ford, *Journals of the Continental Congress*, 5: 424; Washington to President of Congress, 9 Jun 1776, Fitzpatrick, *Washington*, 5: 111–12; Griffenhagen, *Drug Supplies*, p. 118; Gibson, "Role of Disease," p. 124.
27. Quote from Stringer to Gates, 24 Jul 1776, Force, *American Archives*, 5th ser. 1: 651; Beebe, *Journal*, p. 344; John Trumbull to Governor of Connecticut, 12 Jul 1776, Trumbull, *Autobiography*, p. 302; Ltr, Lt Col Israel Shreve to Mary Shreve, 18 Jul 1776, Shreve copybook in the family collection of Mr. and Mrs. Charles J. Simpson, Potomac, Maryland.
28. Quote from Stringer to Potts, 7 Jul 1776, Potts Papers, 1: 70; Stringer to Gates, 24 Jul 1776, Force, *American Archives*, 5th ser. 1: 651–52; Return of the Sick of the General Hospital at Fort George From the 12th to the 26th July 1776 Inclusive, RG 93, M246, roll 135, folder 3–1, item 53.
29. Stringer to Gates, 24 Jul 1776, Force, *American Archives*, 5th ser. 1: 652.
30. Morgan to Potts, 28 Jul 1776, Potts Papers, 1: 77; Griffenhagen, *Drug Supplies*, pp. 118–19; Morgan, *Vindication*, p. 20.
31. Stringer to Potts, 2 Aug 1776, Potts to Morgan, 10 Aug 1776, and Stringer to Potts, 7 Sep 1776, Potts Papers, 1: 84, 87, 98, quote from McHenry to Potts, 21 Aug 1776, 1: 90; Gates to Congress, 29 Jul 1776, Force, *American Archives*, 5th ser. 1: 649; Griffenhagen, *Drug Supplies*, pp. 118–19; McHenry to Potts, 21 Aug 1776, Gibson, *Otto*, p. 110.
32. Quote from Potts to Samuel Adams, 10 Aug 1776, Duncan, *Medical Men*, p. 101; Potts to Morgan, 10 Aug 1776, and Stringer to Potts, 17 Aug 1776, Gibson, *Otto*, pp. 107, 109.
33. Stringer to Potts, 17 Aug 1776, and Gates to Washington, 28 Aug 1776, Gibson, *Otto*, p. 109, quote from p. 103; James W. Gibson, "Smallpox and the American Revolution," *Genealogical Magazine and Historiographical Chronicle* 51 (1948): 56; Ltr, Richard Blanco to author, 22 Apr 1975, p. 2; S.

Adams to J. Adams, 16 Aug 1776, in Samuel Adams, *The Writings of Samuel Adams*, ed. Harry Alonzo Cushing, 4 vols. (New York: Octagon Books, 1968), 3: 310–11.

34. Force, *American Archives*, 5th ser. 1: 1271, quote and data from Gates to Egbert Benson, 22 Aug 1776, 1: 1114; Gates to President of Congress, 2 Sep 1776, Gibson, *Otto*, pp. 101–2.

35. Schuyler to New York Committee of Safety, 9 Sep 1776, Force, *American Archives*, 5th ser. 2: 685; Griffenhagen, *Drug Supplies*, p. 120; Beebe, *Journal*, pp. 345–46, 350, 356; Report of meeting of regimental surgeons of 31 Aug 1776, Force, *American Archives*, 5th ser. 1: 226.

36. Quote from Beebe, *Journal*, p. 358; Griffenhagen, *Drug Supplies*, p. 119.

37. Trumbull to Schuyler, 10 Sep 1776, Force, *American Archives*, 5th ser. 2: 279–80.

38. Dr. Samuel Wigglesworth to New Hampshire Committee of Safety, 27 Sep 1776, and Resolve of Continental Congress, 25 Sep 1776, Force, *American Archives*, 5th ser. 2: 574, 1378; Ford, *Journals of the Continental Congress*, 5: 622, 812; William Williams to Joseph Trumbull, 26 Sep 1776, Burnett, *Letters*, 2: 104.

39. Quote from Elbridge Gerry to John Wendell, 11 Nov 1776, Burnett, *Letters*, 2: 149; Beebe, *Journal*, p. 357; Craigie to Potts, 3 Oct 1776, and Stringer to Potts, 15 Oct 1776, Griffenhagen, *Drug Supplies*, p. 120; Stringer to Gates, 6 Oct 1776, Force, *American Archives*, 5th ser. 2: 923.

40. Stringer to Potts, 29 Oct 1776 and 3 Nov 1776, Potts Papers, 2: 134, 135–38; Thacher, *Journal*, 5 Aug 1776, p. 53.

41. Stringer to Gates, 3 Nov 1776, Force, *American Archives*, 5th ser. 3: 506; John Trumbull to Potts, 8 Aug 1776, Potts Papers, 1: 86.

42. Quote from Report of 27 Nov 1776, Force, *American Archives*, 5th ser. 3: 1584; Ford, *Journals of the Continental Congress*, 6: 990; Pennsylvania Infantry, *5th Regiment Orderly Book of the Northern Army at Ticonderoga and Mt. Independence From October 17th 1776, to January 8th, 1777, With Biographical and Explanatory Notes and an Appendix* (Albany: J. Munsell, 1859), pp. 19–20, 22.

43. Council of Safety to Potts, 6 Dec 1776, Thomas Tillotson to Potts, 18 Feb 1777, and Schuyler to Potts, 22 Mar 1777, Potts Papers, 2: 132, 148, 154; Jordan, "Hospitals," p. 143; Pennsylvania Infantry, *Orderly Book*, pp. 111n–12n; Anthony Wayne to Horatio Gates, 1 Dec 1776, Force, *American Archives*, 5th ser. 3: 1031; Ford, *Journals of the Continental Congress*, 7: 34.

44. Schuyler to Potts, 22 Mar 1777, Potts to Gates, 3 Apr 1777, and Potts to Medical Committee, 3 Apr 1777, Potts Papers, 2: 154, 157, 158; Report of 27 Nov 1776, Force, *American Archives*, 5th ser. 3: 1584; Ford, *Journals of the Continental Congress*, 6: 990.

45. Return of Stringer, 1 Apr 1777, and Potts to Gates, 3 Apr 1777, Potts Papers, 2: 156, 157.

46. Shippen's handwriting is difficult to decipher, but this physician may have been Forgue.

47. Quote from Shippen to Potts, 18 Apr 1777, Potts Papers, 2: 162; Return of the officers of the General Hospital Northern Department, no date, Potts Papers, 1: 12. This document must date after April 1777, when the position of Assistant Director was first created, and before the end of the year, when Potts left the Northern Department (Duncan, *Medical Men*, p. 108). The use of the term "Commissary General" is another example of the casual use of terminology characteristic of the period; Potts was referring to the chief commissary of the Hospital Department, not the Army's Commissary General.

48. Potts announcement of 7 May 1777, Return of the Sick in the General Hospital at Mount Independence, 21 May 1777, and Potts to Committee of Schenectady, 6 May 1777, Potts Papers, 2: 180, 182, 196.

49. Unless otherwise indicated, the section on New York, New Jersey, and Pennsylvania is based on Duncan, *Medical Men*, and Gibson, *Otto*. Also consulted for the preceding paragraph was Risch, *Quartermaster Support*, p. 11.

50. Bell, *Morgan*, p. 189; Morgan to New York Convention, 13 Aug 1776, Force, *American Archives*, 5th ser. 1: 499; Morgan,

Vindication, pp. 19, 96; Byron Polk Stookey, *A History of Colonial Medical Education: In the Province of New York, With Its Subsequent Development (1767–1830)* (Springfield, Ill.: Charles C Thomas, 1962), p. 74; Griffenhagen, *Drug Supplies,* p. 116.

51. For the location of sites mentioned in this section, see Map 3. Morgan, *Vindication,* pp. 55, 116; W. R. Bett, "John Warren (1753–1815), Soldier, Anatomist and Surgeon," *Medical Press* 230 (1953): 137.

52. Morgan, *Vindication,* pp. 108–9, 117.

53. Morgan, *Vindication,* pp. 116–17, quote from p. 118.

54. Morgan, *Vindication,* p. 18; Carrington, *Battles,* pp. 211–12.

55. Morgan, *Vindication,* pp. xxxi–xxxii, 12, 20, 128; Griffenhagen, *Drug Supplies,* p. 117; Washington to New York Legislature, 8 Sep 1776, Fitzpatrick, *Washington,* 6: 35–36.

56. Morgan, *Vindication,* p. 93, quote from p. 124; Washington to New York Legislature, 12 Sep 1776, and Washington to President of Congress, 14 Sep 1776, Fitzpatrick, *Washington,* 6: 48, 54–55.

57. General Orders, 18 Sep 1776, Fitzpatrick, *Washington,* 6: 71.

58. Morgan, *Vindication,* pp. xxxi–xxxii; Griffenhagen, *Drug Supplies,* p. 117; Washington to Shippen, 3 Nov 1776, Fitzpatrick, *Washington,* 6: 239.

59. Morgan, *Vindication,* pp. xxii–xxiv, xxx, 16, 46–47, 142–43, quote from Morgan to Rush, 20 Oct 1776, p. 142; Bell, *Morgan,* p. 200; Washington's General Orders, 2 Sep 1776, Fitzpatrick, *Washington,* 6: 8.

60. *Pennsylvania Journal and Weekly Advertiser,* 17 Jul 1776; Gordon, *Aesculapius,* p. 401; Bell, *Morgan,* p. 197; Van Swieten, *Diseases,* p. 7; Butterfield, *Letters of Rush* 1: 104n. Apparently fewer than 6,000 men ever reported to the flying camp. See also Chapter 2.

61. Data and quote from Ford, *Journals of the Continental Congress,* 5: 808; Mercer to Washington, 16 Jul 1776, and Shippen to Congress, 19 Sep 1776, Force, *American Archives,* 5th ser. 1: 371; 3: 1298.

62. Shippen Report, 1 Nov 1776, William Paca to Maryland Council of Safety, 7 Dec 1776, and Shippen to Washington, 8 Dec 1776, Force, *American Archives,* 5th ser. 3: 463–64, 1094, 1119; Washington to Board of War, 4 Dec 1776, and Washington to Shippen, 12 Dec 1776, Fitzpatrick, *Washington,* 6: 327–28, 362; Bell, *Morgan,* p. 195; David Freeman Hawke, *Benjamin Rush: Revolutionary Gadfly* (Indianapolis: Bobbs-Merrill, 1971), p. 174; Gibson, "Role of Disease," pp. 124–25; Gibson, *Otto,* pp. 120, 123, 199; Rush to Shippen, 28 Nov 1776, *Pennsylvania Packet,* 18 Nov 1780.

63. Gibson does not cite his source for this figure but it would appear to be a weekly report. Gibson, "Role of Disease," pp. 124–25; Morgan, *Vindication,* pp. 19–20; Hawke, *Rush,* p. 174; Ford, *Journals of the Continental Congress,* 7: 51, 70, 143.

64. Thomas Wharton to Richard Peters, 6 Dec 1776, and Shippen to Lee, 17 Dec 1776, Force, *American Archives,* 5th ser. 3: 1094, 1258; Ford, *Journals of the Continental Congress,* 6: 1006; Jordan, "Hospitals," p. 141.

65. Jordan, "Hospitals," pp. 135–41.

66. Jordan, "Hospitals," pp. 135–41, 143; Gibson, *Otto,* p. 140.

67. Jordan, "Hospitals," p. 142; General Orders, 29 Dec 1776, Fitzpatrick, *Washington,* 6: 453–54.

68. Butterfield, *Letters of Rush,* 1: 121n, 2: 1198; Rush to Lee, 14 Jan 1777, 1: 125, 129; Bell, *Morgan,* p. 208; Corner, *Rush,* pp. 128, 130; Hawke, *Rush,* pp. 178–79.

69. Morgan, *Vindication,* pp. 16, 17, 160; Griffenhagen, *Drug Supplies,* p. 117; Morgan to Rush, 20 Oct 1776, Morgan, *Vindication,* pp. 142–43.

70. Morgan, *Vindication,* pp. 17, 18; General Orders, 31 Oct 1776, Fitzpatrick, *Washington,* 6: 235.

71. Morgan, *Vindication,* pp. xxxvi–xxxvii, 19.

72. Morgan, *Vindication,* pp. 136, 137; William Eustis to General Heath, 10 Dec 1776, Force, *American Archives,* 5th ser. 3: 1161–62.

73. Morgan, *Vindication,* pp. xxiv, 133–34, 136, 137; Griffenhagen, *Drug Supplies,* p. 116.

74. Quote from James Tilton, *Economical Observations on Military Hospitals and the Prevention and Cure of Diseases Incident to an Army . . .* (Wilmington, Del.: J. Wilson,

1813), p. 33; Morgan, *Vindication*, pp. 45, 129; Col Isaac Nicoll to John McKesson, 29 Sep 1776, and Gen Nathanael Greene to President of Congress, 10 Oct 1776, Force, *American Archives*, 5th ser. 2: 597, 973.

75. Morgan, *Vindication*, pp. xxxvii, 22, 121–23; General Orders, 5 Nov 1776, Fitzpatrick, *Washington*, 6: 241; Ford, *Journals of the Continental Congress*, 5: 568 (see also Appendix C in this volume); Heath to Morgan, 19 Nov 1776, and Morgan to Heath, 20 Nov 1776, Force, *American Archives*, 5th ser. 5: 769, 781; William Heath, *Heath's Memoirs of the American War*, ed. Rufus Rockwell Wilson (New York: A. Wessels Co., 1904), pp. 94–95.

76. General Orders, 14 Apr 1776, 19 Apr 1776, 20 May 1776, 26 May 1776, Fitzpatrick, *Washington*, 4: 477, 492; 5: 63, 82–83, quote from p. 63; New York Provincial Council Resolution, 26 May 1776, and New York Provincial Congress, 24 May 1776, Force, *American Archives*, 4th ser. 6: 635, 1330–31; Heath, *Memoirs*, pp. 55, 74.

77. Council of Massachusetts to General Artemas Ward, 9 Jul 1776, and Gov Jonathan Trumbull to Washington, 4 Jul 1776, Gibson, *Otto*, pp. 91–92, 99; Brig Gen William Thompson to Washington, 2 Jun 1776, Sparks, *Correspondence*, 1: 209; Maryland Council of Safety to Lieutenant Bracco, 29 Jun 1776, Force, *American Archives*, 4th ser. 6: 1130–31.

78. Lee to Washington, 27 Feb 1777, James Curtis Ballagh, ed., *The Letters of Richard Henry Lee*, 2 vols. (New York: Da Capo Press, 1970 reprint of 1911–14 ed.), 1: 266; William Williams to Jonathan Trumbull, Jr., 6 Nov 1776, Burnett, *Letters*, 2: 142; Washington to Ward, 11 Jul 1776, Fitzpatrick, *Washington*, 5: 256.

79. Washington to Lt Col Robert Hanson Harrison, and to Cochran, 20 Jan 1777, to New York Legislature, and to Gov Nicholas Cooke, 10 Feb 1777, Fitzpatrick, *Washington*, 7: 38, 44–45, 129–30, 131–32, quote from Washington to Shippen, 28 Jan 1777, pp. 75–76; Lee to Patrick Henry, 7 Apr 1777 and 22 Apr 1777, Ballagh, *Letters*, 1: 269, 283; Medical Committee to Washington, 13 Feb 1777, Burnett, *Letters*, 1: 250.

80. Gibson, "Role of Disease," p. 125; Ford, *Journals of the Continental Congress*, 7: 139–40; Washington to Shippen, 6 Jan 1777, and to President of Congress, 5 Feb 1777, Fitzpatrick, *Washington*, 6: 473; 7: 105.

81. Washington to Shippen, 1 Mar 1777, and to Foster, 18 Apr 1777, Fitzpatrick, *Washington*, 7: 220, 432.

82. Washington to Henry, 13 Apr 1777, Fitzpatrick, *Washington*, 7: 409.

83. Ford, *Journals of the Continental Congress*, 7: 317, quote from 292; Nathan G. Goodman, *Benjamin Rush, Physician and Citizen, 1746–1813* (Philadelphia: University of Pennsylvania Press, 1934), p. 86.

84. Richard Henry Lee to Arthur Lee, 20 Apr 1777, Ballagh, *Letters*, 1: 279; Lynn Montross, *Rag, Tag and Bobtail: The Story of the Continental Army, 1775–1783* (New York: Harper & Bros., 1952), p. 184.

85. Corner, *Rush*, p. 131; Victor Leroy Johnson, *The Administraton of the American Commissariat During the Revolutionary War* (Philadelphia, 1941), p. 69.

Chapter 4

1. Peter Shindel, 20 Oct 1845, in C. H. Martin, "The Military Hospital at the Cloister (Ephrata, Pa., 1777)," *Lancaster County (Pa.) Historical Society Papers* 51 (1947): 127.

2. Gibson, *Otto*, p. 140; Isaac Foster to Mary Foster, 31 Jul 1777, in Washington, Library of Congress, Manuscript Division, Papers of Isaac Foster, folder 1.

3. Duncan, *Medical Men*, p. 212. Duncan also refers to an army report for 5 August 1777 and maintains that while it records 14,204 fit for duty from a total of 17,949, it also lists 4,745 sick. It is not clear from the text whether the faulty arithmetic should be laid at the foot of the author or of his source. Lesser contains no report for August 1777 for Washington's army.

4. General Orders, 2, 3, 9, 16, 17 Jun, 19 Oct 1777, Fitzpatrick, *Washington*, 8: 171, 175, 210, 255, 256; 9: 404, quote from Washington to Philip Livingston, Elbridge Gerry, and George Clymer, 19 Jul 1777, 8: 441. A

rather casual attitude was taken at this time toward official designations. General Washington used here the term "Surgeon General," by which he obviously meant the Physician and Surgeon General of the Army, Dr. John Cochran, who supervised the work of the regimental surgeons.

5. General Orders, 1, 9 Jul 1777, Washington to Maj Gen John Sullivan, 7 Jul 1777, Fitzpatrick, *Washington*, 8: 328, 364, 365, 374; Sullivan, *Letters*, 1: 404–5.

6. General Orders, 15, 16, 17 Jun, 4 Sep 1777, Fitzpatrick, *Washington*, 8: 251, 255, 256; 9: 178.

7. Quote from Rush to John Adams, 8 Aug 1777, Butterfield, *Letters of Rush*, 1: 153; J. P. Muhlenberg, "Orderly Book of Gen. John Peter Gabriel Muhlenberg, March 26–December 20, 1777," *Pennsylvania Magazine of History and Biography* 34 (1910): 449.

8. Howard H. Peckham, ed., *The Toll of Independence: Engagements & Battle Casualties of the American Revolution* (Chicago: University of Chicago Press, 1974), pp. 40, 41; John W. Jordan, "Continental Hospital Returns," *Pennsylvania Magazine of History and Biography* 23 (1899): 36–38.

9. Unless otherwise indicated, material in the balance of this chapter is based on Brown, *Medical Department;* Duncan, *Medical Men;* and Gibson, *Otto*. Also consulted for the preceding paragraph were: quote from Tilton, *Observations*, p. 56; James E. Gibson, "John Augustus Otto," *Historical Review of Berks County* 13 (1947): 15; Gibson, "Role of Disease," p. 125; General Orders, 12 Sep 1777, Fitzpatrick, *Washington*, 9: 209.

10. Corner, *Rush*, pp. 132–33; Washington to William Howe, 13 Sep 1777, Fitzpatrick, *Washington*, 9: 217; Butterfield, *Letters of Rush*, 1: 157n; William Shippen, "Just Account of Dr. Alison's Services to the Best of My Remembrance, 15 Dec 1780," in Philadelphia, Historical Society of Pennsylvania, Manuscript Department, Society Miscellaneous Collection, case 19, box 2.

11. Washington to Maj Gen Nathanael Greene, 25 Nov 1777, to William Shippen, 12 Dec 1777, and to Brig Gen Lachlan McIntosh, 4 Apr 1778, Fitzpatrick, *Washington*, 10: 105, 150; 11: 208; Shippen, Just Account; Shippen to John Ettwein, 19 Sep 1777, Jordan, "Hospitals," pp. 144–45, 148; Joseph Mortimer Levering, *A History of Bethlehem, Pennsylvania, 1741–1892, With Some Account of Its Founders and Their Early Activity in America* (Bethlehem, Pa.: Times Publishing Co., 1903), p. 475; John Morgan, Gibson, *Otto*, p. 283; Report of Brig Gen Lachlan McIntosh, 26 Apr 1778, RG 93, M246, roll 135, folder 3–1, item 10; George L. Heiges, "Letters Relating to Colonial Military Hospitals in Lancaster County," *Lancaster County (Pa.) Historical Society Papers* 52 (1948): 74. See Appendix G for data on many of the hospitals not discussed in detail in the text.

12. General Orders, 9 Dec 1777, Fitzpatrick, *Washington*, 10: 141–42; William Shippen to Jonathan Potts, 14 Dec 1777, Potts Papers, 3: 383; Thomas Bond, Jr., to Col John Patten, 13 Dec 1777, in Philadelphia, Historical Society of Pennsylvania, Manuscript Department, Autograph Collection, case 19, box 15; Helen Burr Smith, "Surgeon Jonathan Potts Planned Innoculation [sic] at the Winter Camp," *Picket Post*, April 1947, p. 20.

13. Gibson, "Role of Disease," p. 125; Benjamin Rush to William Shippen, 2 Dec 1777, Maj Gen Nathanael Greene, 2 Dec 1777, William Duer, 13 Dec 1777, and Washington, 26 Dec 1777, Butterfield, *Letters of Rush*, 1: 168–69, 170, 175, 176, 180.

14. Jordan, "Hospitals," pp. 145, 146–47, 150, quote from Shippen to John Ettwein, 19 Sep 1777, pp. 144–45; James A. Beck, *Bethlehem and Its Military Hospital, An Address Delivered at the Unveiling of a Tablet Erected by the Pennsylvania Society of the Sons of the Revolution June 19, 1897* . . . (printed by the Society), pp. 9, 11, 13.

15. Quote from message of 22 Sep 1777, Ballagh, *Letters*, 1: 324; Jordan, "Hospitals," pp. 146–47; Beck, *Bethlehem*, p. 13; Levering, *Bethlehem*, pp. 465, 466, 474, 475.

16. William Shippen to Congress, Oct 1777, Duncan, *Medical Men*, p. 220; Report of Brig Gen Lachlan McIntosh, 27 Apr 1778, RG 93, M246, roll 135, folder 3–1, item 11.

17. Samuel Stringer, report of 1 Apr 1777, Shippen to Potts, 7 Jul 1777, Cutting to Potts, 16 Mar 1778, and Thomas Bond, Jr., to Jonathan Potts, 17 May 1778, Potts Papers, 2: 156, 235; 4: 421, 468; General Orders, 14 Apr 1778, Fitzpatrick, *Washington*, 11: 260; Grif-

fenhagen, *Drug Supplies*, pp. 122, 127; Washington, National Archives, War Department Collection of Revolutionary War Records, Record Group 93, Numbered Record Books, 1775-98, series 5, Microfilm Publication M853, roll 12, pp. 18, 36; Nellie Protsman Waldenmaier, *Some of the Earliest Oaths of Allegiance to the United States of America* (Lancaster, 1944), pp. 22, 23; Bayne-Jones, *Preventive Medicine*, pp. 43-44. The relationship and status of the two apothecaries at this time are not clear. General Washington referred to Cutting as the Apothecary General of the Middle Department and Cutting signed two oaths of allegiance in this capacity in May 1778, but other records of later origin list Cutting as Apothecary General of the Eastern Department during this period.

18. Quote from James Craik to Jonathan Potts, 26 Apr 1778, Gibson, *Otto*, p. 164; Hatch, *Administration*, pp. 92-93.

19. General Orders, 12 Nov 1777, 28 Feb 1778, Washington to the Officers Visiting Hospitals, January 1778, Washington to Col George Gibson, 21 Feb 1778, Fitzpatrick, *Washington*, 10: 47-48, 406, 495-96, 526; George Weedon, *Valley Forge Orderly Book of General George Weedon of the Continental Army Under Command of Gen. George Washington, in the Campaign of 1777-8* (New York: New York Times & Arno Press, 1971 reprint of 1902 edition), p. 128; William Shippen to President of Congress, 24 Nov 1777, Duncan, *Medical Men*, p. 240; Ford, *Journals of the Continental Congress*, 10: 23.

20. General Orders, 15 Jan, 22 Feb, 17 Apr, 29 Apr, and 12 Jun 1778, Fitzpatrick, *Washington*, 10: 306, 499; 11: 270, 271, 319; 12: 50; William Bradford Reed, ed., *Life and Correspondence of Joseph Reed*, 2 vols. (Philadelphia: Lindsay and Blakiston, 1847), 1: 361; Johnson, *American Commissariat*, pp. 107-8; Risch, *Quartermaster Support*, p. 41; Ephraim Blaine to Jonathan Potts, 2 May 1778, and James Craik to Jonathan Potts, 24 May 1778, Potts Papers, 4: 461, 471.

21. Griffenhagen, *Drug Supplies*, pp. 127, 128; Invoice of Medicines Delivered to John Cochran, Esq., Surgeon and Physician General, for the Use of the Middle Department, 6 Feb 1778, Shippen to Potts, 24 Feb, Cutting to Potts, 25 Mar, Craigie to Potts, 27 Mar, 4 Apr, 1 May 1778, Potts Papers, 3: 400; 4: 411, 428, 429, 437, 458.

22. William Browne to Potts, 11 Mar, and Craigie to Potts, 1 May 1778, Potts Papers, 4: 419, 458; John D. Kendig, *A Legendary and Factual Review of the Times of Henry William Stiegel and the Early Days of Manheim* (n.p., 1957), p. 12; William Shainline Middleton, "Medicine at Valley Forge," *Annals of Medical History* 3d ser. 3 (1941); 481; James Hutchinson, "Notes: Valley Forge," *Pennsylvania Magazine of History and Biography* 39 (1915): 221.

23. Quote from James Craik (to Jonathan Potts?), 15 May 1778, Gibson, *Otto*, p. 177; J. B. Cutting to Jonathan Potts, 16 Apr 1778, Gibson, *Otto*, p. 166; General Orders, 14 Apr 1778, Fitzpatrick, *Washington*, 11: 261.

24. Quote from Andrew Craigie to Jonathan Potts, 1 May 1778, Potts Papers, 4: 458; James Craik to Jonathan Potts, 26 Apr 1778, Gibson, *Otto*, p. 164.

25. General Orders, 6 and 8 Jan 1778, Fitzpatrick, *Washington*, 10: 272, quote from p. 276; Hatch, *Administration*, pp. 92-93; Baron de Kalb to Count de Broglio, 21 Dec 1777, and James Craik to Jonathan Potts, 26 Apr 1778, Gibson, *Otto*, pp. 150, 164; Gibson, "Role of Disease," p. 125; Reed, *Joseph Reed*, 1: 362; Alfred Hoyt Bill, *Valley Forge: The Making of an Army* (New York: Harper & Bros., 1952), p. 102.

26. Quote from John Laurens, *The Army Correspondence of Colonel John Laurens in the Years 1777-8* . . . (New York: Bradford Club, 1867), p. 135; William Bell to Jonathan Potts, 22 Apr 1778, Potts Papers, 4: 447; General Washington to Gov George Clinton, 12 Mar 1778, Fitzpatrick, *Washington*, 11: 68; Worthington Chauncey Ford, ed., *General Orders Issued by Major-General Israel Putnam When in Command of the Highlands in the Summer and Fall of 1777* (Boston: Gregg Press, 1972 reprint of 1893 edition), p. 28; Richard Henry Lee to Arthur Lee, 30 Jun 1777, Ballagh, *Letters*, 1: 306; "A Whitemarsh Orderly Book," *Pennsylvania Magazine of History and Biography* 45 (1921): 217-18; Reed, *Joseph Reed*, 1: 361, 362; Weedon, *Valley Forge*, pp. 263-64; Albigence Waldo, "Valley Forge, 1777-1778. Diary of Surgeon Albigence Waldo, of the Connecticut Line," *Pennsyl-*

vania Magazine of History and Biography 21 (1897): 321.

27. Ford, *Journals of the Continental Congress*, 10: 1016; Blanton, *Medicine*, p. 252.

28. James Craik to Jonathan Potts, 22 Mar 1778, 26 Apr 1778, and Tilton to Potts, 8 May 1778, Gibson, *Otto*, pp. 164, 169-70, quote from p. 162; Washington to Officer Commanding at Alexandria, Virginia, 20 Mar 1778, and General Orders, 17 Apr 1778, Fitzpatrick, *Washington*, 11: 116, 271; John Cochran to Jonathan Potts, 22 Mar 1778, Gibson, *Otto*, p. 162; Francis Lightfoot Lee to George Weedon, 31 Mar 1778, Burnett, *Letters*, 3: 147; James Tilton to Jonathan Potts, 22 Apr 1778, Potts Papers, 4: 446.

29. Weedon, *Valley Forge*, p. 294; Fraser Lewis, "Medicine in the Continental Army of the Revolutionary War: 1775-1783," *Philadelphia Medicine* 55 (1959): 257-58; Norwood, "Medicine," p. 399; Shippen, "Plan," pp. 174n, 176; Tilton, *Observations*, p. 16.

30. Waldo, "Valley Forge," p. 316; General Orders, 9, 13 Jan 1778, Fitzpatrick, *Washington*, 10: 284, 300; Edward W. Hocker, "Medical Men Deserve Tribute for Care of Washington's Men at Valley Forge Encampment," *Picket Post* 16 (January 1947): 8; Edward Hand, "Orderly Book of General Edward Hand, Valley Forge, January 1778," *Pennsylvania Magazine of History and Biography* 41 (1917): 223.

31. James Craik to Potts, 26 Apr 1778, and James Fallon to Potts, 22 Apr 1778, Potts Papers, 4: 450, 462, quote from p. 450; Waldo, "Valley Forge," p. 316; General Orders, 21 Jan 1778, Fitzpatrick, *Washington*, 10: 333; Weedon, *Valley Forge*, p. 204.

32. Hand, "Orderly Book," p. 464; General Orders, 29 Jan and 20 Apr 1778, Fitzpatrick, *Washington*, 10: 403; 11: 281; Hocker, "Medical Men," p. 9; Waldo, "Valley Forge," p. 316.

33. General Orders, 26 Dec 1777, 22 Feb 1778, Washington's Instructions to Officers Sent to the Hospital, 28 Feb 1778, General Orders, 25 and 26 May 1778, Fitzpatrick, *Washington*, 10: 207, 499, 526-27; 11: 453, 455; Hand, "Orderly Book," p. 200.

34. James Craik to Potts, 7 Apr and 2 May 1778, Gibson, *Otto*, pp. 162, 173, quote from p. 173; General Orders, 12 Jun 1778, Fitzpatrick, *Washington*, 12: 50.

35. James Craik to Potts, 26 Apr 1778, Gibson, *Otto*, p. 164; Middleton, "Valley Forge," p. 472.

36. Gibson, "Role of Disease," p. 125; James Sproat, "Extracts From the Journal of Rev. James Sproat, Hospital Chaplain of the Middle Department, 1778," ed. John W. Jordan, *Pennsylvania Magazine of History and Biography* 27 (1903): 442; Cyrus T. Fox, ed., *Reading and Berks County Pennsylvania, A History*, 3 vols. (New York: Lewis Historical Publishing Co., 1925), 1: 166; Oaths of Allegiance, RG 93, M853, roll 12, book 165, pp. 52, 78.

37. Sproat, "Extracts," p. 442.

38. James Craik to Potts, 15 May 1778, Potts Papers, 4: 467.

39. Samuel Kennedy to Potts, 27 Apr 1778, and James Fallon to Potts, 27 Apr 1778, Gibson, *Otto*, p. 165, quote from Fallon to Potts; Sproat, "Extracts," pp. 443, 444; Samuel Kennedy to Potts, 22 Apr 1778, Potts Papers, 4: 454.

40. Quote from Bethlehem Diarist in Beck, *Bethlehem*, p. 13; Levering, *Bethlehem*, p. 475; Jordan, "Hospitals," pp. 147-48, 149, 150; John Ettwein, quoted in Raymond Walters, *Bethlehem Long Ago and To-Day* (Bethlehem, Pa.: Carey Printing Co., 1923), p. 52; John Ettwein, quoted in Levering, *Bethlehem*, p. 474; John Ettwein, "A Short Account of the Disturbances in America and of the Brethren's Conduct and Suffering in This Connection," in Kenneth Gardiner Hamilton, *John Ettwein and the Moravian Church During the Revolutionary Period* (Bethlehem, Pa.: Times Publishing Co., 1940), p. 180.

41. Hamilton, *Ettwein*, pp. 180, 181.

42. Various authors chose differing points during the course of the dispersal of the patients of the Bethlehem hospital as the official date of its closing. James Sproat, Journal of James Sproat D.D., 1753, 1757, 1778, 1779, 1780, 1782, 1783, 1784, 1786, held by the Historical Society of Pennsylvania, AM1597, 1778, pp. 1-2, 3-14; Walters, *Bethlehem*, p. 48; John Hill Martin, *Historical Sketch of Bethlehem in Pennsylvania* (New York: AMS Press, 1971 reprint of 1872 edition), p. 31; *Bethlehem of Pennsylvania: The First One Hundred Years, 1741 to 1841* (Bethlehem, Pa., 1968), p. 100; Levering, *Bethlehem*, p. 482; Jordan,

"Hospitals," pp. 150, 151; John Taylor Hamilton, *A History of the Church Known as the Moravian Church, or the Unitas Fratrum or the Unity of the Brethren During the Eighteenth and Nineteenth Centuries,* Transactions of the Moravian Historical Society, vol. 6 (Bethlehem, Pa.: Times Publishing Co., 1900), p. 252.

43. Specific information on the origins of the Lititz pharmacopoeia is sparse. It is usually credited to Brown, who was probably aided by others. The first edition, dated 1778, was unsigned and apparently written in the winter and early spring of 1778, too late to have been used at Valley Forge, although most of the medicines mentioned therein were undoubtedly familiar to the physicians caring for General Washington's men there. Hamilton, *Ettwein,* pp. 184-85; Jordan, "Hospitals," pp. 153-54; Middleton, "Valley Forge," pp. 480-81; Griffenhagen, *Drug Supplies,* pp. 126-27; Lyman F. Kebler, "Andrew Craigie, the First Apothecary General of the United States," *Journal of the American Pharmaceutical Association* 17 (1928): 171; Heiges, "Letters," p. 78; Champe C. McCulloch, "The Scientific and Administrative Achievement of the Medical Corps of the United States Army," *Scientific Monthly* 1 (May 1917): 412; Herbert H. Beck, "The Military Hospital at Lititz, 1777-1778," *Lancaster County Historical Society Papers* 23 (1919): 57.

44. Sisters' House Diary, Beck, "Lititz," pp. 7, 8, quote from p. 8; Jordan, "Hospitals," pp. 154, 155; Jordan, "Returns," p. 41; Return of the Sick and Wounded at Lititz Hospital From Jan. 12 to 22, 1778, in Philadelphia, Historical Society of Pennsylvania, Manuscript Department, Alison Papers, Continental Hospital Returns 1777-78; Samuel X. Radbill, "Francis Alison Jr., a Surgeon of the Revolution," *Bulletin of the History of Medicine* 9 (1941): 247-48; Middleton, "Valley Forge," p. 470.

45. Middleton, "Valley Forge," p. 471; Martin, "Ephrata," pp. 127, 128, 132; Report of Brig Gen Lachlan McIntosh, 26 Apr 1778, RG 93, M246, roll 135, folder 3-1, item 10; "Monument at Ephrata to Brandywine Battle Victims," *Magazine of American History* 30 (1902): 75.

46. Report of Brig Gen Lachlan McIntosh, 26 Apr 1778, RG 93, M246, roll 135, folder 3-1, item 10; Rev Peter Miller to William Shippen, 15 Jul 1779, Gibson, *Otto,* p. 287; Martin, "Ephrata," p. 130.

47. Quote from report of Brig Gen Lachlan McIntosh, 26 Apr 1778, RG 93, M246, roll 135, folder 3-1, item 10; Sproat, 21 Jun 1778, Gibson, *Otto,* p. 329; RG 93, M246, roll 135, folder 3-1, item 11.

48. Report of Brig Gen Lachlan McIntosh, 26 Apr 1778, RG 93, M246, roll 135, folder 3-1, item 10; A Return of the Soldiers in the General Hospital at Reading March 30th 1778, Potts Papers 4: 433; Jordan, "Returns," pp. 38-39; Radbill, "Alison," p. 249; Gibson, "John Augustus," p. 16; "Elijah Fisher's Journal While in the War for Independence and Continued for Two Years After He Came to Maine, 1775-1784," *Magazine of History,* Extra No. 6, entry for 19 Dec 1777, p. 17.

49. Report of Brig Gen Lachlan McIntosh, 26 Apr 1778, RG 93, M246, roll 135, folder 3-1, item 10; Gibson, *Otto,* pp. 159-61; William Shippen to Potts, 24 Mar 1778, Potts Papers, 4: 426; Sproat, "Extracts," p. 441.

50. Jordan, "Hospitals," pp. 155, 156, 157; John Ettwein to George Washington, 25 Mar 1778, Sparks, *Correspondence,* 2: 92; Hamilton, *Ettwein,* pp. 187-89; William Shippen to Potts, 20 and 24 Mar 1778, Potts Papers, 4: 422, 426; Report of Brig Gen Lachlan McIntosh, 26 Apr 1778, RG 93, M246, roll 135, folder 3-1, item 10; Washington to McIntosh, 4 Apr 1778, Fitzpatrick, *Washington,* 11: 206-8.

51. James Tilton to Potts, 8 May 1778, Gibson, *Otto,* p. 170; Tilton to Potts, 22 Apr 1778, Potts Papers, 4: 446; Washington to Brig Gen William Smallwood, 25 Feb 1778, Fitzpatrick, *Washington,* 10: 511, 513; Report of Brig Gen Lachlan McIntosh, 26 Apr 1778, RG 93, M246, roll 135, folder 3-1, item 10.

52. James Craik to Potts, 10 May 1778, Gibson, *Otto,* p. 176.

53. General Orders, 14 and 27 May 1778, Fitzpatrick, *Washington,* 11: 387, 463; Asa B. Gardner, "The New York Continental Line" *Magazine of American History* 7 (1881): 409-10.

54. General Orders, 30, 31 May, 1 and 29 Jun 1778, Fitzpatrick, *Washington,* 11: 487-88, 497; 12: 4, 131.

55. William Shippen to Potts, 16 Jun 1778, Potts Papers, 4: 477.

56. Quote from Samuel Adams to Richard Henry Lee, 22 Jul 1777, in Richard H. Lee, *Memoir of the Life of Richard Henry Lee and His Correspondence With the Most Distinguished Men in America and Europe . . . ,* 2 vols. (Philadelphia: H. C. Carey and I. Lea, 1825), 2: 123; Samuel MacKenzie to Potts, 24 Aug 1777, Potts Papers, 3: 290; Col John Banister to Col Theodorick Bland, Jr., 10 Jun 1777, in Theodorick Bland, *The Bland Papers, Being a Selection From the Manuscripts of Colonel Theodorick Bland, Jr. . . . ,* ed. Charles Campbell, 2 vols. (Petersburg, Va.: E. & J. C. Ruffin, 1840-43), 1: 55; Henry Sewall, "Letters," *Historical Magazine,* 2d ser. 2 (1867): 7, 8.

57. Maj Gen Philip Schuyler to Congress, 25 June 1777, in Philip John Schuyler, "Proceedings of a General Court Martial . . . ," *Collections of the New York Historical Society for the Year 1879,* p. 115.

58. Quote from Sewall, "Letters," p. 7; Gen Philip Schuyler to Congress, 25 Jun 1777, Schuyler, "Court Martial," p. 115; Lesser, *Sinews,* pp. 48, 49. Lesser gives no figures for June 1777 and no breakdown of figures for Ticonderoga and Mount Independence.

59. Thacher, *Journal,* pp. 83-84, 86-87; Walter Steiner, "Dr. James Thacher of Plymouth, Mass., an Erudite Physician of Revolutionary and Post-Revolutionary Fame," *Bulletin of the Institute of the History of Medicine* 1 (1933): 160.

60. Francis Hagan to Potts, 19, 21, 22 Aug and 21 Sep 1777, Nicholas Scull to Potts, 22 Aug 1777, Potts Papers, 3: 281, 285, 286, 287.

61. Samuel MacKenzie to Potts, 27 Aug 1777, Potts Papers, 3: 298.

62. John Bartlett to Potts, 18, 19, 21, 22 Aug 1777, and A Return of the Number of Sick in the Hospital Belonging to the Several Regiments and Companies on the Ground at New York City, 22 Aug 1777, Potts Papers, 3: 278, 280, 284, 288, 289.

63. Maj Gen Philip Schuyler to General Washington, 14 and 28 Jul 1777, Schuyler, "Court Martial," pp. 167, 179; James Wilkinson, *Memoirs of My Own Times,* 3 vols. (Philadelphia: Abraham Small, 1816), 1: 265; Return of the Men Who Died Since March the 1st 1777, General Hospital Northern Department, 29 Aug 1777, Potts Papers, 3: 304.

64. Brig Gen Simon Fraser to Maj Gen Horatio Gates, 1 Sep 1777, Sparks, *Correspondence,* 2: 522-23, quote from Maj Gen Horatio Gates to Brig Gen Simon Fraser, 2 Sep 1777, p. 523; Wilkinson, *Memoirs,* 1: 230; James E. Gibson, "Captured Medical Men and Army Hospitals of the American Revolution," *Annals of Medical History,* n.s. 10 (1938): 385; Return of 15 Aug 1777, Return of the Men Who Died Since March the 1st 1777, General Hospital, Northern Department, 29 Aug 1777, a List of the Sick and Wounded of His Majesty's Troops Left in the Hospital Near Stillwater October the 19th 1777, and a General Return of the Persons of Different Regts Dead in the General Hospl Since the 1st of March 1777 to the 12th Day Nov.r 1777, Potts Papers, 3: 273, 304, 355, 373; Thacher, *Journal,* pp. 103, 112; John McNamara Hayes to Potts, 12 and 15 Oct 1777, Gibson, "Captured," p. 385; Gibson, *Otto,* p. 230.

The report in Lesser for October 1777 for Gates's forces, dated 16 October, indicates that the sick rate in Gates's army was 9 percent as of that date. The accuracy of this figure, however, must be questioned. In Gates's army of the summer of 1777, which was much smaller than that of mid-October, the percentage of the total number of rank and file which was under the care of physicians averaged more than 23 percent, according to the monthly reports for July and August in Lesser. Since during the Revolution the number of patients in the autumn tended to be essentially identical to or greater than that in the summer, a drop of 14 percentage points from summer to fall would have been most unusual; nevertheless, even the sickness rate among the men of the five brigades which were with General Gates during the entire period in question actually dropped almost 15 points, according to the Lesser figures. In absolute terms, furthermore, the number of men sick, despite marked increases in size for three of the five brigades in question, dropped by as much as half or more from August to October, as reported in Lesser. Thus, for example, while Nixon's brigade grew from 1,454 rank and file in August 1777 to 1,481 in October, the number of sick among the rank and file fell from 306 to 142.

A figure of 9 percent sick and wounded for 16 October, furthermore, for units which had very recently seen action is not compatible with a figure of 11 percent (see figures in text) confined to the general hospital alone only twelve days earlier, at which time it might be estimated that another 11 percent might have been under the care of regimental surgeons. The number of sick and wounded in Gates's army on 4 October, therefore, might easily have been as high as 22 percent of the total number of rank and file. It would seem highly unlikely that only 9 percent remained under the care of surgeons less than two weeks later.

65. John McNamara Hayes to Potts, 12, 15 Oct 1777, 10 Feb 1778, Potts Papers, 3: 360, 363, 402; Thacher, *Journal*, p. 110.

66. Thacher, *Journal*, p. 103, quote from p. 103; Wilkinson, *Memoirs*, 1: 323; James Ripley Jacobs, *Tarnished Warrior, Major-General James Wilkinson* (New York: Macmillan Co., 1938), pp. 70-276 *passim*, 296.

67. Thacher, *Journal*, pp. 112, 113-14, quote from p. 112.

68. Malachi Treat to Potts, 20 Oct 1777, A Return of the Patients Now in the Gen. Hosp.l Who Have Been Examined by the Prescribing Physicians and Recommended for Furlows Albany November 13th 1777, A General Return of the Wounded in the Gen. Hospital at Albany in the Service of the United States, 14 Nov 1777, A Return of the Sick in Gen. Hospital Albany Novr 14th 1777, A General Return of the Sick and Wounded in the General Hospitals at Albany and Schenectady December 16th 1777, and Andrew Downe to Potts, 27 Dec 1777, Potts Papers, 3: 357, 374, 379, 380, 384, 389.

69. Dirk Van Ingen to Potts, 16 Aug 1777, A Return of the Sick and Wounded Gen. Hosp.l Schenactady [sic] Nov 10 1777, A General Return of the Sick and Wounded in the General Hospitals at Albany and Schenectady December 16th 1777, A General Return of the Sick and Wounded in the General Hospital Northern Department Albany Febry 16th 1778, and Robert Johnston to Potts, 23 Feb 1778, Potts Papers, 4: 276, 371, 384, 407, 410.

70. A General Return of the Sick and Wounded in the General Hospitals at Albany and Schenectady December 16th 1777, Robert Johnston to Potts, 22 Dec 1777, Malachi Treat to Potts, 23 Dec 1777, A Return of the Present State of the Generl Hospital N. Department at Albany & Schenectady January 1778, and Robert Johnston to Potts, 15 Jan 1778, Potts Papers, 3: 384, 386, 387, 391, 394.

71. Thacher, *Journal*, p. 120; Shippen report of 24 Nov 1777, Duncan, *Medical Men*, p. 239; Smith, "Potts," p. 19; Robert Johnston, Memorial to Congress, 31 May 1786, and Malachi Treat, Statement, 30 May 1786, in Washington, National Archives, Records of the Continental and Confederation Congresses and the Constitutional Convention, Record Group 360, Papers of the Continental Congress, 1774-1789, Microfilm Publication M247, roll 38, items 129, 137.

72. Thacher, *Journal*, pp. 130-31, quote from p. 121; Malachi Treat to Potts, 16 Feb 1778, A General Return of Sick, Wounded, etc., in the General Hospital Northern Department Albany March 16th 1778, Robert Johnston to Potts, 19 Apr 1778, Samuel Stringer to Potts, 20 Apr 1778, Potts Papers, 4: 405, 420, 442, 443, 470.

73. Thacher, *Biography*, p. 153; Joseph Meredith Toner, *The Medical Men of the Revolution With a Brief History of the Medical Department of the Continental Army* (Philadelphia: Collins, 1876), p. 128; Gordon, *Aesculapius*, p. 127; Ford, *Putnam*, p. 22; Washington, National Archives, List of Officers of the Medical Department U.S. Army 1775 to Present Date, Record Group 112, entry 84, room 201. Shippen's report of 24 Nov 1777, Duncan, *Medical Men*, p. 239.

74. Charles B. Graves, "Dr. Philip Turner of Norwich, Connecticut," *Annals of Medical History* 10 (1928): 5, 7, 8; Ford, *Putnam*, pp. 55-56.

75. Quote from Isaac Foster, 2 Oct 1777, Gibson, *Otto*, p. 286; Benjamin Rush to William Shippen, 2 Dec 1777, Butterfield, *Letters of Rush*, 1: 170.

76. Quote from Isaac Foster to Mr. Bartlet, 21 Mar 1778, Foster Papers, folder 1; Ford,

Putnam, p. 21; S. Tenney to Peter Turner, 22 Mar 1778, in Washington, Library of Congress, Manuscript Division, Papers of Peter Turner, 1778–1812.

CHAPTER 5

1. Unless otherwise indicated, passages concerning military operations in this chapter are based on the following: Maurice Matloff, ed., *American Military History* (Washington: Government Printing Office, 1969); Spaulding, *Army;* Christopher Ward, *The War of the Revolution,* ed. John R. Alden, 2 vols. (New York: Macmillan Co., 1952; and Weigley, *Army.*

2. Unless otherwise indicated, material concerning the Hospital Department in this chapter is based on Brown, *Medical Department;* Duncan, *Medical Men;* and Gibson, *Otto.* The preceding paragraph is also based on the following volumes: Quote from Henry Dearborn, *Journals of Henry Dearborn 1776–1783* (Cambridge: John Wilson and Son, 1887), p. 18; Charles Albert Moré, Chevalier de Pontgibaud, *A French Volunteer of the War of Independence,* trans. and ed. Robert B. Douglas (New York: Benjamin Bloom, 1972), p. 56; George Otto Trevelyan, *Saratoga and Brandywine, Valley Forge, England and France at War,* The American Revolution, vol. 4 (London: Longmans, Green and Co., 1929), p. 379; General Orders, 6 and 12 Jul 1778, Fitzpatrick, *Washington,* 12: 160–61, 172; James Craik to Jonathan Potts, 29 Jul 1778, Potts Papers, 4: 479.

3. James Craik to Jonathan Potts, 29 Jul 1778, Potts Papers, 4: 479; General Orders, 7 Aug 1778, Fitzpatrick, *Washington,* 12: 289; A Return of the Sick and Wounded in the Army of the United States Commanded by His Excellency General Washington on September 7, 1778, and Weekly Return of the Sick of the Army of the United States, Commanded by His Excellency General Washington—White Plains August 24, 1778, RG 93, M246, roll 135, folders 3–3, items 54, 55.

4. General Orders, 12 and 13 Sep 1778, and Washington to President of Congress, 4 Dec 1778, Fitzpatrick, *Washington,* 12: 430, 447; 13: 361; RG 93, M246, roll 135, folder 3–3, items 54, 55.

5. Quote from Washington to Dr. James Tillotson, 26 Jul 1778, Fitzpatrick, *Washington,* 12: 235; James Craik to Jonathan Potts, 29 Jul 1778, Potts Papers, 4: 479.

6. Peter Angelakos, "The Army at Middlebrook 1778–1779," *New Jersey Historical Society Proceedings* 70 (1952): 98, 99–100, 112, 116–17, and Barnabas Binney to Gen Nathanael Greene, 18 May 1779, p. 117; General Orders, 10 Mar and 8 Apr 1779, Fitzpatrick, *Washington,* 14: 223, 347.

7. General Orders, 11 Feb 1779, Fitzpatrick, *Washington,* 14: 100–101, quote from p. 101; Angelakos, "Middlebrook," pp. 105, 107; Bayne-Jones, *Preventive Medicine,* pp. 53–54, 58–59.

8. Returns of the Sick in Camp Commanded by His Excellency General Washington, 13 Jul 1779, 2 Aug 1779, 10 Aug 1779, RG 93, M246, roll 135, folder 3–1, items 30, 31, 32; Weekly Return of the Sick in the Army of the United States, Comanded [sic] by His Excelly Genrl Washington, 4 Oct 1779, RG 93, M246, roll 135, folder 3–3, item 61; Angelakos, "Middlebrook," p. 96; General Washington to General Knox, Jun 1779, Fitzpatrick, *Washington,* 15: 214n.

9. Theodore G. Thayer, "The War in New Jersey; Battles, Alarums, and the Men of the Revolution," *New Jersey Historical Society Proceedings,* n. s. 71 (1953): 106; Ricardo Torres-Reyes, *Morristown National Historical Park: 1779–1780 Encampment: A Study of Medical Services* (Washington: Office of History and Historic Architecture, Eastern Service Center, April 1971), pp. 4–5; Don Higginbotham, *The War of American Independence, Military Attitudes, Policies, and Practice, 1763–1789* (New York: Macmillan Co., 1971), p. 356.

10. Unless otherwise indicated, the section concerning Morristown is based on Torres-Reyes, *Study.* The preceding paragraph also contains material from Thayer, "New Jersey," pp. 99, 106; Thacher, *Journal,* pp. 176–77; Journal of Lt Charles Nukerck, in Frederick Cook, ed., *Journals of the Military Expedition of Major General John Sullivan Against the Six Nations of Indians in 1779 With Records of Centennial Celebrations* (Auburn, N.Y.: Knapp, Peck & Thompson, 1887), p. 221.

11. Journal of Rudolphus Van Hovenburgh, Cook, *Journals,* p. 284; S. Sydney Bradford,

"Hunger Menaces the Revolution . . . ," *Maryland Historical Magazine* 61 (1966): 5–6; Risch, *Quartermaster Support*, p. 57; Thacher, *Journal*, p. 181; Reed, *Joseph Reed*, 2: 191.

12. Lesser, *Sinews*, pp. 152–53; RG 93, M246, roll 135, folder 3–1, item 2; Torres-Reyes, *Study*, pp. 8–9, 28–30, 81, 82–84. The figures given by Lesser do not entirely agree with those of Torres-Reyes. The reader should also note that Torres-Reyes concludes that only 416 men at Morristown were sick in February on the basis of a return which, he states, deals with the number of men sick in hospitals and therefore, of course, does not deal with those sick in their own tents. The nature of the returns from this period makes this type of error all too easy. Torres-Reyes also uses the fit-for-duty figure as if it constituted the total enrollment and on this basis gives 3.7 percent as the proportion of the army at Morristown which was sick.

Torres-Reyes does point out that although a reconstruction of a Tilton hut was erected at Jockey Hollow in the 1930's, later investigation has revealed that there was no evidence that as large a building as a Tilton hospital was ever erected there. Tilton himself was stationed at Basking Ridge in the winter of 1779–80, and a reference dated February 1780 has been located which mentions that a hospital was built there for Tilton.

13. Journal of Lt William McKendry, Cook, *Journals*, p. 211; Heath, *Memoirs*, p. 240.

14. James Craik, "A Letter Written by Jas. Craik to Andrew Craigie, Esq., Apy. Genl., August 1780, Relating to the Condition of the Army, Communicated by Nathaniel Paine," *Massachusetts Historical Society Proceedings*, 2d ser. 15 (1901–2): 363.

15. Dr. William Eustis called the unit at Robinson's House a flying hospital (Eustis to Benedict Arnold, 7 Aug 1780, Washington Papers, 4: 69). John Mathews to Medical Committee, 10 Aug 1780, Burnett, *Letters*, 5: 320–21.

16. Shippen to Washington, 4 Jan 1781, Washington Papers, 4: 73.

17. Reports of Mar, May, and Jun 1781, Cochran Letter Book.

18. General Orders, 20 Jun 1781, Fitzpatrick, *Washington*, 22: 238.

19. Reports of Jul, Aug, and Oct 1781, quote from Aug 1781, Cochran Letter Book.

20. Thomas Coffin Amory, *The Military Services and Public Life of Major-General John Sullivan of the American Revolutionary Army* (Port Washington, N.Y.: Kennikat Press, 1968 reprint of 1868 ed.), p. 152; R. W. Vail, ed., *The Revolutionary Diary of Lieut. Obadiah Gore, Jr.* (New York: The New York Public Library, 1929), p. 20n; Order Book of Lt Col Francis Barber, pp. 7, 8, in Louise Wells Murray, ed., *Notes From Craft Collection in Tioga Point Museum on the Sullivan Expedition of 1779 and Its Centennial Celebration of 1879*, . . . (Athens, Pa.: 1929).

21. Quote from Orderly Book, 19 Jun–30 Jul 1779, *Pennsylvania Archives*, 6th ser. 14: 33; Shippen, Just Account; Journal of Lt John L. Hardenburg, Cook, *Journals*, p. 122; Order Book of Lt Col Francis Barber, p. 25, Murray, *Notes*.

22. Journal of Lt William McKendry, Cook, *Journals*, p. 200.

23. Quote from Journal of Rudolphus Van Hovenburgh, Cook, *Journals*, p. 276; "Order of March of Hand's Brigade From Wyoming to Tioga," *Pennsylvania Archives*, 6th ser. 14: 112, 115, 116.

24. Orderly Book, 19 Jun 1779, p. 52; "Order of March," p. 76; Order Book of Lt Col Francis Barber, p. 63, Murray, *Notes*.

25. Order Book of Lt Col Francis Barber, p. 78, Murray, *Notes*; Journal of Sgt Maj George Grant, Cook, *Journals*, p. 110; Jabez Campfield, "Diary of Dr. Jabez Campfield, Surgeon in 'Spencer's Regiment,' While Attached to Sullivan's Expedition Against the Indians From May 23d to Oct 2d, 1779," *New Jersey Historical Society Proceedings*, 2d ser. 3 (1873): 121.

26. James Clinton to George Clinton, 30 Aug 1779, in Henry Steele Commager and Richard B. Morris, eds., *The Spirit of Seventy-Six: The Story of the American Revolution As Told by Participants* (New York: Harper & Row, 1967), p. 1016; Journals of James Norris, George Grant, Moses Fellows, Gookin, Van Hovenburgh, McKendry, Adam Hubley, Burrowes, and Erkuries Beatty, Cook, *Journals*, pp. 30, 34, 43, 47, 89, 106, 110, 160, 166, 233–34, 270; Journal of Lt Robert Parker, in New York (State) University, Divi-

sion of Archives and History, *The Sullivan-Clinton Campaign in 1779. Chronology and Selected Documents* (Albany: The University of the State of New York, 1929), p. 202; "Order of March," p. 100.

27. "Order of March," pp. 112, 115, 116.
28. Journal of James Norris, Cook, *Journals*, p. 237; Albert Hazen Wright, *The Sullivan Expedition of 1779, The Losses*, Studies in History No. 33 of New York Historical Source Studies (1965), pp. 2–21, 28–29.
29. Quote from Dr. James Fallon to Dr. Thomas Burke, 1 Apr 1779, in North Carolina, *The State Records of North Carolina*, 26 vols. (Goldsboro, N.C.: Nash Brothers, 1886–1907), 14: 50; William Shippen to General Washington, 5 Oct 1778, Washington Papers, 4: 32.
30. Sproat, "Extracts," pp. 444, 445; Jordan, "Hospitals," p. 157; Hamilton, *Moravian Church*, p. 252; Hamilton, *Ettwein*, p. 185; Sisters' House Diary, Beck, *Medicine*, p. 12; Return of Stores on Hand in Reading General Hospital the First Day of May 1779, and Thomas Bond, Jr., to Potts, 16 Aug 1781, Potts Papers, 4: 504, 517.
31. Bodo Otto to Medical Committee, 19 May 1780, Gibson, *Otto*, pp. 181, 182, 183, quote from Journal of the Rev. Dr. James Sproat, p. 333; Bodo Otto to Charles Pickering, 26 Aug 1780, RG 93, M859, roll 80; John Cochran to Thomas Bond, 1 Oct 1781, Cochran Letter Book; William Brown to General Washington, 3 Jul 1780, Washington Papers, 4: 67; Gibson, "John Augustus," p. 16; Sproat, "Extracts," p. 445.
32. Quotes from William Brown to General Washington, 3 Jul 1780, Washington Papers, 4: 67; Reports of Aug and Sep 1782, Cochran Letter Book.
33. Sproat, "Extracts," p. 445; Thomas George Morton and Frank Woodbury, *History of the Pennsylvania Hospital 1751–1895* (New York: Arno Press, 1973 reprint of 1895 edition), pp. 60, 61; Francis Randolph Packard, *Some Account of the Pennsylvania Hospital, From Its First Rise to the Beginning of the Year 1938* (Philadelphia: Lea & Febiger, 1938), pp. 72, 73; Francis Randolph Packard, *History of Medicine in the United States* (New York: Paul B. Hoeber, 1931), pp. 570, 572, 573.
34. Minutes of Board Meeting, Morton and Woodbury, *History*, pp. 61–62.
35. Quote from Minutes of Board Meeting, Packard, *History*, pp. 574–75; Morton and Woodbury, *History*, p. 62; Packard, *Hospital*, pp. 74–75; A General Return of the Sick & Wounded in G. Hospitals of the United States, 6 Oct 1779, A General Return of the Sick and Wounded in the Several Hospitals, Belonging to the Army, Commanded by His Excellency General Washington From March 1 to April 1 1780, and A General Return of the Sick and Wounded in the General Hospital Belonging to the Army Under Command of His Excellency General Washington From April 1 to May 1 1778, RG 93, M246, roll 135, folder 3–1, items 2, 3, 12; Shippen Report of 31 Dec 1779, Gibson, *Otto*, p. 180; Chard, "Cochran," p. 374; Thornton Chard, "Illustrations Pertaining to the Medical Life of Doctor John Cochran," *Bulletin of the History of Medicine* 20 (1946): 83; Reports of Feb and Mar 1781, Cochran Letter Book.
36. Reports of Jul, Sep, Oct 1781, Cochran Letter Book; Ford, *Journals of the Continental Congress*, 14: 99.
37. C. Weisenthal to Potts, 6 Sep 1778, Potts Papers, 4: 486.
38. Gibbes, R. W., ed., *Reminiscences, Documentary History of the American Revolution . . .* , 3 vols. (New York: D. Appleton & Co., 1853–57), 2: 259–60, 263; Angelakos, "Middlebrook," pp. 116–17; General Orders, 10 Mar 1779, Fitzpatrick, *Washington*, 14: 223; Shippen Report of 31 Dec 1779, Gibson, *Otto*, p. 180; A General Return of the Sick and Wounded in the Several Hospitals, Belonging to the Army, Commanded by His Excellency General Washington From March 1 to April 1 1780, and From April 1 to May 1780, RG 93, M246, roll 135, folder 3–1, items 2, 3.
39. A Return of the Sick and Wounded in the Gen Hospital at Sunbury From the 31 July to the 22 of Sept 1779, Weekly Returns of 1 Oct, 11–18 Oct, 1–7 Nov, 7–13 Dec 1779, 7 Feb–13 Mar, 17 Apr 1780, Alison Papers; "Order of March," p. 112; Beatty, Cook, *Journals*, p. 35; Weekly Returns of 10–17 Jan, 24–31 Jan, 7–14 Feb, 21–28 Feb. 28 Feb–6 Mar, 6–13 Mar 1780, Jordan, "Returns," pp. 217–19.

40. Quote from Jordan, "Returns," p. 210; Returns of 11–18 Oct, 1–7 Nov 1779, Alison Papers.

41. Report of 17 Apr 1780, Alison Papers; "Order of March," p. 115.

42. Angelakos, "Middlebrook," pp. 102–3, 104–5; General Washington to Director of the Military Hospitals, 3 Jun 1779, and to James Craik, 25 Jun 1779, Fitzpatrick, *Washington*, 15: 220–21, 318; RG 93, M246, roll 135, folder 3–1, item 12.

43. RG 93, M246, roll 135, folder 3–1, items 2, 3; Shippen Report, 31 Dec 1779, Gibson, *Otto*, p. 180; Eliza Susan Quincy, "Basking Ridge in Revolutionary Days. Reprinted From Her Memoirs," *The Somerset County Historical Quarterly* 1 (1912): 35. There is some question about the location of the hospital, since Quincy gives the date of this hospital as 1776, a year when there is no other evidence to indicate that there was a hospital at Basking Ridge. She was, however, by her own account, an infant when the Revolution began and for this part of her story was relying upon the recollections of her mother, who was in her eighties at the time of the writing. The author describes Dr. James Tilton as "director of the medical department" when the hospital was located at Basking Ridge, but in 1776, Tilton was a regimental surgeon in New York; Trenton, New Jersey; and Wilmington, Delaware. (Eliza Susan Morton Quincy, *Memoirs* [Boston: John Wilson and Son, 1861], introduction and p. 17; Phalen, *Chiefs*, pp. 22–23.) Thus it seems likely that the older woman's memory had misled her concerning the date.

44. General Washington through Harrison to Capt William Reily, 21 May 1780, Fitzpatrick, *Washington*, 18: 401n.

45. Quotations from Malachi Treat to General Washington, 27 Jan 1781, Washington Papers, 4: 74; Reports of Mar, May, and Jun 1781, Cochran Letter Book; James Tilton to Timothy Pickering, 3 Oct 1780, RG 93, M859, roll 88, item 25616; General Greene to James Tilton, 27 Sep 1780, in George Washington Greene, *The Life of Nathanael Greene*, 3 vols. (New York: G. P. Putnam and Son, 1867–1871), 2: 229–30.

46. Ford, *Journals of the Continental Congress*, 11: 787–88; Burnett, *Letters*, 4: 249n;
General Washington to Philip Turner, 24 Feb 1780, Fitzpatrick, *Washington*, 18: 49–50; Jabez Hatch to Timothy Pickering, 21 Dec 1780; and Isaac Foster to Timothy Pickering, 21 Dec 1780, RG 93, M859, rolls 82, 85, items 23733, 24798; RG 93, M246, roll 135, folder 3–1, items 1, 2, 3.

47. RG 93, M246, roll 135, folder 3–1, items 1, 2, 3, and A Return of the Sick and Wounded in the Military Hospital Eastern Department, item 14; Isaac Foster to Mr. Peabody, 11 Mar 1780, RG 93, M859, roll 11, item 3610; General Washington to James Wilkinson, 6 Dec 1779, Fitzpatrick, *Washington*, 17: 221; Thacher, *Journal*, p. 152.

48. Reports of Mar, May, and Jun 1781, and John Cochran to Thomas Bond, 5 Jul 1781, Cochran Letter Book.

49. Thacher, *Journal*, p. 131; Shippen, Just Account; Radbill, "Alison," p. 249; General Washington to trustees of church at New Windsor, 31 Jul 1779, Fitzpatrick, *Washington*, 16: 25; RG 93, M246, roll 135, folder 3–1, item 12; A Return of the Sick Sent From Robinson's House to New Windsor, 20 Oct 1778, Alison Papers.

50. A flying hospital and a general hospital could, of course, have shared the same facilities, but this confusion is, perhaps, more likely the result of the casual use of terms common at this time. William Eustis to Benedict Arnold, 7 Aug 1780, Washington Papers 4: 69; Chard, "Cochran," p. 374.

51. Return of 20 Oct 1778, Alison Papers; Chard, "Cochran," p. 374; William Eustis to Benedict Arnold, 7 Aug 1780, Washington Papers, 4: 69; Fisher, "Journal," pp. 38–39.

52. John Cochran to Colonel Hay, 10 Jul 1781, and to Thomas Bond, 5 Jul 1781, Cochran Letter Book.

53. Reports of May–Oct 1781, Cochran Letter Book.

54. RG 93, M246, roll 135, folder 3–1, item 12; *The American Revolution 1775–1783: An Atlas of 18th Century Maps and Charts: Theaters of Operations* (Washington: Government Printing Office, 1972), 139D.

55. General Washington to Dr. William Shippen, 9 Sep 1778, Fitzpatrick, *Washington*, 12: 418; Graves, "Turner," pp. 8, 11; RG 93, M246, roll 135, folder 3–1, item 14.

56. Isaac Foster to Mr. Peabody, 4 Mar 1780, RG 93, M859, roll 11, item 3610; RG 93, M246, roll 135, items 1, 2, 3, 13; Cochrane, "Medical Department," pp. 250–51; General Washington to John Berrien, 25 Feb 1781, Fitzpatrick, *Washington*, 21: 292.

57. While no state was mentioned in this return, General Washington ordered Bedford patients moved east to Danbury, which rules out Bedford, Massachusetts, east of Danbury; Bedford, Pennsylvania, is too far away and in the Middle Department (General Washington to Dr. William Shippen, 9 Sep 1778, Fitzpatrick, *Washington*, 12: 418). William Eustis, 26 Aug 1780, in Edward Warren, *The Life of John Warren, M.D. . . .* (Boston: Noyes, Holmes, & Co., 1874), pp. 187–88 (Edward Warren's assumption that Eustis's hospital was in Pennsylvania is obviously incorrect. The context of the letter makes it clear that the hospital was in the Eastern Department). RG 93, M246, roll 135, folder 3–1, item 14.

58. RG 93, M246, roll 135, folder 3–1, item 14; General Washington to Dr. William Shippen, 9 Sep 1778, Fitzpatrick, *Washington*, 12: 418.

59. Turner to Dr. Timothy Hosmer, 16 Nov 1778, and to William Shippen, 15 Mar 1779, Graves, "Turner," pp. 7, 11; RG 93, M246, roll 135, folder 3–1, item 14; Ford, *Journals of the Continental Congress*, 17: 447; Philip Turner to Hooker, 29 Aug 1780, RG 93, M859, roll 121, item 034827; John Cochran to Peter Turner, 25 Mar 1781, Cochran Letter Book; Thacher, *Journal*, p. 163.

60. Packard, *History*, p. 600; Norwood, *Medical Education*, p. 43; John Warren to Governor and Council of Massachusetts, n.d., Warren, *John Warren*, pp. 193–94; John Cochran to Robert Morris, 26 Jul 1781, Chard, "Cochran," p. 372; John Cochran to Samuel Huntington, 24 May 1781, Cochrane, "Medical Department," p. 248; John Cochran to Thomas Bond, 1 Oct 1781, Reports of Mar and May 1781, Cochran Letter Book; RG 93, M246, roll 135, folder 3–1, items 1, 2, 3, 12, 14.

61. Malachi Treat to Jonathan Potts, 7 May 1778 and 28 Jan 1779, Potts Papers, 4: 442, 498, quote from 498; Washington to Brig Gen James Clinton, 19 Jan 1779, to Malachi Treat, 19 Jan 1779, and to Lord Stirling, 26 Jan 1779, General Orders, 2 Feb 1779, Fitzpatrick, *Washington*, 14: 23, 24, 25, 47, 67; Angelakos, "Middlebrook," p. 117; Thacher, *Journal*, p. 130; Ford, *Journals of the Continental Congress*, 7: 254.

62. General Clinton to Mrs. Clinton, 13 Jun 1779, New York University, *Documents*, p. 96.

63. RG 93, M246, roll 135, folder 3–1, items 2, 7, 12; William Brown to General Washington, 3 Jul 1780, Washington Papers, 4: 67; John Mathews to Medical Committee, 10 Aug 1780, Burnett, *Letters*, 5: 320–21.

64. Malachi Treat to Medical Committee, 21 Aug 1780, Potts Papers, 6: 519.

65. Reports of May–Oct 1781, Cochran Letter Book, quote from May 1781.

66. Quote from John Cochran to Samuel Huntington, 24 May 1781, Cochrane, "Medical Department," p. 248; Return of Medical Department, 23 Jul 1781, Duncan, *Medical Men*, pp. 344–45.

67. Sproat Journal, Gibson, *Otto*, p. 332; General Washington to Malachi Treat, 19 Jan 1779, Washington Papers, 4: 55; Washington to Brig Gen James Clinton, 19 Jan 1779, and General Orders, 3 Feb 1781, Fitzpatrick, *Washington*, 14: 23; 21: 174; Major Wylls to Samuel Blachley Webb, 4 Apr 1781, in James Watson Webb, ed., *Reminiscences of Gen'l Samuel B. Webb . . .*, 2 vols. (New York: privately printed, 1882), 2: 333; Heath, *Memoirs*, p. 296; General Orders, Washington, 8 Jan 1782, RG 93, M853, roll 9, book 57, pp. 111–12; Thacher, *Journal*, pp. 250–51, 298.

68. General Washington to James Craik, 24 May 1780, Washington Papers, 4: 66; Packard, *History*, pp. 590–91, 594; Lafayette to Le Comte de Rochambeau, 19 May 1780, in Marie Joseph Paul Yves Lafayette, *Mémoires, correspondance, et manuscrits du général Lafayette publiées par sa famille*, 2 vols. (Brussels: Société belge de Librairie, 1837), 1: 117; Phalen, *Chiefs*, p. 19.

69. Hall, "Beginnings," p. 123; William Heath to Governor of Rhode Island, 18 Jun 1780, Packard, *History*, pp. 592–93; Maurice Bouvet, *Le Service de santé français pendant la guerre d'indépendance des Etats-Unis* (Paris: Hippocrate, 1933), pp. 31–32, 56, 58–60, 91; Craik to Washington, 21 Jun

1780, Washington Papers, 4: 67; Ludwig von Closen, *The Revolutionary Journal of Baron Ludwig von Closen, 1780–1783*, ed. Evelyn M. Acomb (Chapel Hill: University of North Carolina Press, 1958), pp. 28, 28n, 37; John E. Lane, "Jean-François Coste, Chief Physician of the French Expeditionary Forces in the American Revolution," *Americana* 22 (1928): 54–55; Packard, *History*, p. 594.

70. Unless otherwise indicated, material in this chapter concerning the care of military patients south of Virginia is based on Chalmers Gaston Davidson, *Friend of the People: The Life of Peter Fayssoux of Charleston* (Columbia, S.C.: South Carolina Medical Association, 1950). The preceding paragraph is also based on Ford, *Journals of the Continental Congress*, 19: 292–94.

71. Quote from David Oliphant to Gen William Moultrie, 18 Jul 1778, Davidson, *Fayssoux*, p. 25; Benjamin Mather of the Office of Accounts, Hospital Department, 12 Oct 1786, RG 360, M247, roll 38, item 153.

72. Henry Lee, *Memoirs of the War in the Southern Department of the United States*, 3d ed., 2 vols. (Philadelphia: Bradford and Inskeep, 1812), 1: 139; Gibson, "Role of Disease," p. 126; Hugh Williamson to Dr. Hay, 24 Aug 1780, to Major England, 30 Aug 1780, to Hon Thomas Benbury, Aug and 1 Dec 1780, and Maj William R. Davie to Governor Caswell, 29 Aug 1780, North Carolina, *State Records*, 15: 61–62, 166–67, 370; Gibson, "Captured," pp. 388–89; Banastre Tarleton, *A History of the Campaigns of 1780 and 1781 in the Southern Provinces of North America* (London: T. Cadell, 1787), pp. 31–32; David Hosack, *A Biographical Memoir of Hugh Williamson, M.D., LL.D.* (New York: C. S. Van Winkle, 1820), pp. 56, 57–60; Henry Laurens to Benjamin Lincoln, 9 Oct 1779, Burnett, *Letters*, 4: 479–80; Col Charles C. Pinckney to Moultrie, 1 Jul 1778, Council of War at Camp at Fort Tonyn, 11 Jul 1778, Moultrie to Lieutenant Colonel Balfour, 22 Nov 1780, David Oliphant to Moultrie, 14 Nov 1780, and Peter Fayssoux to David Ramsay, 26 Mar 1785, in William Moultrie, *Memoirs of the American Revolution . . .* , 2 vols. (New York: New York Times & Arno Press, 1968 reprint of 1802 ed.), 1: 229, 235–36; 2: 112, 114, 142, 143, 398.

73. Quote from Horatio Gates to Director of the Hospitals in the Southern Department, Gates, "Letters," p. 284, and Gates to President of Board of War, 20 Jul 1781, p. 288; Lyman C. Draper, *King's Mountain and Its Heroes: History of the Battle of King's Mountain, October 7th 1780, and the Events Which Led to It* (Cincinnati: P. G. Thomson, 1881), p. 306; Joseph Graham, "Narrative of the Revolutionary War in North Carolina in 1780 and 1781," in *Papers of Archibald D. Murphey*, ed. W. H. Hoyt, 3 vols. (Raleigh, 1914), 2: 231n; Surgeon Browne to Major General Gates, 20 Aug 1780, and Gen R. Caswell to Gov Abner Nash, 31 Jul 1780, North Carolina, *State Records*, 14: 562; 15: 11. See also Table 1.

74. Quote from Nathanael Greene to Continental Congress, 28 Dec 1780, in Allen Bowman, *Morale of the American Revolutionary Army* (Washington: American Council on Public Affairs, 1943); Graham, "Narrative," 2: 233, 234; Proceedings of the Board of War, Hillsboro, N.C., 17 Nov 1780, North Carolina, *State Records*, 14: 452.

75. Gen Nathanael Greene to Colonel Marbury, 16 Dec 1780, North Carolina, *State Records*, 15: 181; Theodore Thayer, *Nathanael Greene, Strategist of the American Revolution* (New York: Twayne Publishers, 1960), p. 294; Gibbes, *Reminiscences*, p. 274.

76. General Moultrie to Lieutenant Colonel Balfour, 12 Feb 1781, Moultrie, *Memoirs*, 1: 159.

77. Maj John Armstrong to General Sumter, 1 Jul 1781, and General Sumter to Lt Col John B. Ashe, 14 Jul 1781, North Carolina, *State Records*, 15: 505, 533; Ford, *Journals of the Continental Congress*, 19: 292-94; Norwood, "Medicine," p. 399.

78. Quote from Dr. Robert Wharry to Dr. Reading Beatty, 27 Jul 1781, in Joseph M. Beatty, Jr., "Letters From Continental Officers to Doctor Reading Beatty, 1781–1788," *Pennsylvania Magazine of History and Biography* 54 (1930): 161; Maj John Armstrong to Gen Nathanael Greene, 1781, Greene, *Greene*, 3: 347; Lee, *Memoirs of the War*, 2: 145.

79. Gen Stephen Drayton to General Sumter, 29 Jun 1781, North Carolina, *State Records*, 15: 497.

80. RG 360, M247, roll 30, item 22; Lee, *Memoirs of the War,* 1: 94n; Gibbes, *Reminiscences,* pp. 279, 281.
81. Greene, *Greene,* 3: 407, 408, quote from Greene to President of Congress, n.d., 3: 407; Nathanael Greene, "Report on the 'Battle of Eutaw Springs,'" *Magazine of History,* Extra No. 3, pp. 8–10; Bowman, *Morale,* p. 23.
82. Resolve of the Continental Congress, 25 Ma`  `1, RG 360, M247, roll 30, item 22; Davi. Oliphant to General Moultrie, 7 May 1781, in David Ramsay, *The History of the Revolution in South-Carolina . . . ,* 2 vols. (Trenton: Isaac Collins, 1785), 2: 526–27; 2: 288.
83. Blanton, *Medicine,* p. 273; Robert B. Munford, Jr., "Military Hospital in Williamsburg, 1777," *Virginia Magazine of History* 30 (1922): 389–90.
84. Ford, *Journals of the Continental Congress,* 7: 292, 317; 9: 1016; Blanton, *Medicine,* pp. 252, 274; Goodman, *Rush,* p. 86.
85. A Return of the Sick & in Camp and Fredericksburg and the Vicinity Under the Command of His Excellency George Washington, Oct 25 1778, RG 93, M246, roll 135, folder 3–1, item 29.
86. Quote from General Washington to William Shippen, 10 Oct 1779, Washington Papers, 4: 61; William Shippen to T. Bland, 27 Nov 1780, Duncan, *Medical Men,* p. 322; General Washington to General Scott, 27 Jul 1779, and to William Brown, 22 Apr 1780, Fitzpatrick, *Washington,* 15: 492–93; 18: 291.
87. Report of Mar 1781, Cochran Letter Book; William Rickman to Brig Gen John Peter Gabriel Muhlenberg, 16 May 1780, and William Brown to Washington, 3 Jul 1780, Washington Papers, 4: 66, 67; Bowman, *Morale,* p. 22.
88. Blanton, *Medicine,* pp. 248, 276; William O. Owen, ed., *The Medical Department of the United States Army. Legislative and Administrative History . . .* (New York: P. B. Hoeber, 1920), pp. 164, 165; Commager and Morris, *Seventy-Six,* p. 1230.
89. Blanton, *Medicine,* p. 8; Davidson, *Fayssoux,* pp. 52, 53; Thomas Tudor Tucker to Saint George Tucker, 27 Jul 1781, in Williamsburg, Va., The College of William and Mary in Virginia, Earl Gregg Swem Library, Special Collections Division, Tucker-Coleman Papers, 1780–82, microfilm roll M–13.
90. Quote from John Davis, "The Yorktown Campaign: Journal of Captain John Davis, of the Pennsylvania Line," *Pennsylvania Magazine of History and Biography* 5 (1881): 293; Josiah Atkins, Diary and Letters in Joseph Anderson, ed., *The Town and City of Waterbury, Connecticut, From the Aboriginal Period to the Year Eighteen Hundred and Ninety-Five,* 2 vols. (New Haven: Price & Lee Co., (1896), 1: 476; William Feltman, "The Journal of Lieut. William Feltman, of the First Pennsylvania Regiment, From May 26, 1781, to April 25, 1782, Embracing the Siege of Yorktown and the Southern Campaign," *Pennsylvania Historical Society Collection* 1 (1853): 303–5.
91. Davis, *Journal,* p. 295; William McDowell, "Journal of Lieut William McDowell of the First Penna Regiment, in the Southern Campaign 1781–1782," *Pennsylvania Archives,* 2d ser. 15: 301.
92. Atkins, Diary, Anderson, *Waterbury,* pp. 476, 477, 478, 479; Bouvet, *Service de santé,* pp. 83, 85; Feltman, "Journal," p. 309.
93. Reports of Sep and Oct 1781, Cochran Letter Book; Blanton, *Medicine,* pp. 275–76; Bouvet, *Service de santé,* p. 88; Thacher, *Journal,* pp. 281–82.
94. Bouvet, *Service de santé,* p. 94, and Jean-François Coste to Dr. Cornette, 3 Feb 1786, p. 95; Ebenezer Denny, *Military Journal of Major Ebenezer Denny . . .* (Philadelphia: Historical Society of Pennsylvania, 1859), p. 39.
95. General Orders, 2 Oct 1781, and Washington to Jean-François Coste, 7 Oct 1782, Fitzpatrick, *Washington,* 23: 168; 25: 244; Bouvet, *Service de santé,* pp. 51, 96–97; Packard, *History,* p. 590; Hall, "Beginnings," p. 123; General Gregory to Governor Burke, 22 Aug 1781, North Carolina, *State Records,* 15: 618, Blanton, *Medicine,* pp. 259, 275–76.
96. Blanton, *Medicine,* p. 275; Report of Oct 1781, Cochran Letter Book; Thacher, *Journal,* pp. 286, 293; Bouvet, *Service de santé,* p. 97; James Craik to General Washington, 21 Sep 1781, Washington Papers, 4: 81.
97. Moré, *French Volunteer,* pp. 88–89.
98. General Washington to Col Stephen

Moylan, 31 Oct 1781, Fitzpatrick, *Washington*, 23: 312; General Washington to Gen Arthur St. Clair, 29 Oct 1781, in William Henry Smith, ed., *The St. Clair Papers. The Life and Public Services of Arthur St. Clair ...*, 2 vols. (Cincinnati: Robert Clarke & Co., 1882), 1: 562; General Washington to James Craik, 23 Oct 1781, Washington Papers 4: 81; Denny, *Journal*, p. 45; Blanton, *Medicine*, p. 276; Heath, *Memoirs*, p. 340.

99. Reports for Nov and Dec, 1781, Cochran Letter Book. Duncan suggests that Tilton preceded Treat and that Tilton's term of service was quite brief (Duncan, *Medical Men*, p. 355), but on 2 January 1782, General Washington referred to Tilton as Treat's successor (General Washington to Lt Col Francis Mentges, 2 Jan 1782, Fitzpatrick, *Washington*, 23: 423–24). A letter from Tilton to a friend from Williamsburg is dated 16 December 1781 (Tilton, 16 Dec 1781, Thacher, *Biography*, 2: 140), but one of General Washington's correspondents wrote in a letter dated 29 November 1781 as if Treat were in charge at Williamsburg at that time (Colonel Mentges to General Washington, 29 Nov 1781, Chard, "Cochran," pp. 372–73). A logical assumption would seem to be that Treat directed the hospital at Williamsburg until some time in early December 1781, at which time he was succeeded by Tilton.

100. Washington to Rochambeau, 8 Jan 1782, and to Colonel Mentges, 1 Mar 1782, Fitzpatrick, *Washington*, 23: 435; 24: 34; Colonel Mentges to Washington, 29 Nov 1781, Cochran to Tilton, 1 Jan 1782, and Report of Jan 1782, Cochran Letter Book; Blanton, *Medicine*, pp. 277, 283; Closen, *Journal*, p. 169; Quartermaster General Pickering to Virginia Governor Nelson, 8 Nov 1781, Duncan, *Medical Men*, p. 355.

101. General Greene to General Washington, 25 Oct 1781, Sparks, *Correspondence*, 3: 430.

102. Quotes from Feltman, "Journal," pp. 325, 326, 334; William Addleman Ganoe, *The History of the United States Army* (New York: D. Appleton and Co., 1924), p. 19.

103. Quote from Denny, *Journal*, p. 46; John Bell Tilden, "Extracts From the Journal of Lieutenant John Bell Tilden, Second Pennsylvania Line, 1781–82," *Pennsylvania Magazine of History and Biography* 19 (1895): 226; Doctor Wharry to Dr. Reading Beatty, 12 Mar 1782, Beatty, "Letters," p. 166; McDowell, "Journal," pp. 312–20.

104. McDowell, "Journal," p. 323.

105. McDowell, "Journal," pp. 326–31, quote from p. 328; Tilden, "Journal," p. 227; Greene, *Greene*, 3: 456; Denny, *Journal*, p. 47.

106. McDowell, "Journal," pp. 329–31, 332, quote from p. 331.

107. Quote from General Wayne to Benjamin Rush, 24 Dec 1782, in Charles J. Stille, *Major-General Anthony Wayne and the Pennsylvania Line in the Continental Army* (Philadelphia: J. B. Lippincott Co., 1893), p. 301; General Harmar to St. Clair, 29 Sep 1782, Smith, *St. Clair*, 1: 569; Feltman, "Journals," p. 334.

108. Edward McGrady, *The History of South Carolina in the Revolution 1780–1783*, 2 vols. (New York: Russell & Russell, 1969 reissue of 1902 publication), pp. 676, 701, 702; William Seymour, "Journal of the Southern Expedition, 1780–1783, by William Seymour, Sergeant-Major of the Delaware Regiment," *Pennsylvania Magazine of History and Biography* 7 (1883): 394.

109. Quote from Thacher, *Journal*, p. 281; Heath, *Memoirs*, pp. 341–42, 343, 361; Reports of Feb, May, and Jun, 1782, and Cochran to Thomas Bond, 4 Dec 1781, Cochran Letter Book.

110. General Washington to Pres John Dickinson, 3 Dec 1781, Fitzpatrick, *Washington*, 23: 368–69; Report of Dec 1781 and Cochran to Bond, 4 Dec 1781, Cochran Letter Book; Ltr, Robert Morris to Thomas Bond, 19 Feb 1782, Library of Congress; Daniel Shute, "The Journal of Dr. Daniel Shute, Surgeon in the Revolution 1781–1782," *New England Genealogical Register* 84 (1930): 387, 388.

111. General Orders, 6 Sep and 14 Nov 1782, Fitzpatrick, *Washington*, 25: 132, 345; Samuel Adams to General Heath, 9 Dec 1781, RG 93, M859, roll 101, item 29275.

112. Reports of Dec 1781–Jul 1782, Cochran Letter Book.

113. Reports of Aug, Sep, Nov, Dec 1782, Cochran Letter Book.

114. Reports of Nov 1781, Feb and Mar 1782, Cochran Letter Book; General Washington to William Duer and Daniel Parker, 29 May 1783, Fitzpatrick, *Washington,* 26: 460; Lists of Officers in the Mil. Hostls of the U.S. Exclusive of the Southern Department, 12 Nov 1783, RG 93, M246, roll 135, folder 3–3, item 59.

115. Reports of May–Jul, Sep, Nov, Dec 1782, Cochran Letter Book.

116. Quote from James Craik to Timothy Pickering, 1 May 1782, RG 93, M859, roll 95, item 27685; General Washington to Secretary at War, 18 May 1782, Fitzpatrick, *Washington,* 24: 263.

117. Quote from General Washington to Maj Gen Henry Knox, 11 Nov 1782, Fitzpatrick, *Washington,* 25: 330; William Eustis to Timothy Pickering, 3 Oct and 11 Dec 1782, RG 93, M859, roll 81, items 23505, 23506; Bouvet, *Service de santé,* p. 84; Thacher, *Journal,* pp. 307, 324.

118. General Washington to Maj Gen Henry Knox, 11 Nov 1782, Fitzpatrick, *Washington,* 25: 330; Reports of Aug–Dec 1782, Cochran Letter Book.

119. Reports of Nov and Dec 1781, Cochran Letter Book.

120. Packard, *History,* p. 575; Reports of Nov, Dec 1781, Jan–May 1782, and Cochran to Bond, 4 Dec 1781, Cochran Letter Book.

121. Packard, *History,* p. 575; Reports of Aug, Oct, Nov 1781, Jan, Feb, Jun–Sep, Nov, Dec 1782, Cochran Letter Book.

122. Ford, *Journals of the Continental Congress,* 25: 740; RG 93, M246, roll 135, folder 3–3, item 59; Reports of Feb, Mar, Nov 1781, May–Sep, Nov 1782, Cochran Letter Book; Cochran to James Craik and to John Warren, 10 Oct 1781, Chard, "Cochran," pp. 365, 372; Gibson, *Otto,* p. 314; Cochran, Letters to Binney, 22 Oct 1781, p. 230.

123. General Washington to John Cochran, 18 Jun 1782, Fitzpatrick, *Washington,* 24: 357.

124. Quote from General Orders, 18 May 1782, Fitzpatrick, *Washington,* 24: 265; Ford, *Journals of the Continental Congress,* 25: 740.

125. General Orders, 4 Aug 1782, Fitzpatrick, *Washington,* 24: 464.

CHAPTER 6

1. Unless otherwise indicated, the sections of this chapter concerning the U.S. Army's strength and organization are based on John F. Callan, *The Military Laws of the United States Relating to the Army, Volunteers, Militia, and to Bounty Lands and Pensions, From the Foundation of the Government to the Year 1863* (Philadelphia: George W. Childs, 1863); and Weigley, *Army.* Also consulted for the preceding paragraph was Leonard D. White, *The Federalists: A Study in Administrative History, 1789–1801* (New York: Macmillan Co., 1948), p. 236.

2. Harry M. Ward, *The Department of War, 1781–1795* (Pittsburgh: University of Pittsburgh Press, 1962), p. 187.

3. Unless otherwise indicated, material in this chapter relating to military campaigns is based on Ganoe, *U.S. Army;* Spaulding, *Army;* and Weigley, *Army;* while material describing the work of Army surgeons is based on Brown, *Medical Department.* The preceding paragraph also contains material from Lurton Dunham Ingersoll, *A History of the War Department of the United States, With Biographical Sketches of the Secretaries* (Washington: Francis D. Mohun, 1880), p. 212.

4. U.S. Congress, *American State Papers: Documents, Legislative and Executive of the Congress of the United States. Class V: Military Affairs,* 7 vols. (Washington: Gales and Seaton, 1832–61), 1: 147–51.

5. Quote from J. W. Daniels to Secretary of War, 12 Feb 1810, in Washington, National Archives, Records of the Office of the Secretary of War, Record Group 107, Letters Received by the Secretary of War, Main Series, 1801–1870, Microfilm Publication M221, roll 36; *American State Papers: Military Affairs,* 1: 209, and Henry Dearborn to House of Representatives, 9 Dec 1807, 1: 225; Bernard Devoto, ed., *The Journals of Lewis and Clark* (Boston: Houghton Mifflin, 1953), pp. 489–91.

6. Washington to John Cochran, 10 Aug and 4 Nov 1783, and Washington to Secretary of War, 4 Nov 1783, Fitzpatrick, *Washington,* 27: 95, 230–31; Orderly Book RG 93, M853, roll 9, book 60, pp. 112–15; Ford, *Journals of the Continental Congress,* 25: 740; List of

Officers in the Mil Hostls of the U.S. Exclusive of the Southern Department, 12 Nov 1783, RG 93, M246, roll 135, folder 3-3, item 59.

7. Quote from Oliver Spencer, quoted by Virginius Hall, Forman, *Physicians*; U.S. Congress, Senate, *Journal of the Executive Proceedings of the Senate of the United States, 1789-1901*, 32 vols. (Washington: Govenment Printing Office, 1828-1909), 1: 46-47.

8. Quote from Richard Allison to Brig Gen J. Harmar, 16 Apr 1789, quoted by Virginius C. Hall, "Richard Allison—Surgeon to the Legion," Foreman, *Physicians;* U.S. Congress, Senate, *Executive Proceedings*, 1: 46-47; Josiah Harmar, *The Proceedings of a Court of Inquiry, Held at the Special Request of Brigadier General Josiah Harmar* . . . (Philadelphia, 1791), p. 12.

9. U.S. Congress, Senate, *Executive Proceedings*, 1: 84, 87; Winthrop Sargent, "Winthrop Sargent's Diary While With General Arthur St. Clair's Expedition Against the Indians," *Ohio Archaeological and Historical Quarterly* 33 (1924): 264, 268; Richard C. Knopf, "Biographical Data," Forman, *Physicians;* Smith, *St. Clair*, 2: 200n, and Arthur St. Clair to Secretary of War, 17 Nov 1791, 2: 267n; Frazer E. Wilson, *Arthur St. Clair* (Richmond, Va.: Garrett and Massie, 1944), p. 4. There is some confusion concerning the position of Victor Grasson. Brown and both Tobey and Ashburn, who appear to lean heavily on Brown, classify Grasson as a Regular Army surgeon's mate, one of those whom the President could assign as he saw fit. Grasson is not mentioned in Heitman, however, and contemporary records do not specify his status. It should be noted that volunteer units did, at least on occasion, provide their own surgeons. Brown, *Medical Department*, pp. 73, 271; James Abner Tobey, *The Medical Department of the Army* (Baltimore: Johns Hopkins University Press, 1927), p. 8; Ashburn, *Medical Department*, p. 24; and Francis B. Heitman, *Historical Register and Dictionary of the United States Army From Its Organization, September 29, 1789, to March 2, 1903*, 2 vols. (Washington: Government Printing Office, 1903).

10. Sargent, "Diary," pp. 237, 254, quote from p. 242; Cyrus Townsend Brady, *American Fights and Fighters: Stories of the First Five Wars of the United States From the War of the Revolution to the War of 1812* (New York: McClure, Phillips & Co., 1900), pp. 166-67; Extract from the Diary of Maj Ebenezer Denny, 26 Oct 1791, Smith, *St. Clair*, 2: 255.

11. St. Clair Journal, Wilson, *St. Clair*, p. 71; Frazer E. Wilson, ed., *Journal of Capt. Daniel Bradley: An Epic of the Ohio Frontier* (Greenville, Ohio: Frank H. Jobes & Son, 1935), p. 26; Testimony of Major Zeigler in House Committee Investigation, Smith, *St. Clair*, 2: 290n.

12. Quote from Michael McDonough to Patrick McDonough, 10 Nov 1791, in Washington, Library of Congress, Manuscript Division, Peter Force Collection, Arthur St. Clair Papers, series 7E, box 60, folders 1782, Ag24-1793, Jul6; Sargent, "Diary," pp. 253, 264, 268; Knopf, "Biographical Data," Forman, *Physicians;* Randolph Greenfield Adams and Howard H. Peckham, eds., *Lexington to Fallen Timbers 1775-1794* (Ann Arbor; University of Michigan Press, 1942), p. 37; Wilson, *Bradley*, p. 24.

13. Quote from Michael McDonough to Patrick McDonough, 10 Nov 1791, St. Clair Papers; Wilson, *St. Clair*, p. 82; Extract from the Diary of Maj Ebenezer Denny, Smith, *St. Clair*, 2: 261; Wilson, *Bradley*, p. 34.

14. Wilson, *Bradley*, p. 34.

15. Sargent, "Diary," p. 265, quote from p. 254.

16. Anthony Wayne to Henry Knox, 3 Aug 1792, in Richard C. Knopf, ed., *A Campaign Into the Wilderness: The Wayne-Knox-Pickering-McHenry Correspondence*, 5 vols. (Columbus, Ohio: Anthony Wayne Parkway Board, 1955), 1: 45; U.S. Congress, Senate, *Executive Proceedings*, 1: 117; Harmar, *Inquiry*, pp. 9, 23; Louis Smith, *American Democracy and Military Power: A Study of Civil Control of Military Power in the United States* (Chicago: Unversity of Chicago Press, 1951), p. 177; White, *Federalists*, p. 148. (*See also* Table 7.)

17. Wayne, "Orderly Book," p. 350, quote from p. 361.

18. Quote from Anthony Wayne to Henry Knox, 3 Aug 1792, Knopf, *Campaign*, 1: 45; Wayne, "Orderly Book," p. 350.

19. Wayne, "Orderly Book," p. 390, quote

from p. 363; Henry Knox to Anthony Wayne, 27 Jul and 7 Sep 1792, Knopf, *Campaign,* 1: 38, 76-77.

20. Quote from Wayne, "Orderly Book," p. 403; Richard C. Knopf, ed., "A Surgeon's Mate at Fort Defiance: The Journal of Joseph Gardner Andrews for the Year 1795," *Ohio Historical Quarterly* 66 (1957): 37; Thomas Taylor Underwood, *Journal March 26, 1792, to March 18, 1800. An Old Soldier in Wayne's Army* (Cincinnati, Ohio: Society of Colonial Wars in the State of Ohio, 1945), p. 3n.

21. Underwood, *Journal,* p. 5; Anthony Wayne to Henry Knox, 2 Jul 1793, and Knox to Wayne, 27 Jul 1793, Knopf, *Campaign,* 2: 105-6, 114-15; U.S. Congress, Senate, *Executive Proceedings,* 1: 117, Knopf, "Andrews," pp. 61, 170, 170n; John Boyer, "Daily Journal of Wayne's Campaign," *American Pioneer* 1 (1842): 320.

22. Quotes from Boyer, "Journal," p. 320; Dwight L. Smith, ed., "From Greene Ville to Fallen Timbers," *Indiana Historical Society Publications* 16 (1951-52): 307; Return of the Killed, Wounded and Missing of the Federal Army Commanded by Major General Wayne . . . , in Washington, National Archives, Records of the Office of the Secretary of War, Record Group 107, Copies of War Department Correspondence and Reports, 1791-96, Microfilm Publication T982, p. 454; Richard C. Knopf, ed., "Two Journals of the Kentucky Volunteers, 1793 and 1794," *Filson Club Historical Quarterly* 27 (1953): 266. (*See also* Table 7 on organization of the Legion.)

23. Quote from Smith, "Greene Ville," p. 278; Richard Allison to Anthony Wayne, 23 Jun 1794, cited by Virginius Hall, "Richard Allison—Surgeon to the Legion," Forman, *Physicians.*

24. Boyer, "Journal," pp. 351, 352.

25. Quote from William Clark, "William Clark's Journal of General Wayne's Campaign," *Mississippi Valley Historical Review* 1 (1914-15): 431; Wayne to Knox, 17 Oct 1794, and Wayne to Timothy Pickering, 2 Sep 1795, Knopf, *Campaign,* 3: 73-74; 4: 88.

26. Anthony Wayne to Timothy Pickering, 18 Nov 1795, Knopf, *Campaign,* 4: 88-89, 107, quotes from p. 88, and from Wayne to Timothy Pickering, 5 Oct 1795, p. 106; Wayne, "Orderly Book," p. 619; Charles Whittlesey, "General Wadsworth's Division, War of 1812," *Western Reserve and Northern Ohio Historical Society Tracts* 2 (1879): 119.

27. James McHenry to Anthony Wayne, 16 Jul 1796, and Wayne to McHenry, 28 Aug and 28 Oct 1796, Knopf, *Campaign,* 5: 26, 45, 71, 72.

28. Francis F. Beirne, *War of 1812* (New York: E. P. Dutton & Co., 1949), pp. 60-61; David A. Durfee, ed., *William Henry Harrison 1773-1841. John Tyler 1790-1862. Chronology—Documents—Bibliographical Aids* (Dobbs Ferry, N.Y.: Oceana Publications, 1970), p. 7.

29. William Henry Harrison to Secretary of War, 10 Jul 1811, General Orders, 20 Sep 1811, Harrison to Secretary of War, 13 Oct and 18 Nov 1811, Log of the Army to Tippecanoe, 18 Nov 1811, Report of the Sick, Wounded and Invalids . . . , n.d., in William Henry Harrison, *Governors' Messages and Letters, Messages and Letters of William Henry Harrison,* ed. Logan Esarey, 4 vols. (Indianapolis: Indiana Historical Commission, 1922), 1: 532, 532n, 586, 602, 629, 634, 642-43; Certificates signed by Josiah D. Foster and Hosea Blood, 1811, in Richard C. Knopf, ed., *Document Transcriptions of the War of 1812 in the Northwest,* 8 vols. (Columbus, Ohio: Anthony Wayne Parkway Board, 1957-62), 5: part 1, p. 47.

30. Josiah D. Foster to George Cheyne Shattuck, Jan 1812, Shattuck Papers, 3, Massachusetts Historical Society, quoted in Leonard K. Eaton, "Military Surgery in the Battle of Tippecanoe," *Bulletin of the History of Medicine* 25 (1951): 460.

31. Quote from Adam Walker, *A Journal of Two Campaigns of the Fourth Regiment of U.S. Infantry . . . 1811-1812* (Keene, N.H.: privately printed, 1816), p. 11; General Orders 20 Sep 1811, Harrison to Secretary of War, 25 Sep 1811, and Report of 17 Dec 1811, Harrison, *Messages,* 1: 586, 589, 641.

32. Field Report, Harrison's Army, 12 Oct 1811, and Harrison to Secretary of War, 29 Oct 1811, Harrison, *Messages,* 1: 597-98, 605; Marvin A. Kreidberg and Merton G. Henry, *History of Military Mobilization in the United States Army 1775-1945,* Department of the Army Pamphlet 20-212, June

1955, p. 42; John K. Mahon, *The War of 1812* (Gainesville: University of Florida Press, 1972), pp. 20, 21; Walker, *Journal*, p. 18.

33. Harrison to Secretary of War, 18 Nov 1811, Harrison, *Messages*, 1: 630, 631; Beirne, *War of 1812*, p. 62; Walker *Journal*, p. 85; Eaton, "Tippecanoe," p. 461.

34. Harrison to Secretary of War, 18 Nov 1811, and Log of the Army to Tippecanoe, 13 Nov 1811, Harrison, *Messages*, 1:630, 633, 634, quote from Harrison to Secretary of War, 4 Dec 1811; Walker, *Journal*, pp. 36-37; James Ripley Jacobs, *The Beginning of the U.S. Army 1783-1812* (Port Washington, N.Y.: Kennikat Press, 1947, reissued 1970), p. 362.

35. Henry Knox to Speaker of the House, 28 Nov 1794, RG 107, T982, pp. 505-15.

36. Francis Paul Prucha, *A Guide to the Military Posts of the United States, 1789-1895* (Madison: State Historical Society of Wisconsin, 1964), p. 81; Henry Dearborn to Lyman Spaulding, 9 Apr 1802, in Washington, National Archives, Records of the Office of the Secretary of War, Record Group 107, Letters Sent by the Secretary of War Relating to Military Affairs, 1800-89, Microfilm Publication M6, roll 1, p. 188; Testimony of Capt Christie, Wilkinson, *Memoirs*, 2: 414.

37. Henry Dearborn to Thomas Cushing, 23 Feb 1803, and Dearborn to John Carmichael, 31 Aug 1803, RG 107, M6, roll 1, pp. 373-74; roll 2, p. 54; quote from Dearborn to James Wilkinson, 7 Mar 1803, roll 1, p. 380; Capt John Bowyer and other officers to Secretary of War, 13 May 1804, RG 107, M221, roll 1; U.S. Congress, Senate, *Executive Proceedings*, 1: 414; Knopf, "Biographical Data," Forman, *Physicians;* Thomas H. S. Hamersly, *Complete Army and Navy Register of the United States of America, From 1776 to 1887* (New York: T. H. S. Hamersly, 1888), p. 51; Disposition of Dr. J. F. Carmichael, Wilkinson, *Memoirs*, 2: app. 21.

38. Wilson, *St. Clair,* p. 71; *American State Papers: Military Affairs*, 1: 67; Wilson, *Bradley*, p. 76n; Frazer Ells Wilson, *Fort Jefferson: The Frontier Post of the Upper Miami Valley: A Fascinating Tale of Border Life Gleaned From Authentic Sources and Retold by Frazer Ells Wilson* (Lancaster, Pa., 1950), p. 7; John Heckwelder, "Narrative of His Journey to the Wabash in 1792," *Pennsylvania Magazine of History and Biography* 12 (1888): 12, 42.

39. Prucha, *Guide,* p. 71; Knopf, "Andrews," pp. 57, 60, 69, 75; Henry Dearborn to Jonathan Sparhawk, 18 Oct 1803, RG 107, M6, roll 2, p. 83; Francis LeBaron to Secretary of War, 30 Sep 1810, RG 107, M221, roll 38.

40. All material on Andrews, unless otherwise indicated, is based on Knopf, "Andrews," pp. 60-262, and the quotes in the following paragraphs are from pp. 176, 241, 244, 248, 260, 261, and 262.

41. Unless otherwise indicated, the section on Wilkinson is based on Jacobs, *Wilkinson*. General Wilkinson later wrote a lengthy defense of his conduct at this time, but his memoirs must be considered in the light of the author's reputation for "deviousness" (Weigley, *Army*, p. 107).

42. James Wilkinson to William Eustis, 19 Aug 1809, Report of William Upshaw, Surgeon 5th Infantry, 20 Jul 1809, and Report of Alfred Thruston, Surgeon 7th Infantry, 29 Jul 1809, *American State Papers: Military Affairs*, 1: 270, 292-93; Hamersly, *Register*, p. 55; Kreidberg and Henry, *Mobilization*, p. 41; "Sickness in the Army at New Orleans, in 1809," *Medical Repository* 14 (1811): 85-87; Deposition of Dr. Theodore Elmer, Orders to Brig Gen James Wilkinson from H. Dearborn, 2 Dec 1808, and William Eustis to Dr. Oliver Spencer, Surgeon, Aug 1809, Wilkinson, *Memoirs*, 2: 342, 450-510, app. 109. See also other material, 2: 414, 431, 506, and app. 109.

43. Wilkinson, *Memoirs*, 2: 408-9, 410, 414, 425, and Testimony of Col Electus Backus, app. 108; Hamersly, *Register*, p. 55.

44. Wilkinson, *Memoirs* 2: 346-47, 506, Testimony of Col Electus Backus, app. 108, Deposition of Lieutenant-Colonel Beall, app. 111, and James Wilkinson to Secretary of War, 19 Apr 1809, 2: 349, quote from p. 350; William Eustis to James Wilkinson, 30 Apr 1809, *American State Papers: Military Affairs*, 2: 269.

45. Wilkinson, *Memoirs*, 2: 371, 375-76; William Eustis to James Wilkinson, 30 Apr 1809, *American State Papers: Military Affairs*, 1: 269; "Sickness in the Army," p. 86.

46. Jacobs, *The Beginning*, pp. 346, 347; James Wilkinson to Secretary of War, 20 May 1809, *American State Papers: Military Affairs*, 1: 269; Wilkinson, *Memoirs*, 2: 367–68, 390; "Sickness in the Army," p. 85; Jabez W. Heustis, "Observations on the Disease Which Prevailed in the Army at Camp Terre-aux-Boeufs, in June, July, and August of the Year 1809," *Medical Repository*, 2d ser. 3 (1817): 38.

47. Wilkinson, *Memoirs*, 2: 372.

48. "Sickness in the Army," p. 87; James Wilkinson to William Eustis, 19 Aug 1809, and William Upshaw Report, 20 Jul 1809, *American State Papers: Military Affairs*, 1: 220, 292–93; Heustis, "Observations," p. 38; Wilkinson, *Memoirs*, 2: app. 108.

49. Jacobs, *The Beginning*, pp. 349, 352–53; Wilkinson, *Memoirs*, 2: 430, 483–84, 485; Eustis to Spencer, Aug 1809, pp. 450–51; Eustis to Dr. John M. Daniel, 1809, p. 479.

50. Wilkinson to Eustis, 18 Jun 1809, and Eustis to Wilkinson, 22 Jun 1809, *American State Papers: Military Affairs*, 1: 269; Wilkinson, *Memoirs*, 2: 386.

51. Wilkinson, *Memoirs*, 2: 406, 407, 417; Jacobs, *The Beginning*, p. 351; Report of Alfred Thruston, 29 Jul 1809, *American State Papers: Military Affairs*, 1: 293.

52. Wilkinson, *Memoirs*, 2: 417, Testimony of Col Electus Backus, app. 108, and Deposition of Captain Dale, app. 111.

53. Wilkinson, *Memoirs*, 2: 480 and app. 108.

54. William Eustis to James Wilkinson, 10 Sep 1809, Wilkinson, *Memoirs*, 2: app. 110, data and quote from Deposition of Doctor Dow, app. 109.

55. Quote from William Upshaw Report, 20 Jul 1809, *American State Papers: Military Affairs*, 1: 292–93; Heustis, "Observations," pp. 34, 36; "Sickness of the Army," pp. 86–87; Deposition of Lieutenant-Colonel Beall, Wilkinson, *Memoirs*, 2: app. 111.

56. Medical Department, United States Army, *Communicable Diseases, Preventive Medicine in World War II*, vol. 6 (Washington: Government Printing Office, 1963), chart 1, p. 14, and table 9, p. 112; Wilkinson, *Memoirs*, 2: 427.

57. Wilkinson, *Memoirs*, 2: 347; Depositions of Captain Dale and Lieutenant-Colonel Beall, app. 111; data and quote from John Smith, for Secretary of War, to Abraham D. Abrahams, 20 Aug. 1808, 2: 435.

58. Heustis, "Observations," pp. 33, 37, quote from pp. 33–34.

59. Heustis, "Observations," pp. 35, 36.

60. Heustis, "Observations," pp. 35, 36, 39, quotes from pp. 37, 38, 41.

61. Heustis, "Observations," pp. 36, 40, 41, quote from p. 40. After studying contemporary accounts of the condition of Wilkinson's men at this time, Col Robert J. T. Joy, MC, in 1976 Director of the Walter Reed Army Institute of Research in Washington, D.C., commented that "these troops were the victims of a combination of events—any one or two of which would have been enough to cripple a force; in combination, the force was destroyed." Colonel Joy believed that their condition resulted from "A combination of vitamin deficiency, starvation, and malaria as the common substrate upon which diarrhea, dysentery, hepatitis, typhoid, and pneumonia were laid, all being helped along by poor housing, poor clothing, and demands for hard physical labor, with a shortage of moderately effective medicine and the overuse of a useless, or dangerous therapy. Any one man didn't have to have everything—just a few would kill him." The only effective medicines available to these men were opium for diarrhea and bark for malaria. The oral lesions, Colonel Joy noted, resulted from the overuse of mercury and possibly from scurvy as well. (Letter to the author, 11 Jun 1976.)

62. Risch, *Quartermaster Support*, pp. 76–84; General Orders, Harrison, *Messages*, 1: 586; Clark, "Journal," p. 431; White, *Federalists*, p. 148; Boyer, "Journal," p. 351; Wayne to Henry Knox, 2 Jul 1793, Timothy Pickering, 2 Sep and 5 Oct 1795, and James McHenry, 28 Oct 1796, Knopf, *Campaign*, 2: 105–6; 4: 88, 106, 107; 5: 71; Dittrick, "Medical Agents," Forman, *Physicians*; Francis LeBaron to Secretary of War, 20 Jun 1802, 30 Sep 1810, and Will Stewart to Secretary of War, 30 Mar 1812, RG 107, M221, rolls 38 and 40; Dearborn to Maj Constant Freeman, 27 Jun 1801, Wilkinson, 17 Jul 1801, Thomas Cushing, 20 Mar 1802, Israel Whelen, 27 Mar 1802, and Secretary of War to Smith Cutler, 14 Jan 1809, RG 107, M6, roll 1, pp. 91, 95, 165–66, 171–75; roll 4, p. 12.

63. William Eustis to Benjamin Rush, 2 Jan 1810, 31 May 1810, Eustis to Dr. James Mease, 31 May 1810, RG 107, M6, roll 4, pp. 254, 363, quote from Secretary of War to Smith Cutler, 14 Jan 1809, p. 12; Dittrick, "Medical Agents," Forman, *Physicians;* James Mease to Secretary of War, 28 Jan and 28 May 1810, RG 107, M221, roll 38.

64. Quote from Secretary of War to Tench Coxe, 12 Feb 1812, RG 107, M6, roll 5, p. 273; Francis LeBaron to Adjutant General, 30 Jun and 4 Dec 1812, in Washington, National Archives, Records of the Adjutant General's Office, 1780s–1917, Record Group 94, Letters Received by the Adjutant General 1805–21, Microfilm Publication M566, roll 12; Francis LeBaron to Secretary of War, 26 Feb 1812, RG 107, M221, roll 46.

65. Francis LeBaron to Secretary of War, 13 Feb and Apr 1812, RG 107, M221, roll 46.

66. Secretary of War to Francis LeBaron, 14 Jul and 24 Aug 1812, quote from Secretary of War to Francis LeBaron, 20 Aug 1812, RG 107, M6, roll 6, pp. 25, 95, 96, 100; LeBaron to Secretary of War, 26 Feb 1812, RG 107, M221, roll 46.

67. William Atherton, *Narrative of the Suffering & Defeat of the Northwestern Army Under General Winchester* . . . (Frankfort, Ky., 1842), p. 39.

CHAPTER 7

1. Unless otherwise indicated, the material in this chapter is based on Beirne, *War of 1812;* Brown, *Medical Department,* pp. 81–100; James Ripley Jacobs and Glenn Tucker, *The War of 1812: A Compact History* (New York: Hawthorn Books, 1969); Weigley, *Army,* pp. 97–133, 566; and Charles Maurice Wiltse, *The New Nation, 1800–1845* (London: Macmillan, 1965).

2. Secretary of War to Henry Dearborn, 26 Aug 1812, RG 107, M6, roll 6, p. 100, quote from Secretary of War to Francis LeBaron, 24 Aug 1812, p. 95.

3. Secretary of War to Francis LeBaron, 29 Aug 1812, RG 107, M6, roll 6, p. 104.

4. LeBaron to Secretary of War, 17 Oct 1812, RG 107, M221, roll 46; Secretary of War to LeBaron, 25 Aug 1812, RG 107, M6, roll 6, p. 96.

5. Secretary of War to Francis LeBaron, 4 and 9 Oct 1812, RG 107, M6, roll 6, pp. 181, 188; Francis LeBaron to Secretary of War, 17 Oct 1812, RG 107, M221, roll 46.

6. Francis LeBaron to Secretary of War, 13 Nov 1812, RG 107, M221, roll 46; Secretary of War to Francis LeBaron, 16 Oct 1812 and 12 May 1813, RG 107, M6, roll 6, pp. 195, 413–14.

7. Francis LeBaron to Adjutant and Inspector, Washington City, 8 Dec 1812, RG 94, M566, roll 12, quotes from Francis LeBaron to Adjutant General, 5 Oct 1812.

8. Unless otherwise indicated, Callan, *Military Laws* has formed the basis of discussions of the laws governing the activities of the Medical Department.

9. *American State Papers: Military Affairs,* 1: 428, 432–33, 435, quote from p. 434; Thomas H. Palmer, ed., *Historical Register of the United States,* 4 vols. (Philadelphia, 1814–16), 3: 7; Marguerite McKee, "Service of Supply in the War of 1812," *Quartermaster Review* 6 (1927): 51.

10. *Niles' Weekly Register* (Baltimore) 6: 36; *American State Papers: Military Affairs,* 1: 384–85; Wolfe, "Genesis," pp. 842–43.

11. James Mann, *Medical Sketches of the Campaigns of 1812, 13, 14* . . . (Dedham, Mass.: H. Mann and Co., 1816), p. 75; Secretary of War to Francis LeBaron, 6 Aug 1813 and 6 Jul 1814, RG 107, M6, roll 7, pp. 31, 252.

12. Regulations for the Medical Department, Dec 1814, Brown, *Medical Department,* pp. 94–98; Palmer, *Historical Register,* 3: 709; Tilton to Assistant Inspector General, 4 Jun 1814, RG 94, M566, roll 59.

13. Quote from T. R. Adams, "The Medical and Political Activities of Dr. James Tilton," *Annual Report of the John Carter Brown Library* (Providence, R.I.: The John Carter Brown Library, Brown University and the Colonial Society of Massachusetts) 7 (1972): 30; Tilton, *Observations.*

14. Quote from James Tilton to Secretary of War, 23 Aug 1814, RG 107, M221, roll 66; Benjamin Waterhouse to Secretary of War, 12 Jul 1815, RG 107, M221, roll 67.

15. Quote from James Tilton to Secretary of War, 19 Sep 1814, in Washington, National

Archives, Records of the Office of the Secretary of War, Record Group 107, Letters Received by the Secretary of War, Unregistered Series, 1789–1861, Microfilm Publication M222, roll 10. Brown states that the leg was amputated in 1814 but Phalen maintains that the operation was performed 7 December 1815 (*Chiefs*, p. 25). Neither his letters nor those of his colleagues in late 1814 and 1815 refer even obliquely to his having undergone major surgery (see letters of Tilton for this period in RG 94, M566, rolls 59 and 82; RG 107, M221, rolls 66 and 67; and RG 107, M222, roll 10; as well as Benjamin Waterhouse to Secretary of War, 12 Jul 1815, RG 107, M221, roll 67). Thus it seems safe to assume that Brown was mistaken as to the date of the amputation (see p. 98 in *Medical Department*). Tilton's frequent presence in Wilmington is established by the many letters he sent from that city (see James Tilton to Adjutant General, 5 Feb, 4, 7, 9, 30 Jun, 15 Aug, 19 Sep, 4, 15 Oct, 3, 8 Nov, and 5 Dec 1814, RG 94, M566, roll 59).

16. *American State Papers: Military Affairs*, 1: 591; Francis LeBaron to Secretary of War, 17 Jun 1813, and to Adjutant General, 20 Dec 1814, RG 94, M566, roll 12; Francis LeBaron to Secretary of War, 2 June 1814, RG 107, M221, roll 63; McKee, "Service of Supply," p. 51.

17. Office of Adjutant General to James Tilton, 29 May 1814, in Washington, National Archives, Records of the Adjutant General's Office, 1780s–1917, Record Group 94, Letters Sent by the Office of the Adjutant General, Main Series, 1800–1890, Microfilm Publication M565, roll 4, vol. 3, p. 547.

18. Quote from James Tilton to Assistant Inspector General, 4 Jun 1814, RG 94, M566, roll 59.

19. James Tilton to Secretary of War, 10 Feb 1815, RG 107, M221, roll 66.

20. Quote from James Tilton to Secretary of War, 20 Aug 1814, RG 107, M221, roll 66; Statement of Dr. Catlett, 1814, *American State Papers: Military Affairs*, 1: 584; William M. Marine, *The British Invasion of Maryland, 1812–1815* (Baltimore: Society of the War of 1812 in Maryland, 1913), p. 174; Office of Adjutant General to Dr. John R. Martin, 26 Jun 1813, 21 and 23 Feb, 15 Mar, and 26 Jun 1814, RG 94, M565, roll 4, 3: 216, 373, 379, 412, 543.

21. James Ewell, *The Medical Companion* . . . , 3d ed. (Philadelphia: privately printed, 1817), pp. 690–91.

22. Tilton to Secretary of War, 27 Oct 1814, RG 107, M221, roll 66, quotes from roll 59; Mann, *Sketches*, pp. 255–56.

23. James Mann to James Tilton, 14 Feb 1814, Brown, *Medical Department*, p. 93.

24. Benjamin Waterhouse to Tilton, 13 Aug 1814, RG 107, M221, roll 82, quotes from Waterhouse to Secretary of War, 13 Aug 1814, roll 67; A. Hays to James Tilton, 2 Oct 1814 and 2 Jan 1815, RG 94, M566, rolls 59, 82; Tilton to Secretary of War, 19 Sep 1814, RG 107, M222, roll 10. A black cockade, worn on the hat, was a part of the Army's uniform (*American State Papers: Military Affairs*, 1: 434).

25. Tilton to Secretary of War, 20 Aug 1814 and 10 Feb 1815, RG 107, M221, roll 66; Charles Smart, *The Connection of the Army Medical Department With the Development of Meteorology in the United States*, U.S. Department of Agriculture, Weather Bureau, Report of the International Meteorological Congress held at Chicago, Ill., 21–24 Aug 1893, Bulletin No. 11, part 2 (1895): 208; Palmer, *Historical Register*, 3: 8.

26. Tilton to Secretary of War, 20 Aug 1814, RG 107, M221, roll 66; Palmer, *Historical Register*, 3: 7–8.

27. Tilton to Secretary of War, 10 Feb 1815, RG 107, M221, roll 66.

28. McKee, "Service of Supply," p. 51; Kreidberg and Henry, *Mobilization*, pp. 58–59; Jabez W. Heustis, *Physical Observations and Medical Tracts and Researches on the Topography and Diseases of Louisiana* (New York: T. and J. Swords, 1817), pp. 105n–106n; Brereton Greenhous, "A Note on Western Logistics in the War of 1812," *Military Affairs* 34 (1970): 43.

29. Office of Adjutant General to Members of the General Staff, 29 Oct 1814, RG 94, M565, roll 5, vol. 3½; Secretary of War to LeBaron, 21 Jun 1813, RG 107, M6, roll 6, pp. 468–69; LeBaron to Secretary of War, 28 Jul 1813, RG 107, M221, roll 54.

30. Secretary of War to LeBaron, 24 Mar 1813, RG 107, M6, roll 6, p. 336.

31. Quotes and data from Secretary of War to LeBaron, 16 Oct 1813, RG 107, M6, roll 7, pp. 93, 94; LeBaron to Secretary of War, 29 Jun 1814, RG 94, M566, roll 12; LeBaron to Secretary of War, 18 Sep 1814, RG 107, M221, roll 63.

32. LeBaron to Secretary of War, 30 Mar 1813, RG 107, M221, roll 54, quote from Dr. Shaw to Secretary of War, 21 Apr 1813, roll 57; Secretary of War to LeBaron, 24 May 1813, RG 107, M6, roll 6, p. 336.

33. Joseph Lovell to Secretary of War, 18 May 1813, LeBaron to Secretary of War, 30 Mar and 9 Jun 1813, RG 107, M221, roll 54; Secretary of War to Francis LeBaron, 12 May and 25 Jun 1813, RG 107, M6, roll 6, pp. 413–14, 474.

34. LeBaron to Secretary of War, Dec and 30 Mar 1813, 21 Mar 1814, RG 107, M221, roll 54, quote from Dec 1813; James Mann to LeBaron, n.d., Mann, *Sketches*, p. 259; Secretary of War to LeBaron, 12 May 1813 and 11 Apr 1814, RG 107, M6, roll 6, pp. 413–14; roll 7, p. 160.

35. James Cutbush to Adjutant General, 31 Dec 1814, RG 94, M566, roll 4.

Chapter 8

1. Except where otherwise noted, all military and political material is based on Beirne, *War of 1812*; Harry L. Coles, *The War of 1812* (Chicago: University of Chicago Press, 1965); Jacobs and Tucker, *The War of 1812*; Kreidberg and Henry, *Mobilization*; and Mahon, *The War of 1812*.

2. James Mann to Secretary of War, 17 Aug 1812, RG 107, M221, roll 47; Mann, *Sketches*, p. vi.

3. Mann, *Sketches*, pp. vi, 12, 45–46; James Mann to Secretary of War, 17 Aug and 5 Oct 1812, RG 107, M221, roll 47; William Beaumont, *William Beaumont's Formative Years: Two Early Notebooks, 1811–1821*, ed. Genevieve Miller (New York: Henry Schuman, 1946), p. 10.

4. Mann, *Sketches*, p. vi; James Mann to Secretary of War, 17 Aug and 5 Oct 1812, RG 107, M221, roll 47.

5. James Mann to Secretary of War, 5 Oct 1812, RG 107, M221, roll 47.

6. Mann, *Sketches*, pp. 13, 14, 15, 19, 20; James Mann to Secretary of War, 5 Oct 1812, RG 107, M221, roll 47.

7. Mann, *Sketches*, pp. 15–16.

8. Mann, *Sketches*, pp. 13–14, 20, 34, quotes from p. 13.

9. Mann, *Sketches*, pp. 15, 19, quote from p. 14.

10. Beaumont, *Notebooks*, pp. xii, 11, quotes from p. 11; Secretary of War to Mr. Leib, 27 Nov 1812, in Washington, Library of Congress, Manuscript Division, William Eustis Papers, II–33–N.H.; Ashburn, *Medical Department*, pp. 50–53.

11. Mann, *Sketches*, pp. 4, 14, quotes from pp. 14, 35–36.

12. Mann, *Sketches*, pp. 25, 44, quote from p. 44.

13. Mann, *Sketches*, pp. 43, 45; Brown, *Medical Department*, p. 83; Phalen, *Chiefs*, p. 27.

14. Mann, *Sketches*, pp. 45, 47, quote from p. 45.

15. Louis L. Babcock, *The War of 1812 on the Niagara Frontier* (Buffalo, N.Y.: Buffalo Historical Society, 1927), pp. 64–65, letter of 11 Nov 1812, published in the *New York Evening Post* of 25 Nov 1812, quote from letter of 8 Nov 1812, published in the *New York Evening Post* of 25 Nov 1812; John Brannan, *Official Letters of the Military and Naval Officers of the United States During the War With Great Britain* (Washington: Way & Gideon, 1823), p. 100.

16. Report of the State of the 14th Regiment of Infantry, Babcock, *Niagara*, pp. 62–63; Amos Stoddard, Maj 1st Regt. Artillery, to Secretary of War, 16 Sep 1812, Knopf, *Documents*, 6, part 3: 160; Brannan, *Letters*, p. 95.

17. Elijah D. Efner, "The Adventures and Enterprises of Elijah D. Efner," *Publications of the Buffalo Historical Society* 4 (1896): 44; John C. Parish, ed., *The Robert Lucas Journal of the War of 1812* (Iowa City, Iowa: The State Historical Society of Iowa, 1906), p. 18; Extract of letter of Dr. James Reynolds from Detroit, 7 Jul 1812, Knopf, *Documents*, 5, part 1: 112; William Stanley Hatch, *A Chapter of the History of the War of 1812 in*

the Northwest . . . (Cincinnati: Miami Printing and Publishing Co., 1872), p. 25.

18. William Hull, *Memoirs of the Campaign of the Northwestern Army of the United States, 1812* (Boston: True & Greene, 1824), pp. 3, 10; Parish, *Lucas Journal*, p. 19; Walker, *Journal*, p. 48; Samuel R. Brown, *An Authentic History of the Second War for Independence* . . . , 2 vols. (Auburn, N.Y.: J. G. Hathaway, 1815), 1: 37n; Efner, "Adventures," p. 44.

19. Parish, *Lucas Journal*, pp. 19, 63-64; Walker, *Journal*, p. 48; Brown, *Authentic History*, 1: 37n; John Miller to Gen Thomas Worthington, 24 Nov 1812, Knopf, *Documents*, 3: 123; William Kennedy Beall, "Journal of William K. Beall, July-August 1812," reprinted from *American Historical Review* 17 (1912): 785-86; Clarence Stewart Peterson, *Known Military Dead During the War of 1812* (Baltimore, April 1955), p. 55; G. M. Fairchild, Jr., ed., *Journal of an American Prisoner at Fort Malden and Quebec in the War of 1812* (Quebec: privately printed, 1909), p. 304.

20. William Hull to Secretary of War, 26 Aug 1812, Brannan, *Letters*; Fanny J. Anderson, "Medical Practices During the War of 1812," *Bulletin of the History of Medicine* 16 (1944): 268; Brown, *Authentic History*, 1: 68; U.S. Congress, Senate, *Executive Proceedings*, 1: 473; Orders, Brig Gen William Hull, 7 Aug 1812, in Milo Milton Quaife, ed., *War on the Detroit, The Chronicles of Thomas Verchères de Boucherville and the Capitulation by an Ohio Volunteer* (Chicago: Lakeside Press, 1940), pp. 195n-196n, 275-76; Abraham W. Beth to Gen Thomas Worthington, 8 Jan 1812, H. Johnson to Secretary of War, 16 and 18 Aug 1812, and A. Edwards to Secretary of War, 17 Sep 1812, Knopf, *Documents*, 3: 37; 6, part 3: 36, 39, 162; Fairchild, *Journal*, p. 7.

21. Coles, *1812*, p. 55.

22. Letter from Captain Heald, 23 Oct 1812, and T. Forsythe to Governor Howard, 7 Sep 1812, Knopf, *Documents*, 5: part 1: 269; 6, 118; Peterson, *Dead*, p. 68; William Jay, "Table of the Killed and Wounded in the War of 1812. Compiled During the War," *Collections of the New York Historical Society*, 2d ser. 2 (1849): 449; John Kinzie, "Narrative of the Ft. Dearborn Massacre," *Illinois State Historical Society* 46 (1953): 349.

23. Brown, *Authentic History*, 2: 85, 87-88; Atherton, *Narrative*, pp. 18-19; Samuel Hopkins to Governor Shelby, 27 Nov 1812, and Lt Col John B. Campbell to Gen W. H. Harrison, 25 Dec 1812, Brannan, *Letters*, pp. 97, 115-16.

24. Elias Darnell, "A Journal Containing an Accurate and Interesting Account of the Hardships, Sufferings, Battles, Defeat, and Captivity of Those Heroic Kentucky Volunteers and Regulars, Commanded by General Winchester, in the Years 1812-13 . . . ," *Magazine of History*, Extra No. 31 (New York: W. Abbatt, 1914 reprint of 1854 ed.), p. 203, quote from p. 210; Winchester's General Orders, Camp Defiance, 1 and 9 Oct 1812, James Winchester, "Papers and Orderly Book of Brigadier General J. Winchester," *Michigan Pioneer and Historical Society Collections* 31 (1901): 259, 264-65; Harrison's Orders, 3 Oct 1812, in Washington, Library of Congress, Manuscript Division, microfilm of William Henry Harrison Papers, roll 1, series 1; Charles E. Slocum, "Some Errors Corrected: Fort Winchester, at Defiance, Ohio," *Ohio Archeological and Historical Quarterly* 10 (1901-2): 483; Atherton, *Narrative*, pp. 18-19.

25. Atherton, *Narrative*, p. 19.

26. Hull, *Memoirs*, p. 3; William Henry Harrison to James Winchester, 4 Oct 1812, and to Secretary of War, 20 Jan 1813, Harrison, *Messages*, 2: 162, 316.

27. Brown, *Authentic History*, 1: 89-90; Thomas P. Dudley, "Battle and Massacre at Frenchtown, Michigan, January 1813, by Rev. Thomas P. Dudley, One of the Survivors," *Western Reserve and Northern Ohio Historical Society Publications* No. 1 (1870): 1-2, 3; James Winchester to William Henry Harrison, 17 and 19 Jan 1813, William Lewis to James Winchester, 20 Jan 1813, and McClanahan to William Henry Harrison, 26 Jan 1813, Harrison, *Messages*, 2: 314, 315, 321, 339; Atherton, *Narrative*, p. 39; Statement of Capt. R. Matson of 13 Feb 1813, and Statement of James Garrard, Jr., Brigade Inspector, 11 Mar 1813, Knopf, *Documents*, 5: part 2: 27, 40; Garrett Glenn Clift, *Remember the Raisin:*

Kentucky and Kentuckians in the Battles and Massacre at Frenchtown, Michigan Territory, in the War of 1812 (Frankfort: Kentucky Historical Soc., 1961), pp. 127, 128, 129, 131–32, 134–35.

28. Atherton, *Narrative*, pp. 53–54, 61; Darnell, "Journal," pp. 220, 222, 223; Brown, *Authentic History*, 1: 92.

29. William Henry Harrison to Governor Meigs, 24 Jan 1813; Harrison, *Messages*, 2: 329–30.

30. Register of the Army for 1813, *American State Papers: Military Affairs*, 1: 391.

31. William Henry Harrison to Secretary of War, 9 Jul 1813, Harrison, *Messages*, 2: 485, quote from p. 486.

32. Jay, "Table," p. 452; Eleazer D. Wood, "Journal of the Northwestern Campaign of 1812–13 Under Major-General William Harrison," in G. W. Cullum, ed., *Campaigns of the War of 1812–15* (New York: Miller, 1879), p. 402, quotes from pp. 402, 403.

33. Cullum, *Campaigns*, p. 403, quote from p. 401; William Henry Harrison to Secretary of War, 5 May 1813, Brannan, *Letters*, p. 158.

34. William Henry Harrison to Secretary of War, 5 May 1813, Brannan, *Letters*, p. 158.

35. Cullum, *Campaigns*, p. 402.

36. Robert Yost, "His Book," *Ohio Archaeological and Historical Quarterly* 23 (1914): 154–55; Duncan McArthur to Secretary of War, 6 Oct 1813, Brannan, *Letters*, p. 230.

37. Yost, "Book," pp. 156–57, quote from p. 157; Anderson, "Medical Practices," p. 269; William Henry Harrison to Secretary of War, 9 Oct 1813, Brannan, *Letters*, p. 238.

38. James Wilkinson to Secretary of War, 16 Nov 1813, *American State Papers: Military Affairs*, 1: 476; Wilkins Report, 3 Nov 1813, and Major Birdsall Statement, 6 Nov 1813, in John Armstrong, *Notices of the War of 1812*, 2 vols. (New York: Wiley & Putnam, 1840), 2: 9, 211–12.

39. Register, Rules and Regulations of the Army for 1813, *American State Papers: Military Affairs*, 1: 384–85; James Tilton to Secretary of War, 20 Aug 1814, RG 107, M221, roll 66.

40. Mann, *Sketches*, pp. 64–65, 248, 249, quote from p. 248.

41. Jesse S. Myer, *Life of William Beaumont* (St. Louis: C. V. Mosby Co., 1939), pp. 44–45, 53–54; Mann, *Sketches*, pp. 94, 95, 126, quote from p. 250; Beaumont, *Notebooks*, pp. 16, 47, 48; W. E. Horner, quoted in Brown, *Medical Department*, p. 92; Greenhous, "Logistics," p. 43.

42. Winfield Scott, *Memoirs of Lieut.-General Scott, LL.D.*, 2 vols. (New York: Sheldon & Co., 1864), 1: 145.

43. Mann, *Sketches*, pp. 241, 242, 246–47; Brown, *Medical Department*, p. 89.

44. Register of the Army for 1813, *American State Papers: Military Affairs*, 1: 391; Mann, *Sketches*, p. 45.

45. Quote from Beaumont, *Notebooks*, p. 44; Mann, *Sketches*, p. 117; Secretary of War to Major General Hampton, 25 Sep 1813, in Ernest A. Cruikshank, *Documentary History of the Campaign Upon the Niagara Frontier*, 4 vols. (Welland, Ont.: Arno Press & New York Times, 1971 reprint of 1896–1908 edition), 2: 107.

46. Beaumont, *Notebooks*, pp. 15, 43, 44; Mann, *Sketches*, p. 58, quote from p. 57.

47. Beaumont, *Notebooks*, p. 15.

48. Mann, *Sketches*, pp. 57, 58; Lewis Potter Bush, *The Delaware State Medical Society and Its Founders in the Eighteenth Century* (New York, 1886), p. 9.

49. Secretary of War to Dr. Ross, 22 Jun 1813, RG 107, M6, roll 6, p. 472; Wilkinson, *Memoirs*, 3: app. 9 #2 and 26, and Remarks on the Weekly Sick Report Made by Order of Brigadier General Brown, Commanding at Sackett's Harbor, Saturday, September 18, 1813, app. 9 #2 (there are two appendixes 9 in this volume); *American State Papers: Military Affairs*, 1: 387; Jay, "Table," p. 452.

50. Mann, *Sketches*, pp. 62–63, 89; Armstrong, *War of 1812*, 2: 22.

51. Mann, *Sketches*, p. 70, Joseph Lovell quoted in Mann, p. 67, quotes from pp. 65–66, 71; Colonel Scott to Wilkinson, 11 Oct 1813, *American State Papers: Military Affairs*, 1: 483.

52. Colonel Scott to James Wilkinson, 11 Oct 1813, *American State Papers: Military Affairs*, 1: 483; Francis LeBaron to Secretary of War, 12 Sep 1813, RG 107, M221, roll 54; Mann, *Sketches*, pp. 62–63, 66.

53. Mann, *Sketches*, pp. 62–63, 64–65, 252; Beaumont, *Notebooks*, p. 51; Francis LeBaron

to Secretary of War, 6 May 1813, RG 107, M221, roll 54.

54. Mann, *Sketches*, pp. 64–65, 93–94, 241, quote from p. 64; Scott, *Memoirs*, 1: 136.

55. Mann, *Sketches*, p. 63, quote from p. 89.

56. Colonel Scott to James Wilkinson, 11 Oct 1813, *American State Papers: Military Affairs*, 1: 483; Mann, *Sketches*, pp. 94, 95, quote from p. 94.

57. Secretary of War to Major General Hampton, 25 Sep 1813, Cruikshank, *Documents*, 2: 107; Mann, *Sketches*, pp. 95, 96–97, 117, quote from pp. 96–97. Joseph Lovell's report of the summer of 1814 states that a hospital was *established* at Williamsville on 1 August 1814, implying that for some time before that date, there was no hospital in operation there (Lovell report, Mann, *Sketches*, p. 162).

58. Beaumont, *Notebooks*, pp. 16, 46, 47, quotes from pp. 16, 46; Stephen H. Moore to his brother, 5 May 1813, Brannan, *Letters*, p. 151.

59. Beaumont, *Notebooks*, pp. 16, 47, 48, 51.

60. Quote from Colonel Purdy's Report, fall 1813, Brannan, *Letters*, 277–78; Mann, *Sketches*, p. 119; Dr. Ross to Inspector General, 8 Dec 1813, Wilkinson, *Memoirs*, 3: app. 9 #1.

61. Dr. Ross to Inspector General, 8 Dec 1813, Wilkinson, *Memoirs*, 3: app. 9 #1.

62. Joseph Lovell quoted in Mann, *Sketches*, p. 119.

CHAPTER 9

1. Unless otherwise indicated, material concerning military activities in this chapter is based upon Beirne, *War of 1812*; Coles, *1812*; Mahon, *The War of 1812*; Matloff, *Military History*; and Spaulding, *Army*.

2. Unless otherwise indicated, material concerning the Medical Department in this chapter is based on Brown, *Medical Department*. The preceding paragraph is also based on Henry Huntt, "An Abstract Account of the Diseases Which Prevailed Among the Soldiers, Received into the General Hospital, at Burlington, Vermont, During the Summer and Autumn of 1814," *Medical Recorder* 1 (1818): 179; Register of the Army for 1813, *American State Papers: Military Affairs*, 1: 391; Mann, *Sketches*, pp. 127, 144, 246–47, 256–57.

3. Mann, *Sketches*, p. 261, Mann to General Smith, Apr 1814, and to Colonel Smith, 21 Apr 1814, quote from Mann to Brigadier General Smith, 28 Apr 1818, pp. 261, 265–66, 267; George Izard to Secretary of War, 19 Jul 1814, in George Izard, *Official Correspondence With the Department of War Relative to the Military Operations of the American Army Under the Command of Major General Izard on the Northern Frontier of the United States in the Years 1814 and 1815* (Philadelphia: Thomas Dobson, 1816), pp. 54–55.

4. Data and quote from Huntt, "Burlington," p. 177; Purcell report, Mann, *Sketches*, p. 153. Comments by Mann, in an essay written several years before the war, suggested that in the early nineteenth century physicians believed that the difference between diarrhea and dysentery lay in the fact that the latter was characterized by cramps and tenesmus, even though the "evacuations are small," while the former involved copious bowel movements without tenesmus (Mann, *Sketches*, p. 280, quote from p. 279).

5. Data and quote from Huntt, "Burlington," pp. 177–78; Report of the Killed, Wounded and Missing at Plattsburgh, From the 6th to the 11th of September 1814, Brannan, *Letters*, p. 419; Mann, *Sketches*, p. 153.

6. Quote from George Izard to Secretary of War, 25 Jun 1814, Izard, *Correspondence*, p. 38; Mann, *Sketches*, pp. 116, 267, 270, and James Mann to Adjutant General, 17 Aug 1814, p. 267.

7. Mann, *Sketches*, pp. 145, 271.

8. James Mann to James Tilton, Nov 1814, Brown, *Medical Department*, pp. 99–100, quote from p. 100.

9. James Mann to Elbridge Gerry, 6 Nov 1814, Mann, *Sketches*, p. 272; James Tilton to Secretary of War, 10 Feb 1815, RG 107, M221, roll 66.

10. Mann, *Sketches*, pp. 125, 262–63, James Mann to Major General Brown, 1 Feb 1814, p. 266.

11. Mann, *Sketches*, p. 126; James M. Phalen, "Surgeon James Mann's Observations on

Battlefield Amputations," *Military Surgeon* 87 (1940): 464.

12. Mann, *Sketches*, pp. 125, 144, quote from p. 125.

13. James Tilton to Secretary of War, 7 Jun 1814, RG 94, M566, roll 59; Report of a Case of Amputation, by J. B. Whitridge, M.D., Hospital Surgeon's Mate, 28 Jun 1814, Mann, *Sketches*, p. 215; LeBaron to Secretary of War, 8 Jan 1814, and Tilton to Secretary of War, 20 Aug 1814, RG 107, M221, rolls 54 and 66; A List of Deaths . . . at Sackett's Harbor From 23d October 1813 to the 20th January 1814 and at Brownville From the Last to the Present Date, in Washington, National Archives, Post Revolutionary War Records, Record Group 98, book 566.

14. Tilton to Dr. William M. Ross, 7 Jun 1814, and to the Secretary of War, 10 Feb 1815, RG 94, M566, rolls 59, 66; Mann, *Sketches*, p. 56; RG 98, book 566.

15. A. Hays to Tilton, 7 Mar 1814, and Tilton to Secretary of War, 20 Aug 1814 and 10 Feb 1815, RG 107, M221, rolls 59 and 66; Mann, *Sketches*, pp. 94, 179; U.S. War Department, *Subject Index, General Orders*, p. 99.

16. Major General Izard to Secretary of War, 8 Nov 1814, Cruikshank, *Documents*, 4: 298.

17. Quote from Major General Izard to Secretary of War, 26 Nov 1814, Izard, *Correspondence*, p. 121; Major General Izard to Secretary of War, 8 Nov 1814, Cruikshank, *Documents*, 4: 298.

18. Quote from Eber D. Howe, "Recollections of a Pioneer Printer," *Buffalo Historical Society Publications* 9 (1906): 398; Clayton Tiffin to Major General Izard, 6 Dec 1814, RG 94, M566, roll 59; Scott, *Memoirs*, 1: 147, 148; Report of Hospital Surgeon Lovell, 1 Aug 1814, Cruikshank, *Documents*, 4: 452–53; Louis L. Babcock, *The Siege of Fort Erie, An Episode of the War of 1812* (Buffalo: Peter Paul Book Co., 1899), p. 44n; W. E. Horner, "Surgical Sketches," *Medical Examiner and Record of Medical Science*, new ser. 8 (1952): 761, 764, 768, 791; Jacob Brown to Secretary of War, 6 Jul 1814, in Herman Allen Fay, *Collection of the Official Accounts, in Detail, of All the Battles Fought by Sea and Land Between the Navy and Army of the United States and the Navy and Army of Great Britain During the Years 1812, 13, 14, & 15* (New York, 1817), p. 210.

19. James Tilton to Secretary of War, 20 Aug 1814, RG 107, M221, roll 66; Major General Jacob Brown reported that 249 were wounded at the Battle of Chippewa ("Report of the Killed and Wounded of the Left Division Commanded by Major General Brown in the Action of 5th July 1814, on the Plains of Chippewa, Upper Canada," Brannan, *Letters*, p. 372).

20. Effner, "Adventures," pp. 51–52, quote from p. 52; E. P. Gaines to Secretary of War, 7 and 23 Aug 1814, Brannan, *Letters*, pp. 384, 399; Mann, *Sketches*, pp. 70, 111.

21. E. W. Ripley to Brigadier General Gaines, 17 Aug 1814, Brannan, *Letters*, p. 392.

22. James Tilton to Secretary of War, 10 Feb 1815, RG 107, M211, roll 66.

23. Nathan Boulden to James Tilton, 9 Oct 1814, RG 94, M566, roll 59.

24. A. Hays to Tilton, 11 Dec 1814 and 2 Jan 1815, RG 94, M566, roll 82, quote from 11 Dec 1814.

25. Tilton to Secretary of War, 17 Jan 1815, RG 94, M566, roll 82.

26. Mann, *Sketches*, p. 111.

27. Report of Hospital Surgeon Lovell on the State of Diseases Among the Troops on the Niagara Frontier During the Campaign of 1814, Cruikshank, *Documents*, 4: 452.

28. Tilton to Secretary of War, 10 Feb 1815, RG 107, M221, roll 66.

29. Hamersly, *Register*, pp. 133–34; Register, and Rules and Regulations of the Army for 1813, *American State Papers: Military Affairs*, 1: 386–87.

30. Emory Upton, *Military Policy of the United States* (Washington: Government Printing Office, 1904), p. 126; Albert Kimberley Hadel, "The Battle of Bladensburg," *Maryland Historical Magazine* 1 (1906): 157, 160, 167; Marine, *British Invasion*, p. 76, and Report of Lieutenant Colonel Armistead to Secretary of War, pp. 167, 169; Statement of General Walter Smith, in John S. Williams, *The Invasion and Capture of Washington* (New York: Harper & Bros., 1857), p. 346; William H. Winder to Secretary of War, 27 Aug 1814, Brannan, *Letters*, p. 402; Statement

of Dr. Catlett, *American State Papers: Military Affairs*, 1: 584; John M. Stahl, *The Invasion of the City of Washington, A Disagreeable Study in and of Military Unpreparedness* (Argos, Ind.: Van Trump Co., 1918), p. 224; Jay, "Table," p. 456.

31. Tilton to Secretary of War, 23 Aug 1814, RG 107, M221, roll 66; Office of Adjutant General to W. N. Miner, Esq, 24 Nov 1814, RG 94, M565, roll 5, vol. 3½, p. 208; A Requisition of Medicine Instruments &c Wanting for the Military Post & Hospital at Washington, City, 6 Nov 1813, RG 107, M222, roll 7; James Blake to Tilton, 5 Nov 1814, and J. O. Tyler to Secretary of War, 19 Oct 1814, RG 94, M566, roll 48, frame 0619, and roll 54, frame 0166; Office of Adjutant General to Dr. W. Jones, 19 Jul 1814, RG 94, M565, roll 5, vol. 3½, p. 85; Constance McLaughlin Green, *Washington, Village and Capital, 1800–1878* (Princeton, N.J.: Princeton University Press, 1962), p. 3; Register, and Rules and Regulations of the Army for 1813, *American State Papers: Military Affairs*, 1: 386.

32. Register, and Rules and Regulations of the Army for 1813, and Statement of Dr. Catlett, *American State Papers: Military Affairs*, 1: 396, 585, quote from Report of R. M. Johnson to the House of Representatives, 1: 530; Hamersly, *Register*, pp. 95, 147.

33. Statement of Dr. Catlett, *American State Papers: Military Affairs*, 1: 583. Catlett's status at this time is not clear. He wished to resign as surgeon of the 1st Infantry and, although his resignation appears to have been rejected initially, it was accepted in mid-June 1814. By early August, however, Catlett had not yet been notified of this fact and by the time he received the notice, he had begun to believe that his reputation had been blackened and asked to be kept in the Army until he could clear his name. In September he accepted another appointment with the Army. Hanson Catlett to Lieutenant Colonel Nicholas, 4 Jun 1814, to Secretary of War, 9 Aug 1814, and to Acting Secretary of War, 9 Sep 1814, RG 94, M566, roll 39, frames 0634–0635, 0638, 0640–0642, 0648; Office of Adjutant General to Catlett, 15 Jun 1814, RG 94, M565, roll 5, vol. 3½, p. 35.

34. Catlett to Adjutant and Inspector General, 2 Sep 1814, RG 107, M221, roll 60; Catlett Statement, *American State Papers: Military Affairs*, 1: 584; Marine, *British Invasion*, p. 174; Catlett to Secretary of War, 30 Aug 1814, RG 94, M566, roll 39, frame 0646; Statement of Dr. Catlett, Armstrong, *War of 1812*, 2: 226; Hadel, "Bladensburg," p. 167; Office of Adjutant General to Catlett, 12 Sep 1814, RG 94, M565, roll 5, vol. 3½, p. 145.

35. Green, *Washington*, p. 51; Albert Alleman, "Experiences of an American Physician at the Capture of Washington by the British in 1814," *Medical Library and Historical Journal* 4 (1906): 187; Ewell, *Medical Companion*, pp. 690–91.

36. Office of Adjutant General to Dr. A. Elzy, 17 Jan 1815, RG 94, M565, roll 5, vol. 3½, p. 295, quote from Office of Adjutant General to H. Huntt, 13 Jan 1815, p. 292; Tilton to Secretary of War, 10 Feb 1815, RG 107, M221, roll 66.

37. Register, and Rules and Regulations of the Army for 1813, and A Report of the Army, Its Strength and Distribution, Previous to the 1st of July 1814, *American State Papers: Military Affairs*, 1: 387, 535; Nathaniel Claiborne, *Notes on the War in the South* (New York: Arno Press & The New York Times, 1971 reprint of 1819 edition), p. 47.

38. Andrew Jackson to Secretary James Monroe, 27 Dec 1814, in John S. Bassett, ed., *Correspondence of Andrew Jackson*, 7 vols. (Washington: Carnegie Institution of Washington, 1926–35), 2: 127; Stanley Clisby Arthur, *The Story of the Battle of New Orleans* (New Orleans: Louisiana Historical Society, 1915), p. 248; William McCarty, *History of the American War of 1812, From the Commencement Until the Final Termination . . .*, 2d ed. (Freeport, N.Y.: Books for Libraries Press, 1970 reprint of 1816 edition), p. 229; A. S. Colyar, *Life and Times of Andrew Jackson, Soldier, Statesman, President*, 2 vols. (Nashville, Tenn.: Marshall & Bruce Co., 1904), 1: 239; Arsène Lacarrière Latour, *Historical Memoir of the War in West Florida and Louisiana in 1814–15*, trans. H. P. Nugent (Gainesville: University of Florida Press, 1964 version of 1816 original), p. 45.

39. Latour, *Memoir*, p. 148; Andrew Jackson to Secretary of War, 19 Jan 1815, Bassett, *Jackson*, 2: 148.

Reports on American casualties vary, but from 55 to 62 were killed and from 175 to 185 wounded. Report of the American Loss in Several Actions Below New Orleans, Brannan, *Letters*, p. 461; Bassett, *Jackson*, 2: 143n; Arthur, *New Orleans*, p. 247; Latour, *Memoir*, pp. lix, 122–23, 135; Howell Tatum, *Major Howell Tatum's Journal . . .*, ed. John Spencer Bassett (Northampton, Mass.: Smith College Studies in History, 1922), pp. 117–18, 122, 130.

40. Hamersly, *Register*, pp. 84, 133, 134; Register, and Rules and Regulations of the Army for 1813, *American State Papers: Military Affairs*, 1: 387, 391.

41. Register, and Rules and Regulations of the Army for 1813, *American State Papers: Military Affairs*, 1: 418.

42. Quotes from A. G. Goodlet to Secretary of War, Jun 1815, RG 107, M221, roll 61; O. H. Spencer to Secretary of War, 10 May 1814, RG 107, M221, roll 66.

43. Secretary of War to Commanding Officers at New Orleans, 17 Jun 1815, RG 107, M6, roll 8, p. 166.

44. Quote from Statement of David C. Kerr, Hosp. Surgeon, Bassett, *Jackson* 2: 203; James Parton, *Life of Andrew Jackson*, 3 vols. (Boston: Fields, Osgood & Co., 1870), 2: 121; *American State Papers: Claims*, 5 Feb 1790–3 Mar 1823, p. 752; Arthur, *New Orleans*, pp. 81, 240–41; Alcée Fortier, *A History of Louisiana*, 4 vols. (New York: Manzi, Joyant, & Co., 1904), 3: 167.

45. Bassett, *Jackson*, 2: 163n; Office of Adjutant General to Dr. David C. Kerr, 4 Feb 1813, RG 94, M565, roll 4, vol. 3, p. 93; Tilton to Secretary of War, 10 Feb 1815, RG 107, M221, roll 66.

46. Quote from Stephen Simpson to George Simpson, 9 Jan 1815, *American Historical Review* 2 (1896): 268; Daniel Patterson to Secretary of Navy, 27 Jan 1815, and General Orders, 21 Jan 1815, Brannan, *Letters*, pp. 462–63, 480; Andrew Jackson to Secretary Monroe, 27 Dec 1814, Bassett, *Jackson*, 128; Colonel Bartholomew Shaumburg to William C. C. Claiborne, 30 Oct 1815, in W. C. C. Claiborne, *Official Letter Books of W. C. C. Claiborne, 1801–1816*, ed. Dunbar Rowland, 6 vols. (Jackson, Miss.: State Dept. of Archives and History, 1917), 6: 380; Eron Opha Rowland, *Andrew Jackson's Campaign Against the British, or the Mississippi Territory in the War of 1812 . . .* (Freeport, N.Y.: Books for Libraries Press, 1971 reprint of 1926 edition), pp. 81, 81n; Latour, *Memoir*, p. 184; Office of Adjutant General to Dr. O. H. Spencer, 10 Jul 1814, and Francis LeBaron to Adjutant and Inspector General, 20 Dec 1814, RG 94, M565, roll 5, vol 3½, p. 82; M566, roll 12; Hamersly, *Register*, p. 272; Jane Lucas de Grummond, *The Baratarians and the Battle of New Orleans* (Baton Rouge: Louisiana State University Press, 1961), p. 100.

47. Latour, *Memoir*, pp. 163, 177, 225, quote from p. 225; Parton, *Jackson*, 2: 221, 229–30; L'Ami des Lois, 16 Jan 1815, in Reed Adams, "New Orleans and the War of 1812," *Louisiana Historical Quarterly* 17 (1934): 362; Arthur, *New Orleans*, pp. 219–20; Alexander Walker, *Jackson and New Orleans . . .* (New York: J. C. Derby, 1856), p. 347; John Henry Cooke, *A Narrative of Events in the South of France and of the Attack on New Orleans, in 1814 and 1815* (London: T. & W. Boone, 1835), pp. 263–64; Resolution of the Legislature of Louisiana, Fortier, *Louisiana*, 3: 167.

48. Andrew Jackson to Major-General Lambert, 8 Jan 1815, Bassett, *Jackson*, 2: 134.

49. Quote from Andrew Jackson to Col Robert Hays, 17 Feb 1815, Bassett, *Jackson* 2: 172; Parton, *Jackson* 2: 226; General Orders, D. Parker, Adjutant and Inspector General, 6 Jan 1815, *Niles' Weekly Register* (Baltimore) 7: 317.

50. General Orders, Headquarters 7th Military District, 21 Jan 1815, Brannan, *Letters*, p. 480.

51. Prucha, *Guide*, p. 94; Hamersly, *Register*, p. 134; Tilton to Secretary of War, 20 Aug 1814, RG 107, M221, roll 66.

52. Quote from Tilton to Secretary of War, 20 Aug 1814, RG 107, M221, roll 66; Joseph Wheaton, *Appeal to the Senate and House of Representatives of the United States of America* (District of Columbia, 1820), p. 29.

53. Wheaton, *Appeal*, pp. 19–20, 21–22, quote from p. 19.

54. Tilton to Secretary of War, 20 Aug 1814, RG 107, M221, roll 66; Register, Rules and Regulations of the Army for 1813, *American State Papers: Military Affairs*, 1: 386.

CHAPTER 10

1. William Eustis to Secretary of War, 21 Mar 1815, RG 94, M566, roll 12.

2. Quote and data from Crawford to Chairman of Military Committee, 27 Dec 1815, *American State Papers: Military Affairs*, 1: 636; Army Register for 1816, *American State Papers: Military Affairs*, 1: 628, 635; Ingersoll, *War Department*, p. 216; Henry C. Corbin and Raphael P. Thian, eds., *Legislative History of the General Staff of the Army of the United States* (Washington: Government Printing Office, 1901), p. 409; Francis LeBaron to William Eustis, 16 Mar 1815, Eustis Papers; James Mann to James Tilton, 18 Mar 1815, Francis LeBaron to Secretary of War, 18 Mar 1815, James Tilton to Secretary of War, 28 Apr 1815, James Mann to President Madison, 7 Sep 1815, and James Mann to Colonel Conner, 14 Dec 1815, RG 94, M566, rolls 75, 82.

3. Unless otherwise indicated, all material in this section is based on Ganoe, *U.S. Army*; Spaulding, *Army*; and Weigley, *Army*. Also consulted for the preceding paragraph were John Caldwell Calhoun, *The Papers of John C. Calhoun*, ed. W. Edwin Hemphill, 2 vols. to date (Columbia: University of South Carolina Press for the South Carolina Society, 1963), 2: lxi; Corbin and Thian, *Legislative History*, p. 409; Army Register for 1816, *American State Papers: Military Affairs*, 1: 635.

4. Quote from "Review of Circular Letter of Benjamin Waterhouse to His Surgeons in the 2nd Military District, September 1817," *Medical Repository* 19 (1818): 395–96; Corbin and Thian, *Legislative History*, p. 410; Bayne-Jones, *Preventive Medicine*, pp. 79–80.

5. Tilton to Secretary of War, 28 Apr and 8 May 1815, quote from Joseph Eaton to James Tilton, 22 Apr 1815, RG 94, M566, roll 82; Office of the Adjutant General to J. H. Sackett, 13 Jan 1816, RG 94, M565, roll 5, vol. 3½, pp. 491–92; Register for 1816, *American State Papers: Military Affairs*, 1: 627–28, 631–32, 633, 634, 635.

6. Quote from James Tilton to Secretary of War, 28 Apr 1815, RG 94, M566, roll 82; James Mann to President Madison, 7 Sep 1815, Mann to Secretary of War, 14 Apr 1815, Mann to Colonel Conner, 14 Dec 1815, Francis LeBaron to Secretary of War, 18 Mar 1815, Morgan Lewis and Jabez C. [illegible] to Secretary of War, 21 Mar 1815, RG 94, M566, roll 75; Office of Adjutant General to T. Watkins, 11 May 1816, RG 94, M565, roll 5, vol. 4, p. 30.

7. Francis LeBaron to Adjutant and Inspector General, 18 Apr 1815, RG 94, M566, roll 12; Francis LeBaron to Secretary of War, 5 and 10 Feb, 3 Apr, and 6 Jun 1815, RG 107, M221, rolls 63, 64; George Graham to Francis LeBaron, 27 Jul 1815, RG 107, M6, roll 8, pp. 243–44.

8. Quotes from Francis LeBaron to Adjutant and Inspector General, 28 May 1816, RG 94, M566, roll 12; and to Secretary of War, 8 May 1817, RG 107, M221, roll 74.

9. Francis LeBaron to Secretary of War, 7 Mar 1815, and Benjamin Waterhouse to Secretary of War, 12 Jul 1815, RG 107, M221, rolls 63, 67; Joseph Lovell to Adjutant General, 30 Oct 1817, RG 94, M566, roll 98; Office of Adjutant General to Henry Huntt, 15 Jun 1815, RG 94, M565, roll 5, vol. 3½, p. 386.

10. Francis LeBaron to Secretary of War, 13 Jan 1816, to Adjutant and Inspector General, 31 Mar 1817, and to Inspector General, 19 Jun 1817, RG 94, M566, roll 12; LeBaron to Secretary of War, 26 Jul 1816, RG 107, M221, roll 70.

11. Francis LeBaron to Secretary of War, 28 May and 26 Jul 1816, RG 107, M221, roll 70; Secretary of War to Dr. W. P. Jones, 14 Jan 1815, RG 107, M6, roll 8, pp. 25–26.

12. Quote from Francis LeBaron to Secretary of War, 14 Sep 1816, RG 107, M221, roll 70; LeBaron to Secretary of War, 6 Jun 1815, and to Adjutant and Inspector General, 28 May 1816, RG 107, M221, rolls 12, 64; James Cutbush to Adjutant General, 5 Jun 1816, RG 94, M566, roll 41.

13. Quote from Francis LeBaron to Adjutant and Inspector General, 7 Nov 1816, RG 94, M566, roll 12; LeBaron to Secretary of War, 26 Jul and 14 Sep 1816, RG 107, M221, roll 70.

14. Secretary of War to LeBaron, 5 Feb 1817, RG 107, M6, roll 8, p. 243.

15. Francis LeBaron to Secretary of War, 7 Mar 1815, RG 107, M221, roll 63, quote

from James Tilton to Secretary of War, 10 Feb 1815, roll 66; Office of Adjutant General to Dr. J. H. Sackett, 23 Oct 1817, and to Dr. F. Swift, 22 Oct 1817, RG 94, M565, roll 5, vol. 4, p. 262.

16. James Tilton to Secretary of War, 17 Jan 1815, RG 94, M566, roll 82, quote from James Mann to Secretary of War, 14 Apr 1815, roll 75; Office of Adjutant General to Henry Huntt, 7 Feb and 15 Jun 1815, RG 94, M565, roll 5, vol. 3½, pp. 318, 386.

17. Remarks on the Sick Report of the Northern Division for the Year Ending 30 Jun 1817, Brown, *Medical Department*, p. 102.

18. I. M. McKay to Maj Perrin Willis, 30 Oct 1817, RG 94, M566, roll 98.

19. Remarks on the Sick Report of the Northern Division for the Year Ending 30 Jun 1817, Brown, *Medical Department*, p. 102.

20. Francis LeBaron to Secretary of War, 25 Apr and 4 May 1813, RG 107, M221, roll 54.

21. Quote from George Izard to Secretary of War, 1 Jun 1814, Izard, *Correspondence*, pp. 21–22; James Tilton to Secretary of War, 12 Jul 1813, RG 107, M221, roll 57.

22. General Committee of Defense, *Observations*; Heustis, *Diseases of Louisiana*, pp. 130–31; James Mann to Secretary of War, 14 Apr 1815, RG 94, M566, roll 75; Brown, *Medical Department*, p. 105.

23. Brown, *Medical Department*, p. 104.

24. James Tilton to Secretary of War, 20 Aug 1814, RG 107, M221, roll 66.

25. Mann, *Sketches*, pp. 122, 124.

26. Quote from RG 98, vol. 683, 1st and 9th Regiments; Brown, *Medical Department*, p. 102; RG 98, vols. 680, 683; Samuel Akerly, "Medical Topography of the Military Positions in the Third United States Military District: Together With a Summary Report on the Diseases of the Army . . . ," *Medical Repository*, 2d ser. 3 (1817): 294.

27. Heustis, *Diseases of Louisiana*, p. 138.

28. Brown, *Medical Department*, pp. 88, 102, 103, quote from p. 88; Mann, *Sketches*, p. 76; Heustis, *Diseases of Louisiana*, p. 136; Benjamin Waterhouse, *Circular Letter From Dr. Benjamin Waterhouse to the Surgeons of the Different Posts in the Second Military Department* (Cambridge, Mass., 1817), pp. 12–13.

29. Waterhouse, *Letter*, pp. 8–9, 10, 15, quotes from pp. 10, 15; Heustis, *Diseases of Louisiana*, pp. 136, 137.

30. Mann, *Sketches*, pp. 130–31.

31. Waterhouse, *Letter*, p. 16.

32. Quote from Waterhouse, *Letter*, p. 14; Heustis, *Diseases of Louisiana*, p. 136.

33. Heustis, *Diseases of Louisiana*, pp. 138, 139, quote from p. 139 (Heustis's preferences in fruit may seem exotic, but, of course, he was writing of his experience in Louisiana); Waterhouse, *Letter*, pp. 12, 17, 19–20.

34. Mann, *Sketches*, p. 76.

35. Quote from Heustis, *Diseases of Louisiana*, p. 114; Warren, *Mercurial Practice*, pp. 45–46, 92. The term *typhoid* has apparently often been used to mean "resembling typhus" [see first definition of typhoid in *Dorland's Illustrated Medical Dictionary*, 24th ed. (Philadelphia: W. B. Saunders Co., 1965), p. 1640] and the two diseases were not clearly distinguished until 1837. [See Hume, *Victories*, pp. 99–100; and Leonard G. Wilson, "The Clinical Definition of Scurvy and the Discovery of Vitamin C," *Journal of the History of Medicine and Allied Sciences* 30 (1975): 59.]

36. Purcell Report, Mann, *Sketches*, p. 153. Sordes is "The dark-brown, foul matter which collects on the lips and teeth in low fevers" (*Dorland*, p. 1406).

37. Data and quote from Waterhouse, *Letter*, p. 5; Brown, *Medical Department*, p. 105; James Thacher, *American Modern Practice; Or, a Simple Method of Prevention and Cure of Diseases* . . . (Boston: Ezra Read, 1817), p. 173.

38. Joseph Lovell Report, Mann, *Sketches*, pp. 163–64.

39. Quote from Joseph Lovell Report, Mann, *Sketches*, p. 103; Warren, *Mercurial Practice*, p. 98.

40. Thomas, *Modern Practice*, p. 43.

41. Mann, *Sketches*, pp. 68, 128, 160–61, quote from p. 90.

42. Brown, *Medical Department*, pp. 102, 104–5, quote from p. 102; Army Register for 1816, *American State Papers: Military Affairs*, 1: 635.

43. Mann, *Sketches*, p. 129.

44. Hanson Catlett to Major McClelland, 17 Jan 1815, RG 94, M566, roll 67.

45. Waterhouse, *Letter*, p. 22.

46. Mann, *Sketches*, pp. 186–98.
47. Waterhouse, *Letter*, pp. 14, 15.
48. Mann, *Sketches*, pp. 130–31, 134, 136, quotes from pp. 134, 136.
49. Mann, *Sketches*, pp. 80–81.
50. Quotes from Waterhouse, *Letter*, pp. 6–7; Mann, *Sketches*, pp. 88–89.
51. Mann, *Sketches*, p. 206; "Diseases of the Army of the Third United States Military District," *Medical Repository*, new ser. 3 (1817): 407; John Shaw, "Narrative of John Shaw: Dictated to Lyman C. Draper," *Wisconsin State Historical Society Publications* 2 (1855): 217.
52. Horner, "Surgical Sketches," 9: 1, 2.
53. Horner, "Surgical Sketches," 9: 3, 71, quote from p. 71.
54. Horner, "Surgical Sketches," 9: 78.
55. Horner, "Surgical Sketches," 9: 7.
56. Barton became the first Surgeon-General of the Navy in 1842. William Paul Crillon Barton, *A Treatise Containing a Plan for the Internal Organization and Government of Marine Hospitals in the United States; Together With Observations on Military and Flying Hospitals . . .* , 2d ed. (Philadelphia, 1817), pp. 131, 132, quotes from pp. 131, 132; Mann, *Sketches*, pp. 240–41.
57. Mann, *Sketches*, p. 240.
58. Mann, *Sketches*, pp. 238–39, 243, quote from p. 238.
59. Mann, *Sketches*, p. 250.
60. Mann, *Sketches*, pp. 244, 246; Brown, *Medical Department*, p. 106.
61. Mann, *Sketches*, pp. 235–36; Office of the Adjutant General to James Mann, 16 Jul, 14 Nov 1816, and to Dr. W. P. C. Barton, 15 Oct 1816, RG 94, M565, roll 5, vol. 4, pp. 66, 117, 124.

Appendixes

1. Unless otherwise indicated, material in this appendix is based on Gibson, *Otto*. Washington's General Orders, 20 Nov 1777, Fitzpatrick, *Washington*, 10: 88; Weedon, *Valley Forge*, p. 135; Robert Kirkwood, *The Journals and Order Book of Captain Robert Kirkwood of the Delaware Regiment of the Continental Line*, ed. Joseph Brown Turner (Port Washington, N.Y.: Kennikat Press, 1910), p. 248; Shippen report of 24 Nov 1777, Duncan, *Medical Men*, p. 239.
2. Quote from Sproat, "Extracts," p. 443, Rev Henry Melchior Mühlenberg to Halle Fathers in Germany, Gibson, *Otto*, pp. 153–54.
3. Duncan, *Medical Men*, p. 226; Jordan, "Returns," pp. 36–38; A Return of the Wounded Belonging to Different Regiments and Their Respective Companies, Lancaster, 11 Oct 1777, Alison Papers; Gen George Washington to Lt Col William Stephens Smith, 27 Jan 1778, Fitzpatrick, *Washington*, 10: 356–57; Ebenezer David, *A Rhode Island Chaplain in the Revolution, Letters of Ebenezer David to Nicholas Brown, 1775–1778*, eds. Jeannette D. Black and William Greene Roelker (Providence: The Rhode Island Society of the Cincinnati, 1949), p. 75; Report of Brig Gen Lachlan McIntosh, 26 Apr 1778, RG 93, M246, roll 135, folder 3–1, item 10.
4. Butterfield, *Letters of Rush*, 1: 158.
5. Griffenhagen, *Drug Supplies*, p. 127; James Craik to Jonathan Potts, 7 Apr 1778, Gibson, *Otto*, p. 162; Heiges, "Letters," pp. 74, 77; Shippen report of 24 Nov 1777, Duncan, *Medical Men*, p. 239. Duncan's book contains neither footnotes nor bibliography and the original of this report has not been located. His version of the document lists "Mendham" rather than Manheim, but because it is not likely that the Mendham hospital was still open, because, although no state is mentioned, the hospital is listed with those in Pennsylvania, and because Duncan has been known to misread the city names in eighteenth century reports, it seems obvious that Manheim is the name intended by Shippen.
6. Weedon, *Valley Forge*, pp. 109–10; Shippen report of 24 Nov 1777, Duncan, *Medical Men*, p. 239.
7. Middleton, "Valley Forge," p. 485.
8. Jordan, "Returns," p. 40; Radbill, "Alison," p. 252; A Return of the Sick & Wounded in the Hospital at Plumstead, 10 Dec 1777, Alison Papers; Shippen, Just Account.
9. Sproat Journal, Gibson, *Otto*, p. 329.
10. Sproat Journal, Gibson, *Otto*, p. 326; Report of Brig Gen Lachlan McIntosh, 27 Apr 1778, RG 93, M246, roll 135, folder 3–1, item 11.

11. Report of Brig Gen Lachlan McIntosh, 26 Apr 1778, RG 93, M246, roll 135, folder 3-1, item 10.

12. Quote from Report of Brig Gen Lachlan McIntosh, 25 Apr 1778, RG 93, M246, roll 135, folder 3-1, item 10; Heiges, "Letters," p. 77.

13. Matthew Irwine to Jonathan Potts, 22 Mar 1778, Potts Papers, 4: 423; Report of Brig Gen Lachlan McIntosh, 27 Apr 1778, RG 93, M246, roll 135, folder 3-1, item 11; Sproat Journal, Gibson, *Otto*, p. 328.

14. Washington's General Orders, 17 Jun 1777, Fitzpatrick, *Washington*, 8: 251; Accounts of John Dunn, 1777-78, RG 93, M859, roll 124, frame 989, item 035501.

15. Washington's General Orders, 17 Jun 1777, Fitzpatrick, *Washington*, 8: 257; Ella W. Mockridge, *Our Mendham* (Ann Arbor, Mich., 1961), p. 56; Mendham, New Jersey, Mayor's Tercentenary Committee, *The Mendhams*, (Brookside, N.J., 1964), p. 32.

16. Butterfield, *Letters of Rush*, 1: 167n; Benjamin Rush to Julia Rush, 10 Nov 1777, and Benjamin Rush to James Searle, 19 Nov 1777, Butterfield, *Letters of Rush*, 1: 166.

Bibliography

Ackerknecht, Erwin Heinz. *Malaria in the Upper Mississippi Valley, 1760-1900.* Baltimore: Johns Hopkins Press, 1945.

———. *A Short History of Medicine.* New York: Ronald Press Co., 1955.

Adams, John. *Letters of John Adams Addressed to His Wife.* Edited by Charles Francis Adams. 2 vols. Boston: Charles C. Little and James Brown, 1841.

Adams, Randolph Greenfield, and Peckham, Howard H., eds. *Lexington to Fallen Timbers 1775-1794.* Ann Arbor: University of Michigan Press, 1942.

Adams, Reed. "New Orleans and the War of 1812." *Louisiana Historical Quarterly* 16 (1933): 221-34, 479-503, 681-703; 17 (1934): 169-82, 349-63, 502-23.

Adams, Samuel. *The Writings of Samuel Adams.* Edited by Harry Alonzo Cushing. 4 vols. New York: Octagon Books, 1968.

Adams, T. R. "The Medical and Political Activities of Dr. James Tilton." *Annual Report of the John Carter Brown Library* (Brown University and the Colonial Society of Massachusetts, Providence, R.I.) 7 (1972): 30-32.

Aiken, John. *Thoughts on Hospitals.* London: Joseph Johnson, 1771.

Akerly, Samuel. "Medical Topography of the Military Positions in the Third United States Military District: Together With a Summary Report on the Diseases of the Army ...." *Medical Repository,* 2d ser. 3 (1817): 293-300, 405-7.

Alison Papers. See under Philadelphia, Pa.

Alleman, Albert. "Experiences of an American Physician at the Capture of Washington by the British in 1814." *Medical Library and Historical Journal* 4 (1906): 185-88.

The American Revolution 1775-1783: An Atlas of 18th Century Maps and Charts: Theaters of Operations. Washington: Government Printing Office, 1972.

American State Papers. See under U.S. Congress.

Amory, Thomas Coffin. *The Military Services and Public Life of Major-General John Sullivan of the American Revolutionary Army,* Port Washington, N.Y.: Kennikat Press, 1968 reprint of 1868 edition.

Anderson, Fanny J. "Medical Practices During the War of 1812." *Bulletin of the History of Medicine* 16 (1944): 261-75.

Anderson, Joseph, ed. *The Town and City of Waterbury, Connecticut, From the Aboriginal Period to the Year Eighteen Hundred and Ninety-Five.* 2 vols. New Haven: Price & Lee Co., 1896.

Angelakos, Peter. "The Army at Middlebrook 1778-1779." *New Jersey Historical Society Proceedings* 70 (1952): 97-120.

Applegate, Howard Lewis. "The American Revolutionary War Hospital Department." *Military Medicine* 126 (1961): 296-306.

———. "The Medical Administrators of the American Revolutionary Army." *Military Affairs* 25 (1961): 1-10.

———. "Preventive Medicine in the American Revolutionary Army." *Military Medicine* 126 (1961): 379-82.

———. "Remedial Medicine in the American Revolutionary Army." *Military Medicine* 126 (1961): 450-53.

Armstrong, John. *Notices of the War of 1812.* 2 vols. New York: Wiley & Putnam, 1840.

Arnold, Benedict. *The Present State of the American Rebel Army, Navy and Finances, Transmitted to the British Government, October 1780.*

Arthur, Stanley Clisby. *The Story of the Battle of New Orleans.* New Orleans: Louisiana Historical Society, 1915.

Ashburn, P. M. *A History of the Medical*

Department of the United States Army. Boston: Houghton Mifflin Co., 1929.

Atherton, William. *Narrative of the Suffering & Defeat of the Northwestern Army Under General Winchester* .... Frankfort, Ky., 1842.

Babcock, Louis L. *The Siege of Fort Erie, An Episode of the War of 1812.* Buffalo, N.Y.: Peter Paul Book Co., 1899.

———. *The War of 1812 on the Niagara Frontier.* Buffalo, N.Y.: Buffalo Historical Society, 1927.

Ballagh, James Curtis, ed. *The Letters of Richard Henry Lee.* 2 vols. New York: Da Capo Press, 1970 reprint of 1911–14 edition.

Bartlett, Josiah. *A Dissertation on the Progress of Medical Science in the Commonwealth of Massachusetts.* Boston: T. B. Wait and Co., 1810.

Barton, William Paul Crillon. *A Treatise Containing a Plan for the Internal Organization and Government of Marine Hospitals in the United States; Together With Observations on Military and Flying Hospitals, and a Scheme for Amending and Systematizing the Medical Department of the Navy.* 2d ed. Philadelphia, 1817.

Bassett, John S., ed. *Correspondence of Andrew Jackson.* 7 vols. Washington: Carnegie Institution of Washington, 1926–35.

Bayne-Jones, Stanhope. *The Evolution of Preventive Medicine in the United States Army, 1607–1939.* Washington: Government Printing Office, 1968.

Beall, William Kennedy. "Journal of William K. Beall, July–August 1812." Reprinted from *American Historical Review* 17 (1912): 783–808.

Beatty, Joseph M., Jr. "Letters From Continental Officers to Doctor Reading Beatty, 1781–1788." *Pennsylvania Magazine of History and Biography* 54 (1930): 155–74.

Beaumont, William. *William Beaumont's Formative Years: Two Early Notebooks, 1811–1821.* Edited by Genevieve Miller. New York: Henry Schuman, 1946.

Beck, Herbert H. "The Military Hospital at Lititz, 1777–1778." *Lancaster County Historical Society Papers* 23 (1919): 5–14.

Beck, James A. *Bethlehem and Its Military Hospital, An Address Delivered at the Unveiling of a Tablet Erected by the Pennsylvania Society of the Sons of the Revolution, June 19, 1897, in Memory of the Soldiers of the Continental Army, Who Suffered and Died at the Military Hospital at Bethlehem, Pennsylvania.* Printed by the Society.

Beck, John B. *Medicine in the American Colonies: An Historical Sketch of the State of Medicine in the American Colonies, From Their First Settlement to the Period of the Revolution.* Albuquerque, N. Mex.: Horn & Wallace, 1966 reprint of 1850 edition.

Beebe, Lewis. *Journal of Dr. Lewis Beebe.* The New York Times & Arno Press, 1971.

Beirne, Francis F. *War of 1812.* New York: E. P. Dutton & Co., 1949.

Bell, Whitfield Jenks, Jr. *John Morgan, Continental Doctor.* Philadelphia: University of Pennsylvania Press, 1965.

———. "Medical Practice in Colonial America." *Bulletin of the History of Medicine* 31 (1957): 442–53.

———. "Philadelphia Medical Students in Europe, 1750–1800." *Pennsylvania Magazine of History and Biography* 67 (1943): 1–29.

Bernardo, C. Joseph, and Bacon, Eugene R. *American Military Policy: Its Development Since 1775.* Harrisburg: Stackpole, 1955.

Bethlehem of Pennsylvania: The First One Hundred Years: 1741 to 1841. Bethlehem, Pa., 1968.

Bett, W. R. "John Warren (1753–1815), Soldier, Anatomist and Surgeon." *Medical Press* 230 (1953): 137.

Bick, Edgar M. "French Influences on Early American Medicine and Surgery." *Journal of the Mount Sinai Hospital* 24 (1957): 499–509.

Bill, Alfred Hoyt. *Valley Forge: The Making of an Army.* New York: Harper & Bros., 1952.

Billings, John S. "The History and Literature of Surgery." In *System of Surgery*, vol. 1, edited by Frederic Shephard Dennis. Philadelphia: Lea Bros. & Co., 1895.

Billroth, Theodor. "Historical Studies on the Nature and Treatment of Gunshot Wounds From the Fifteenth Century to the Present Time." Translated by C. P. Rhoads. *Yale*

Journal of Biology and Medicine 4 (1931-32): 3-36, 119-48, 225-57.

Blake, John Ballard. *Benjamin Waterhouse and the Introduction of Vaccination, a Reappraisal.* Philadelphia: University of Pennsylvania Press, 1957.

———. "Diseases and Medical Practice in Colonial America." In "Symposium on the History of American Medicine." *International Record of Medicine* 171 (1958): 350-63.

———. *Public Health in the Town of Boston, 1630-1822.* Cambridge: Harvard University Press, 1959.

Blanco, Richard L. *Physician of the American Revolution: Jonathan Potts.* New York: Garland STPM Press, 1979.

———. To author, letter, 22 April 1975.

Bland, Theodorick. *The Bland Papers, Being a Selection From the Manuscripts of Colonel Theodorick Bland, Jr., of Prince George County, Virginia, to Which Are Prefixed an Introduction, and a Memoir of Colonel Bland.* Edited by Charles Campbell. 2 vols. Petersburg, Va.: E. & J. C. Ruffin, 1840-43.

Blanton, Wyndham Bolling. *Medicine in Virginia in the Eighteenth Century.* Richmond: Garrett & Massie, 1931.

Bouvet, Maurice. *Le Service de santé français pendant la guerre d'indépendance des Etats-Unis.* Paris: Hippocrate, 1933.

Bowman, Allen. *Morale of the American Revolutionary Army.* Washington: American Council on Public Affairs, 1943.

Boyd, Mark F. "An Historical Sketch of the Prevalence of Malaria in North America." *American Journal of Tropical Medicine* 21 (1941): 223-44.

Boyer, John. "Daily Journal of Wayne's Campaign." *American Pioneer* 1 (1842): 315-22, 351-57.

Bradford, S. Sydney. "Hunger Menaces the Revolution, December 1779-January 1780." *Maryland Historical Magazine* 61 (1966): 1-23.

Brady, Cyrus Townsend. *American Fights and Fighters: Stories of the First Five Wars of the United States From the War of the Revolution to the War of 1812.* New York: McClure, Phillips & Co., 1900.

Brannan, John. *Official Letters of the Military and Naval Officers of the United States During the War With Great Britain.* Washington: Way & Gideon, 1823.

Brasch, Frederick E. "The Royal Society of London and Its Influence Upon Scientific Thought in the American Colonies." *Scientific Monthly* 33 (1931): 336-55, 448-69.

Brocklesby, Richard. *Oeconomical and Medical Observations, in Two Parts, From the Year 1758 to the Year 1763, Inclusive . . . .* London: T. Becket and P. A. De Hondt, 1764.

Brown, Harvey E. *The Medical Department of the United States Army From 1775 to 1873.* Washington: The Surgeon General's Office, 1873.

Brown, Samuel R. *An Authentic History of the Second War for Independence . . . .* 2 vols. Auburn, N.Y.: J. G. Hathaway, 1815.

Buchan, William. *Domestic Medicine; Or, the Family Physician . . . .* 2d American ed. Philadelphia: Joseph Crukshank, 1774.

———. *Observations Concerning the Diet of the Common People . . . .* London: A. Steahan, T. Cadell, Jr., and W. Davies, J. Balfour and W. Creich, 1797.

———. *Observations Concerning the Prevention and Cure of the Venereal Disease Intended to Guard the Ignorant and Unwary Against the Baneful Effects of That Insidious Malady.* Dublin: P. Wogan, J. Millikin, W. Sleater, J. Rice, P. Moore, 1796.

Burnett, Edmund Cody, ed. *Letters of Members of the Continental Congress.* 8 vols. Washington: Carnegie Institution of Washington, 1921-36.

Bush, Lewis Potter. *The Delaware State Medical Society and Its Founders in the Eighteenth Century.* New York, 1886.

Butterfield, Lyman H. "Benjamin Rush: A Physician As Seen in His Letters." *Bulletin of the History of Medicine* 20 (1946): 138-56.

Butterfield, Lyman H., ed. *Letters of Benjamin Rush: Memoirs of the American Philosophical Society.* 2 vols. Princeton: Princeton University Press, 1951.

Calhoun, John Caldwell. *The Papers of John C. Calhoun.* Edited by W. Edwin Hemphill. 2 vols. to date. Columbia: University of South Carolina Press for the South Carolina Society, 1963.

Callan, John F. *The Military Laws of the United States Relating to the Army, Volunteers, Militia, and to Bounty Lands and Pensions, From the Foundation of the Government to the Year 1863.* Philadelphia: George W. Childs, 1863.

Campfield, Jabez. "Diary of Dr. Jabez Campfield, Surgeon in 'Spencer's Regiment,' While Attached to Sullivan's Expedition Against the Indians From May 23d to Oct 2d, 1779." *New Jersey Historical Society Proceedings,* 2d ser. 3 (1873): 115-36.

Cantlie, Neil. *A History of the Army Medical Department.* 2 vols. Edinburgh: Churchill Livingstone, 1974.

Carney, Sydney H., Jr. "Some Medical Men in the Revolution." *Magazine of History* 21 (1915): 183-96.

Carrington, Henry B. *Battles of the American Revolution, 1775-1781: Historical and Military Criticism With Topographical Illustration.* 6th ed., rev. New York: A. S. Barnes & Co., 1968.

Carson, Joseph. *A History of the Medical Department of the University of Pennsylvania, From Its Foundation in 1765.* Philadelphia: Lindsay and Blakiston, 1869.

Casey, Powell A. *Louisiana in the War of 1812.* 1963.

Cash, Philip. *Medical Men at the Siege of Boston, April, 1775-April, 1776: Problems of the Massachusetts and Continental Armies.* Philadelphia: American Philosophical Society, 1973.

Chard, Thornton. "Excerpts From the Private Journal of Doctor John Cochran." *New York History* 42 (1944): 360-78.

———. "Illustrations Pertaining to the Medical Life of Doctor John Cochran." *Bulletin of the History of Medicine* 20 (1946): 76-84.

Claiborne, Nathaniel. *Notes on the War in the South.* New York: Arno Press & The New York Times, 1971 reprint of 1819 edition.

Claiborne, W. C. C. *Official Letter Books of W. C. C. Claiborne, 1801-1816.* Edited by Dunbar Rowland. 6 vols. Jackson, Miss.: State Department of Archives and History, 1917.

Clark, William. "William Clark's Journal of General Wayne's Campaign." *Mississippi Valley Historical Review* 1 (1914-15): 418-43.

Clendening, Logan, ed. *Source Book of Medical History.* New York: Dover Publications, 1942.

Clift, Garrett Glenn. *Remember the Raisin: Kentucky and Kentuckians in the Battles and Massacre at Frenchtown, Michigan Territory, in the War of 1812.* Frankfort: Kentucky Historical Society, 1961.

Closen, Ludwig von. *The Revolutionary Journal of Baron Ludwig von Closen, 1780-1783.* Edited by Evelyn M. Acomb. Chapel Hill: University of North Carolina Press, 1958.

Cochran, John. Five Letters to Barnabas Binney. *Pennsylvania Magazine of History and Biography* 5 (1881): 229-31.

Cochran Letter Book. *See under* Morristown, N.J.

Cochrane, John. "Medical Department of the Revolutionary Army." *Magazine of American History* 12 (1884): 241-60.

Codman, John. *Arnold's Expedition to Quebec.* New York: Macmillan Co., 1902.

Coles, Harry L. *The War of 1812.* Chicago: University of Chicago Press, 1965.

Colyar, A. S. *Life and Times of Andrew Jackson, Soldier, Statesman, President.* 2 vols. Nashville, Tenn.: Marshall & Bruce Co., 1904.

Commager, Henry Steele, and Morris, Richard B., eds. *The Spirit of Seventy-Six: The Story of the American Revolution As Told by Participants.* New York: Harper & Row, 1967.

Comrie, John D. *History of Scottish Medicine.* 2d ed. 2 vols. London: Baillière, Tindall, & Cox, 1932.

Cook, Frederick, ed. *Journals of the Military Expedition of Major General John Sullivan Against the Six Nations of Indians in 1779 With Records of Centennial Celebrations.* Auburn, N.Y.: Knapp, Peck & Thompson, 1887.

Cooke, John Henry. *A Narrative of Events in the South of France and of the Attack on New Orleans, in 1814 and 1815.* London: T. & W. Boone, 1835.

Corbin, Henry C., and Thian, Raphael P., eds. *Legislative History of the General Staff of the Army of the United States.* Washington: Government Printing Office, 1901.

Corner, Betsy Copping. *William Shippen, Jr.:*

Pioneer in American Medical Education. Philadelphia: American Philosophical Society, 1951.

Corner, George W., ed. *The Autobiography of Benjamin Rush: His "Travels Through Life" Together With His "Commonplace Book" for 1789–1813.* Princeton, N.J.: Princeton University Press, 1948.

Craik, James. "A Letter Written by Jas. Craik to Andrew Craigie, Esq., Apy. Genl., August 1780, Relating to the Condition of the Army, Communicated by Nathaniel Paine." *Massachusetts Historical Society Proceedings,* 2d ser. 15 (1901–2): 362–64.

Cross, Trueman. *Military Laws of the United States; to Which Is Prefixed the Constitution of the United States.* Washington: Edward de Krafft, 1825.

Cruikshank, Ernest A. *The Battle of Lundy's Lane.* Welland, Ontario: Lundy's Lane Historical Society, 1893.

——. *Documentary History of the Campaign Upon the Niagara Frontier.* 4 vols. Arno Press & The New York Times, 1971 reprint of 1896–1908 edition.

Cullum, G. W., ed. *Campaigns of the War of 1812–15.* New York: Miller, 1879.

Cutbush, Edward. *Observations on the Means of Preserving the Health of Soldiers and Sailors; and on the Duties of the Medical Departments of the Army and Navy: With Remarks on Hospitals and Their Internal Arrangements.* Philadelphia: Fry and Kammerer, 1808.

Dalton, R. H. "A Glance at the American Medical Profession Since the Beginning of the Present Century." *Journal of the American Medical Association* 21 (1893): 953–55.

Darnell, Elias. "A Journal Containing an Accurate and Interesting Account of the Hardships, Sufferings, Battles, Defeat, and Captivity of Those Heroic Kentucky Volunteers and Regulars, Commanded by General Winchester, in the Years 1812–1813 . . . ." *Magazine of History,* Extra No. 31. New York: W. Abbatt, 1914 reprint of 1854 edition.

David, Ebenezer. *A Rhode Island Chaplain in the Revolution, Letters of Ebenezer David to Nicholas Brown, 1775–1778.* Edited by Jeannette D. Black and William Greene Roelker. Providence: The Rhode Island Society of the Cincinnati, 1949.

Davidson, Chalmers Gaston. *Friend of the People: The Life of Peter Fayssoux of Charleston.* Columbia, S.C.: South Carolina Medical Association, 1950.

Davis, John. "The Yorktown Campaign: Journal of Captain John Davis, of the Pennsylvania Line." *Pennsylvania Magazine of History and Biography* 5 (1881): 290–310.

Davis, Nathan Smith. *Contributions to the History of Medical Education and Medical Institutions in the United States of America, 1776–1876.* Washington: Government Printing Office, 1877.

——. *History of Medical Education and Institutions in the United States From the First Settlement of the British Colonies to the Year 1850.* Chicago: S. C. Griggs & Co., 1851.

Dawson, Henry Barton. *Battles of the United States.* 2 vols. New York: Johnson, Fry and Co., 1858.

Dearborn, Henry. *Journals of Henry Dearborn, 1776–1783.* Cambridge: John Wilson and Son, 1887.

De Grummond, Jane Lucas. *The Baratarians and the Battles of New Orleans.* Baton Rouge: Louisiana State University Press, 1961.

D'Elia, D. J. "Dr. Benjamin Rush and the American Medical Revolution." *Proceedings of the American Philosophical Society* 110 (1966): 227–34.

Denny, Ebenezer. *Military Journal of Major Ebenezer Denny,. An Officer in the Revolutionary and Indian Wars, With the Introductory Memoir.* Philadelphia: Historical Society of Pennsylvania, 1859.

Devoto, Bernard, ed. *The Journals of Lewis and Clark.* Boston: Houghton Mifflin Co., 1953.

Diller, Theodore. *Franklin's Contribution to Medicine.* Brooklyn, N.Y.: Albert T. Huntington, 1912.

"Diseases of the Army of the Third United States Military District." *Medical Repository,* new ser. 3 (1817): 407.

Dorland's Illustrated Medical Dictionary. 24th ed. Philadelphia: W. B. Saunders Co., 1965.

Draper, Lyman C. *King's Mountain and Its*

Heroes: History of the Battle of King's Mountain, October 7th, 1780, and the Events Which Led to It. Cincinnati: P. G. Thomson, 1881.

Drinker, Cecil Kent. Not So Long Ago. New York: Oxford University Press, 1937.

Drowne, Solomon. "Original Letters." Pennsylvania Magazine of History and Biography 5 (1881): 110-14.

Dudley, Thomas P. "Battle and Massacre at Frenchtown, Michigan, January 1813, by Rev. Thomas P. Dudley, One of the Survivors." Western Reserve and Northern Ohio Historical Society Publications No. 1 (1870).

Duffy, John. Epidemics in Colonial America. Baton Rouge: Louisiana State University Press, 1953.

Duncan, Louis C. Medical Men in the American Revolution, 1775-1783. Army Medical Bulletin No. 25. Carlisle Barracks, Pa.: Medical Field Service School, 1931.

Durfee, David A., ed. William Henry Harrison 1773-1841; John Tyler 1790-1862; Chronology — Documents — Bibliographical Aids. Dobbs Ferry, N.Y.: Oceana Publications, 1970.

Eaton, Leonard K. "Military Surgery in the Battle of Tippecanoe." Bulletin of the History of Medicine 25 (1951): 460-63.

Efner, Elijah D. "The Adventures and Enterprises of Elijah D. Efner." Publications of the Buffalo Historical Society 4 (1896): 35-54.

Eliot, Ephraim. "Account of the Physicians of Boston." Proceedings of the Massachusetts Historical Society 6 (1863-64): 177-84.

Elliott, Charles Winslow. Winfield Scott. New York: Macmillan Co., 1937.

Eustis Papers. See under Washington, D.C., Library of Congress, Manuscript Division.

Ewell, James. The Medical Companion: Treating, According to the Most Successful Practice, I. The Diseases Common to Warm Climates and on Ship Board; II. Common Cases in Surgery, as Fractures, Dislocations &c.; III. The Complaints Peculiar to Women and Children, With a Dispensatory and Glossary . . . . 3d ed. Philadelphia: privately printed, 1817.

Fairchild, G. M., Jr., ed. Journal of an American Prisoner at Fort Malden and Quebec in the War of 1812. Quebec: privately printed, 1909.

Farmer, Laurence. "The Early Directors of the Medical Services of the American Revolutionary Army." Bulletin of the New York Academy of Medicine 36 (1960): 765-76.

Fay, Herman Allen. Collection of the Official Accounts, in Detail, of All the Battles Fought by Sea and Land Between the Navy and Army of the United States and the Navy and Army of Great Britain During the Years 1812, 13, 14, & 15. New York, 1817.

Feltman, William. "The Journal of Lieut. William Feltman, of the First Pennsylvania Regiment, From May 26, 1781, to April 25, 1782, Embracing the Siege of Yorktown and the Southern Campaign." Pennsylvania Historical Society Collections 1 (1853): 303-48.

Fisher, Elijah. "Elijah Fisher's Journal While in the War for Independence and Continued for Two Years After He Came to Maine, 1775-1784." Magazine of History, Extra No. 6.

Fitz, Reginald H. "Zabdiel Boylston, Inoculator, and the Epidemic of Smallpox in Boston in 1721." Bulletin of the Johns Hopkins Hospital 22 (1911): 315-27.

Fitzpatrick, John C. The Spirit of the Revolution. Boston: Houghton Mifflin Co., 1924.

Fitzpatrick, John C., ed. The Diaries of George Washington, 1748-1799. 4 vols. Boston: Houghton Mifflin Co., 1925.

―――――. The Writings of George Washington From the Original Manuscript Sources, 1745-1799. 39 vols. Washington: Government Printing Office, 1931-44.

Force, Peter, ed. American Archives: Fourth and Fifth Series, Containing a Documentary History of the United States of America From March 7, 1774 to the Definitive Treaty of Peace With Great Britain, September 3, 1783. 9 vols. Washington: M. St. Clair Clarke and Peter Force, 1848-53.

Ford, Worthington Chauncey, ed. General Orders Issued by Major-General Israel Putnam When in Command of the Highlands in the Summer and Fall of 1777. Boston: Gregg Press, 1972 reprint of 1893 edition.

Ford, Worthington Chauncey; Hunt, Gaillard; and others, eds. Journals of the Continental

Congress. 34 vols. Washington: Government Printing Office, 1904–37.

Forman, Jonathan, comp. *Physicians and the Indian Wars.* Columbus: Ohio State Medical Association, 1953.

Fortier, Alcée. *A History of Louisiana.* 4 vols. New York: Manzi, Joyant & Co., 1904.

Foster Papers. *See under* Washington, D.C., Library of Congress, Manuscript Division.

Fox, Cyrus T., ed. *Reading and Berks County Pennsylvania, A History.* 3 vols. New York: Lewis Historical Publishing Co., 1925.

Fox, Richard Hingston. *Dr. John Fothergill and His Friends, Chapters in Eighteenth Century Life.* London: Macmillan and Co., 1919.

Freeman, Douglas Southall. *Victory With the Help of France.* George Washington, A Biography, vol. 5. New York: Charles Scribner's Sons, 1952.

French, Allen. *General Gage's Informers.* Ann Arbor: University of Michigan Press, 1932.

Friedman, Reuben. "Scabies in Colonial America." *Annals of Medical History,* 3d ser. 2 (1940): 401–3.

Gahn, Bessie W. Brown. "Dr. William Brown, Physician-General to the American Army." *Journal of the American Pharmaceutical Association* 16 (1927): 1090–91.

Galdston, Iago. "The Rise of Modern Research." *Ciba Symposia* 8 (1946): 354–61.

Gale, Benjamin. "Historical Memoirs, Relating to the Practice of Inoculation for the Small Pox, in the British American Provinces, Particularly in New England." *Philosophical Transactions of the Royal Society of London* 55 (1765): 193–204.

Ganoe, William Addleman. *The History of the United States Army.* New York: D. Appleton and Co., 1924.

Gardner, Asa B. "The New York Continental Line." *Magazine of American History* 7 (1881): 401–19.

Garrison, Fielding H. *History of Medicine.* Philadelphia: W. B. Saunders Co., 1914.

———. "Notes on the History of Military Medicine." *Military Surgeon* 49–51 (1921–22), reprinted by the Association of Military Surgeons, 1922.

Gates, Horatio. "Letters of General Gates on the Southern Campaign." *Magazine of American History* 5 (1880): 281–310.

General Committee of Defense. *Observations Relative to the Means of Preserving Health in Armies.* 7 September 1814.

Gibbes, R. W., ed. *Reminiscences, Documentary History of the American Revolution . . . .* 3 vols. New York: D. Appleton & Co., 1853–57.

Gibson, James E. "Captured Medical Men and Army Hospitals of the American Revolution." *Annals of Medical History,* new ser. 10 (1938): 382–89.

———. *Dr. Bodo Otto and the Medical Background of the American Revolution.* Baltimore: Charles C Thomas, 1937.

———. "John Augustus Otto." *Historical Review of Berks County* 13 (1947): 14–18.

———. "The Role of Disease in the 70,000 Casualties in the American Revolutionary Army." *Transactions and Studies of the College of Physicians of Philadelphia,* 4th ser. 17 (1949): 121–27.

———. "Smallpox and the American Revolution." *Genealogical Magazine and Historiographical Chronicle* 51 (1948): 55–57.

Gilman, C. M. B. "Military Surgery in the American Revolution." *Journal of the Medical Society of New Jersey* 57 (1960): 491–96.

Godfrey, Carlos E. *Organization of the Provisional Army of the United States in the Anticipated War With France, 1789–1800.* Pennsylvania Magazine of History and Biography 38 (1914): 129–82.

Gooch, Benjamin. *A Practical Treatise on Wounds and Other Chirurgical Subjects; to Which is Prefixed a Short Historical Account of the Rise and Progress of Surgery and Anatomy, Addressed to Young Surgeons.* 2 vols. Norwich: W. Chase, 1767.

Goodman, Nathan G. *Benjamin Rush, Physician and Citizen, 1746–1813.* Philadelphia: University of Pennsylvania Press, 1934.

Gordon, Maurice B. *Aesculapius Comes to the Colonies.* Ventnor, N.J.: Ventnor Publishers, 1949.

———. "Medicine in Colonial New Jersey and Adjacent Areas." *Bulletin of the History of Medicine* 17 (1945): 38–60.

Gore, Albert A. *The Story of Our Services Under the Crown: A Historical Sketch of* the *Army Medical Staff*. London: Baillière, Tindall, & Cox, 1879.

Graham, Harvey. *The Story of Surgery*. Garden City, N.Y.: Doubleday, Doran & Co., 1939.

Graham, Joseph. "Narrative of the Revolutionary War in North Carolina in 1780 and 1781." In *Papers of Archibald D. Murphey*. Edited by W. H. Hoyt. 3 vols. Raleigh, 1914.

Graves, Charles B. "Dr. Philip Turner of Norwich, Connecticut." *Annals of Medical History* 10 (1928): 1-24.

Green, Constance McLaughlin. *Washington, Village and Capital, 1800-1878*. Princeton, N.J.: Princeton University Press, 1962.

Greene, George Washington. *The Life of Nathanael Greene*. 3 vols. New York: G. P. Putnam and Son, 1867-1871.

Greene, Nathanael. "Report on the 'Battle of Eutaw Springs.'" *Magazine of History*, Extra No. 3.

Greenhous, Brereton. "A Note on Western Logistics in the War of 1812." *Military Affairs* 34 (1970): 41-44.

Gregorie, Anne King. *Thomas Sumter*. Columbia, S.C.: R. L. Bryan Co., 1931.

Griffenhagen, George B. *Drug Supplies in the American Revolution*. U.S. National Museum Bulletin 225. Washington: Smithsonian Institution, 1961.

Hadel, Albert Kimberley. "The Battle of Bladensburg." *Maryland Historical Magazine* 1 (1906): 155-67.

Hales, Stephen. *A Treatise on Ventilators*. London: Manby, 1758.

Hall, Courtney Robert. "The Beginnings of American Military Medicine." *Annals of Medical History*, 3d ser. 4 (1942): 122-31.

Hamersly, Thomas H. S. *Complete Army and Navy Register of the United States of America, From 1776 to 1887*. New York: T. H. S. Hamersly, 1888.

Hamilton, John Taylor. *A History of the Church Known as the Moravian Church, or the Unitas Fratrum or the Unity of the Brethren During the Eighteenth and Nineteenth Centuries*. Transactions of the Moravian Historical Society, vol. 6. Bethlehem, Pa.; Times Publishing Co., 1900.

Hamilton, Kenneth Gardiner. *John Ettwein and the Moravian Church During the Revolutionary Period*. Bethlehem, Pa.: Times Publishing Co., 1940.

Hamilton, Robert. *Observations on the Marsh Remittent Fever* . . . . London: T. Gillet, 1801.

Hand, Edward. "Orderly Book of General Edward Hand, Valley Forge, January 1778." *Pennsylvania Magazine of History and Biography* 41 (1917): 198-223, 257-73, 458-68.

Harmar, Josiah. *The Proceedings of a Court of Inquiry, Held at the Special Request of Brigadier General Josiah Harman* . . . . Philadelphia, 1791.

Harris, David. "Medicine in Colonial America." *California and Western Medicine* 50 (1939): 355-58, 415-18; 51 (1939): 35-38.

Harrison, William Henry. *Governors' Messages and Letters, Messages & Letters of William Henry Harrison*. Edited by Logan Esarey. 4 vols. Indianapolis: Indiana Historical Commission, 1922.

Harvey, Samuel Clark. *The History of Hemostasis*. New York: Paul B. Hoeber, 1929.

Hatch, Louis Clinton. *The Administration of the American Revolutionary Army*. Harvard Historical Studies, vol. 10. New York: Lenox Hill, 1904.

Hatch, William Stanley. *A Chapter of the History of the War of 1812 in the Northwest. Embracing the Surrender of the Northwestern Army and Fort, at Detroit, August 16 1812. With a Description and Biographical Sketch of the Celebrated Indian Chief Tecumseh*. Cincinnati: Miami Printing and Publishing Co., 1872.

Hawke, David Freeman. *Benjamin Rush: Revolutionary Gadfly*. Indianapolis: Bobbs-Merrill, 1971.

Heart, Jonathan. *Journal of Capt. Jonathan Heart* . . . . Edited by Consul Willshire Butterfield. Albany, N.Y.: Joel Munsell's Sons, 1885

Heath, William. *Heath's Memoirs of the American War*. Edited by Rufus Rockwell Wilson. New York: A. Wessels Co., 1904.

Heaton, Claude Edwin. "Medicine in New York During the English Colonial Period, 1664-1775." *Bulletin of the History of Medicine* 17 (1945): 9-37.

Heckwelder, John. "Narrative of His Journey to the Wabash in 1792." *Pennsylvania Magazine of History and Biography* 11 (1887): 466-75; 12 (1888): 34-54.

Heiges, George L. "Letters Relating to Colonial Military Hospitals in Lancaster County." *Lancaster County (Pa.) Historical Society Papers* 52 (1948): 73-96.

Heitman, Francis Bernard. *Historical Register and Dictionary of the United States Army From Its Organization, September 29, 1789, to March 2, 1903.* 2 vols. Washington: Government Printing Office, 1903.

———. *Historical Register of Officers of the Continental Army During the War of the Revolution, April 1775 to December 1783.* Washington, 1892-93.

Hess, Alfred. *Scurvy, Past and Present.* Philadelphia: J. B. Lippincott, 1920.

Heustis, Jabez W. "Observations on the Disease Which Prevailed in the Army at Camp Terreaux-Boeufs, in June, July, and August of the Year 1809." *Medical Repository*, 2d ser. 3 (1817): 33-41.

———. *Physical Observations, and Medical Tracts and Researches on the Topography and Diseases of Louisiana.* New York: T. and J. Swords, 1817.

Higginbotham, Don. *The War of American Independence, Military Attitudes, Policies, and Practice, 1763-1789.* New York: Macmillan Co., 1971.

Hindle, Brooke. *The Pursuit of Science in Revolutionary America, 1735-1789.* Chapel Hill: University of North Carolina Press, 1956.

Hocker, Edward W. "Medical Men Deserve Tribute for Care of Washington's Men at Valley Forge Encampment." *Picket Post* 16 (1947): 7-14.

Horner, W. E. "Surgical Sketches." *Medical Examiner and Record of Medical Science*, new ser. 8 (1852): 753-74; 9 (1852): 1-24, 69-85.

Hosack, David. *A Biographical Memoir of Hugh Williamson, M.D., LL.D.* New York: C. S. Van Winkle, 1820.

———. *Observations on the Laws Governing the Communication of Contagious Diseases and the Means of Arresting Their Progress.* New York: Van Winkle and Wiley, 1815.

Howe, Eber D. "Recollections of a Pioneer Printer." *Buffalo Historical Society Publications* 9 (1906): 375-406.

Hull, William. *Memoirs of the Campaign of the Northwestern Army of the United States, 1812.* Boston: True & Greene, 1824.

Hume, Edgar Erskine. *Victories of Army Medicine: Scientific Accomplishments of the Medical Department of the United States Army.* Philadelphia: J. B. Lippincott Co., 1943.

Hunter, John. *Hunterian Reminiscences; Being the Substance of a Course of Lectures on the Principles and Practice of Surgery, Delivered by the Late Mr. John Hunter, in the Year 1785.* Edited by J. W. K. Parkinson. London: Sherwood, Gilbert, and Pepir, 1833.

———. *Observations on the Diseases of the Army in Jamaica and on the Best Means of Preserving the Health of Europeans in the Climate. Also, Observations on the Hepatitis of the East Indies.* 3d ed. London: T. Payne, 1808.

———. *Treatise on the Blood, Inflammation and Gunshot Wounds.* London: John Richardson, 1794.

———. *A Treatise on the Venereal Disease.* Abridged by William Currie. Philadelphia: Charles Cist, 1787.

Huntt, Henry. "An Abstract Account of the Diseases Which Prevailed Among the Soldiers, Received into the General Hospital, at Burlington, Vermont, During the Summer and Autumn of 1814." *Medical Recorder* 1 (1818): 176-79.

Hutchinson, James. "Notes: Valley Forge." *Pennsylvania Magazine of History and Biography* 39 (1915): 221.

Ingersoll, Lurton Dunham. *A History of the War Department of the United States, With Biographical Sketches of the Secretaries.* Washington: Francis D. Mohun, 1880.

Izard, George. *Official Correspondence With the Department of War Relative to the Military Operations of the American Army Under the Command of Major General Izard on the Northern Frontier of the United States in the Years 1814 and 1815.* Philadelphia: Thomas Dobson, 1816.

Jackson, Robert. *A System of Arrangement*

and *Discipline for the Medical Department of Armies.* London: John Murray, 1805.

Jacobs, James Ripley. *The Beginning of the U.S. Army, 1783–1812.* Port Washington, N.Y.: Kennikat Press, 1947, reissued 1970.

———. *Tarnished Warrior, Major-General James Wilkinson.* New York: Macmillan Co., 1938.

Jacobs, James Ripley, and Tucker, Glenn. *The War of 1812: A Compact History.* New York: Hawthorn Books, 1969.

James, Marquis. *Andrew Jackson: The Border Captain.* Indianapolis: Bobbs-Merrill, 1933.

Jay, William. "Table of the Killed and Wounded in the War of 1812: Compiled During the War." *Collections of the New York Historical Society,* 2d ser. 7 (1849): 447–66.

Johnson, Victor Leroy. *The Administration of the American Commissariat During the Revolutionary War.* Philadelphia, 1941.

———. "Robert Morris and the Provisioning of the American Army During the Campaign of 1781." *Pennsylvania History* 5 (1938): 7–20.

Jones, Edward Alfred. *The Loyalists of Massachusetts: Their Memorials, Petitions and Claims.* Baltimore: Genealogical Publ. Co., 1969.

Jones, John. *The Surgical Works of the Late John Jones, M.D.* 3d ed. Edited by James Mease. Philadelphia: Wrigley and Berriman, 1795.

Jones, Joseph. *Letters of Joseph Jones of Virginia, 1777–1787.* Edited by Worthington Chauncey Ford. New York: New York Times, 1971 reprint of 1889 edition.

Jordan, John W. "Continental Hospital Returns." *Pennsylvania Magazine of History and Biography* 23 (1899): 35–50, 210–33.

———. "The Military Hospitals at Bethlehem and Lititz During the Revolution." *Pennsylvania Magazine of History and Biography* 20 (1896): 137–57.

Joy, Col Robert J. T., to author, letters, 25 March 1976 and 11 June 1976.

Kebler, Lyman F. "Andrew Craigie, the First Apothecary General of the United States." *Journal of the American Pharmaceutical Association* 17 (1928): 63–74, 167–78.

Kendig, John D. *A Legendary and Factual Review of the Times of Henry William Steigel and the Early Days of Manheim.* n.p., 1957.

King, L. S. *The Medical World of the Eighteenth Century.* Chicago: University of Chicago Press, 1958.

Kinzie, John. "Narrative of the Ft. Dearborn Massacre." Edited by Mentor L. Williams. *Illinois State Historical Society Collections* 46 (1953): 343–62.

Kirkwood, Robert. *The Journals and Order Book of Captain Robert Kirkwood of the Delaware Regiment of the Continental Line.* Edited by Joseph Brown Turner. Port Washington, N.Y.: Kennikat Press, 1910.

Klebs, Arnold C. "The Historic Evolution of Variolation." *Bulletin of Johns Hopkins Hospital* 24 (1913): 69–83.

Knollenberg, Bernard, ed. "The Correspondence of John Adams and Horatio Gates." *Proceedings of the Massachusetts Historical Society* 67 (1941–44): 135–51.

Knopf, Richard C., ed. *Campaign Into the Wilderness: The Wayne-Knox-Pickering-McHenry Correspondence.* 5 vols. Columbus, Ohio: Anthony Wayne Parkway Board, 1955.

———. *Document Transcriptions of the War of 1812 in the Northwest.* 8 vols. Columbus, Ohio: Anthony Wayne Parkway Board, 1957–62.

———. "A Surgeon's Mate at Fort Defiance: The Journal of Joseph Gardner Andrews for the Year 1795." *Ohio Historical Quarterly* 66 (1957): 57–86, 159–86, 238–68.

———. "Two Journals of the Kentucky Volunteers, 1793 and 1794." *Filson Club Historical Quarterly* 27 (1953): 247–81.

Kraus, Michael. "American and European Medicine in the Eighteenth Century." *Bulletin of the History of Medicine* 8 (1940): 679–95.

Kreidberg, Marvin A., and Henry, Merton G. *History of Military Mobilization in the United States Army 1775–1945.* Department of the Army Pamphlet 20-212, June 1955.

Kremers, E., and Urdang, G. *History of Pharmacy.* 2d ed. Philadelphia: J. B. Lippincott Co., 1951.

Ladenheim, Jules Calvin. "The Doctors' Mob of 1788." *Journal of the History of Medicine and Allied Sciences* 5 (1950): 23–43.

Lafayette, Marie Joseph Paul Yves. *Mémoires, correspondance, et manuscrits du général Lafayette publiées par sa famille.* 2 vols. Brussels: Société belge de Librairie, 1837.

Lane, John E. "Jean-François Coste, Chief Physician of the French Expeditionary Forces in the American Revolution." *Americana* 22 (1928): 51-80.

Latour, Arsène Lacarrière. *Historical Memoir of the War in West Florida and Louisiana in 1814-15.* Gainesville: University of Florida Press, 1964 reprint of 1816 edition.

Laurens, John. *The Army Correspondence of Colonel John Laurens in the Year 1777-8, Now First Printed From Original Letters Addressed to His Father, Henry Laurens, President of Congress, With a Memoir by William Gilmore Simms.* New York: The Bradford Club, 1867.

Le Dran, Henri François. *The Operations in Surgery of Mons. Le Dran.* Translated by Thomas Gataker. London: C. Hitch and R. Dodsby, 1749.

Lee, Henry. *Memoirs of the War in the Southern Department of the United States.* 2 vols. Philadelphia: Bradford and Inskeep, 1812.

Lee, Richard H. *Memoir of the Life of Richard Henry Lee and His Correspondence With the Most Distinguished Men in America and Europe. Illustrations of Their Characters and of the Events of the American Revolution.* 2 vols. Philadelphia: H. C. Carey and I. Lea, 1825.

Leikind, Morris C. "Vaccination in Europe." *Ciba Symposia* 3 (1942): 1102-13, 1124.

Lesser, Charles H., ed. *The Sinews of Independence: Monthly Strength Reports of the Continental Army.* Chicago: University of Chicago Press, 1976.

Levering, Joseph Mortimer. *A History of Bethlehem, Pennsylvania, 1741-1892, With Some Account of Its Founders and Their Early Activity in America.* Bethlehem, Pa.: Times Publishing Co., 1903.

Lewis, Fraser. "Medicine in the Continental Army of the Revolutionary War: 1775-1783." *Philadelphia Medicine* 55 (1959): 254-55, 257-59.

Lind, James. *An Essay on Diseases Incidental in Europeans in Hot Climates With the Method of Preventing Their Fatal Consequences.* London: T. Becket & P. A. De Hondt, 1768.

——. *A Treatise of the Scurvy: In Three Parts. Containing an Inquiry Into the Nature, Causes, and Cure of That Disease; Together With a Critical and Chronological View of What Has Been Published on the Subject.* Edinburgh: Sands, Murray, and Cochran for A. Kincaid & A. Donaldson, 1753.

Lucia, Salvatore P. *A History of Wine as Therapy.* Philadelphia: J. B. Lippincott Co., 1963.

Mahon, John K. *The War of 1812.* Gainesville: University of Florida Press, 1972.

Major, R. H. *A History of Medicine.* Springfield, Ill.: Charles C Thomas, 1954.

Mann, James. *Medical Sketches of the Campaigns of 1812, 13, 14* . . . . Dedham, Mass.: H. Mann and Co., 1816.

Marine, William M. *The British Invasion of Maryland, 1812-1815.* Baltimore: Society of the War of 1812 in Maryland, 1913.

Martin, C. H. "The Military Hospital at the Cloister (Ephrata, Pa., 1777)." *Lancaster County (Pa.) Historical Society Papers* 51 (1947): 127-33.

Martin, John Hill. *Historical Sketch of Bethlehem in Pennsylvania.* New York: AMS Press, 1971 reprint of 1872 edition.

Massachusetts (Colony) Provincial Congress. *The Journals of the Provincial Congress of the Massachusetts Bay Colony in 1774 and 1775 and of the Committee of Safety* . . . . Boston: Dutton and Wentworth, 1838.

Matloff, Maurice, ed. *American Military History.* Washington: Government Printing Office, 1969.

McCarty, William. *History of the American War of 1812, From the Commencement, Until the Final Termination Thereof, on the Memorable Eighth of January, 1815, at New Orleans.* 2d ed. Freeport, N.Y.: Books for Libraries Press, 1970 reprint of 1816 edition.

McCulloch, Champe C. "The Scientific and Administrative Achievement of the Medical Corps of the United States Army." *Scientific Monthly* 1 (1917): 410-27.

McDowell, William. "Journal of Lieut William McDowell of the First Penna Regiment, in the Southern Campaign 1781-1782." *Pennsylvania Archives*, 2d ser. 15: 296-340.

McGrady, Edward. *The History of South Carolina in the Revolution 1780–1783.* 2 vols. New York: Russell & Russell, 1969 reissue of 1902 edition.

McKee, Marguerite. "Service of Supply in the War of 1812." *Quartermaster Review* 6 (1927): 45–55.

Medical Department, U.S. Army. *Communicable Diseases.* Preventive Medicine in World War II, vol. 6. Washington: Government Printing Office, 1963.

———. *Infectious Diseases.* Internal Medicine in World War II, vol. 2. Washington: Government Printing Office, 1963.

"Medical History of Louis XIV (Editorial)." *Annals of Medical History,* 1st ser. 8 (1926): 202–3.

Mendham, New Jersey, Mayor's Tercentenary Committee. *The Mendhams.* Brookside, N.J., 1964.

Middleton, Peter. *A Medical Discourse, or an Historical Inquiry Into the Ancient and Present State of Medicine; the Substance of Which Was Delivered at Opening the Medical School, in the City of New York.* New York: Hugh Gaine, 1769.

Middleton, William Shainline. "John Morgan, Father of Medical Education in North America." *Annals of Medical History,* 1st ser. 9 (1927): 13–26.

———. "Medicine at Valley Forge." *Annals of Medical History,* 3d ser. 3 (1941): 461–86.

———. "William Shippen, Junior." *Annals of Medical History,* n. s. 4 (1932): 442–52, 538–49.

Miller, Genevieve. "Medical Schools in the Colonies." *Ciba Symposia* 8 (1947): 522–32.

Miller, Samuel. *A Brief Retrospect of the Eighteenth Century.* 2 vols. New York: T. and J. Swords, 1803.

Mitchell, Silas Weir. *The Early History of Instrumental Precision in Medicine.* New Haven: Tuttle, Morehouse & Taylor, 1892.

Mockridge, Ella W. *Our Mendham.* Ann Arbor, Mich., 1961.

Monro, Donald. *An Account of the Diseases Which Were Most Frequent in the British Military Hospitals in Germany, From January 1761 to the Return of the Troops to England in March 1763* . . . . London: A. Millar, D. Wilson, T. Durham, and T. Payne, 1764.

Montross, Lynn. *Rag, Tag and Bobtail: The Story of the Continental Army, 1775–1783.* New York: Harper & Bros., 1952.

"Monument at Ephrata to Brandywine Battle Victims." *Magazine of American History* 30 (1902): 75.

Moré, Charles Albert, Chevalier de Pontgibaud. *A French Volunteer of the War of Independence.* Translated and edited by Robert B. Douglas. New York: Benjamin Bloom, 1972.

Morgan, John. "A Discourse Upon the Institution of Medical Schools in America." In *Publications of the Institute of the History of Medicine.* Johns Hopkins University, ser. 4, Bibliotheca Medica Americana, vol. 2. Reprinted facsimile from the first edition (Philadelphia: William Bradford, 1765) with introduction by Abraham Flexner. Baltimore: Johns Hopkins Press, 1937.

———. *A Recommendation of Inoculation, According to Baron Dimsdale's Method.* Boston: J. Gill, 1776.

———. *A Vindication of His Public Character in the Station of Director-General of the Military Hospitals, and Physician in Chief to the American Army, Anno 1776.* Boston: Powars and Willis, 1777.

Morris, Robert, to Thomas Bond, letters, 19 February 1782 and 19 June 1783, Xeroxes held by Library of Congress, obtained from Miss Elizabeth Thomson.

Morristown, N.J. Morristown National Historical Park. John Cochran Letter Book, microfilm 5168.

Morton, Thomas George, and Woodbury, Frank. *History of the Pennsylvania Hospital 1751–1895.* New York: Arno Press, 1973 reprint of 1895 edition.

Moultrie, William. *Memoirs of the American Revolution* . . . . 2 vols. New York: New York Times & Arno Press, 1968 reprint of 1802 edition.

Muhlenberg, J. P. "Orderly Book of Gen. John Peter Gabriel Muhlenberg, March 26–December 20, 1777." *Pennsylvania Magazine of History and Biography* 34 (1910): 21–40, 336–60, 438–77.

Multhauf, Robert P. *A Catalogue of Instruments and Models in the Possession of the*

American Philosophical Society. Philadelphia: American Philosophical Society, 1961.
Mumford, James Gregory. *A Narrative of Medicine in America.* Philadelphia: J. B. Lippincott Co., 1903.
Munford, Robert B., Jr. "Military Hospital in Williamsburg, 1777." *Virginia Magazine of History* 30 (1922): 388-90.
Murray, Louise Wells, ed. *Notes From Craft Collection in Tioga Point Museum on the Sullivan Expedition of 1779 and Its Centennial Celebration of 1879, Including Order Book of General Sullivan Never Before Published.* Original Manuscript in the New Jersey Historical Society. Athens, Pa., 1929.
Myer, Jesse S. *Life of William Beaumont.* St. Louis: C. V. Mosby Co., 1939.
National Archives Record Groups. *See under* Washington, D.C.
New York (State) University. Division of Archives and History. *The Sullivan-Clinton Campaign in 1779. Chronology and Selected Documents.* Albany: University of the State of New York, 1929.
Niles' Weekly Register. Baltimore, Md.
North Carolina. *The State Records of North Carolina.* 26 vols. Goldsboro, N.C.: Nash Bros., 1886-1907.
Norwood, William Frederick. "The Enigma of Dr. Benjamin Church, A High-Level Scandal in the American Colonial Army Medical Service." *Medical Arts and Sciences* 10 (1956): 71-93.
———. *Medical Education in the United States Before the Civil War.* Philadelphia: University of Pennsylvania Press, 1944.
———. "Medicine in the Era of the American Revolution." *International Record of Medicine* 171 (1958): 391-407.
"Order of March of Hand's Brigade From Wyoming to Tioga." *Pennsylvania Archives,* 6th ser. 14: 67-121.
"Orderly Book, June 19 1779--July 30 1779." *Pennsylvania Archives,* 6th ser. 14: 21-65.
Original Papers Relating to the Siege of Charleston, 1780, Mostly Selected From the Papers of General Benjamin Lincoln, in the Thomas Addis Emmet Collection, Lenox Library, New York, and Now First Published. Charleston, S.C.: Walker, Evans & Cogwell Co., 1898.

Owen, William O. *A Chronological Arrangement of Congressional Legislation Relating to the Medical Corps of the United States Army From 1785 to 1917.* Chicago: American Medical Association, 1918.
Owen, William O., ed. *The Medical Department of the United States Army (Legislative and Administrative History). During the Period of the Revolution (1776-1786). Compiled From the Journals of the Provincial Congress of Massachusetts Bay, 1775, and From the Journals of the Continental Congress, 1774-1783.* New York: Paul B. Hoeber, 1920.
Packard, Francis Randolph. "Editorial: Washington and the Medical Affairs of the Revolution." *Annals of Medical History,* n.s. 4 (1932): 306-12.
———. *History of Medicine in the United States.* New York: Paul B. Hoeber, 1931.
———. "How London and Edinburgh Influenced Medicine in Philadelphia in the Eighteenth Century." *Annals of Medical History,* n.s. 4 (1932): 227-28.
———. *Some Account of the Pennsylvania Hospital, From Its First Rise to the Beginning of the Year 1938.* Philadelphia: Lea & Febiger, 1938.
Palmer, Thomas H., ed. *Historical Register of the United States.* 4 vols. Philadelphia, 1814-16.
Parish, John C., ed. *The Robert Lucas Journal of the War of 1812.* Iowa City, Iowa: State Historical Society of Iowa, 1906.
Parton, James. *Life of Andrew Jackson.* 3 vols. Boston: Fields, Osgood & Co., 1870.
Peckham, Howard H., ed. *The Toll of Independence: Engagements & Battle Casualties of the American Revolution.* Chicago: University of Chicago Press, 1974.
Pennsylvania Infantry. *5th Regiment Orderly Book of the Northern Army at Ticonderoga and Mt. Independence From October 17th, 1776, to January 8th, 1777, With Biographical and Explanatory Notes and an Appendix.* Albany: J. Munsell, 1859.
Pennsylvania Packet. Philadelphia, Pa.
Pepper, O. H. Perry. "Benjamin Rush's Theories on Blood Letting After One Hundred and Fifty Years." *Transactions of the College of Physicians of Philadelphia,* 4th ser. 14 (1946): 121-26.

Pepper, William. *The Medical Side of Benjamin Franklin.* Philadelphia: William J. Campbell, 1911.

Peterson, Clarence Stewart. *Known Military Dead During the War of 1812.* Baltimore, 1955.

Phalen, James M. *Chiefs of the Medical Department, United States Army, 1775–1940.* Army Medical Bulletin No. 52. Carlisle Barracks, Pa.: Medical Field Service School, April 1940.

———. "Surgeon James Mann's Observations on Battlefield Amputations." *Military Surgeon* 87 (1940): 463–66.

Philadelphia, Pa. Historical Society of Pennsylvania. Manuscript Department. Alison Papers, Continental Hospital Returns, 1777–78.

———. Autograph Collection, case 19, box 15, Papers of Thomas Bond, Jr.

———. Journal of James Sproat, D.D., 1753, 1757, 1778, 1779, 1780, 1782, 1783, 1784, 1786.

———. Papers of Jonathan Potts.

———. Society Miscellaneous Collection, case 19, box 2.

Pilcher, James Evelyn. "Benjamin Church, Director General and Chief Physician of the Hospital of the Army, 1775." *Journal of the Association of Military Surgeons* 13 (1903): 320–24.

Postell, William Dosite. "Medical Education and Medical Schools in Colonial America." *International Record of Medicine* 171 (1958): 364–70.

Potts Papers. *See under* Philadelphia, Pa.

Power, D'Arcy. *Selected Writings: 1877–1930.* Oxford: Clarendon Press, 1931.

Pringle, John. *Observations on the Diseases in the Army, in Camp and Garrison.* London: A. Millar, D. Wilson, and T. Payne, 1752.

———. *Six Discourses, Delivered by Sir John Pringle, Bart. . . . , To Which Is Prefixed the Life of the Author by Andrew Kippis, D. D. F. R. S. and S. A.* London: W. Strahan and T. Cadell, 1783.

Prucha, Francis Paul. *A Guide to the Military Posts of the United States, 1789–1895.* Madison: State Historical Society of Wisconsin, 1964.

Quaife, Milo Milton, ed. *War on the Detroit, the Chronicles of Thomas Verchères de Boucherville and the Capitulation by an Ohio Volunteer.* Chicago: Lakeside Press, 1940.

Quincy, Eliza Susan Morton. "Basking Ridge in Revolutionary Days. Reprinted From Her Memoirs." *The Somerset County Historical Quarterly* 1 (1912): 34–43.

———. *Memoirs.* Boston: John Wilson and Son, 1861.

Radbill, Samuel X. "Francis Alison Jr., a Surgeon of the Revolution." *Bulletin of the History of Medicine* 9 (1941): 243–57.

Ramsay, David. *The History of the Revolution in South-Carolina . . . .* 2 vols. Trenton: Isaac Collins, 1785.

———. *A Review of the Improvements, Progress and State of Medicine in the XVIIIth Century.* Charleston: W. P. Young, 1801.

Ratcliffe, A. W. "The Historical Background of Malaria—a Reconsideration." *Journal of the Indiana Medical Association* 39 (1946): 339–47.

Ravaton, Hugues. *Chirurgie d'armée ou traité des plaies d'armées à feu.* Paris: Didot le jeune, 1768.

Record Groups in National Archives. *See under* Washington, D.C.

Reed, John Frederick. *Campaign to Valley Forge, July 1, 1777–December 19, 1777.* Philadelphia: University of Pennsylvania Press, 1965.

Reed, William Bradford, ed. *Life and Correspondence of Joseph Reed.* 2 vols. Philadelphia: Lindsay and Blakiston, 1847.

"Review of Circular Letter of Benjamin Waterhouse to His Surgeons in the 2nd Military District, September 1817." *Medical Repository* 19 (1818): 395–96.

RG (Record Group). *See under* Washington, D.C., National Archives.

Risch, Erna. *Quartermaster Support of the Army: A History of the Corps, 1775–1939.* Washington: Government Printing Office, 1962.

Roberts, Kenneth Lewis, ed. *March to Quebec: Journals of the Members of Arnold's Expedition.* New York: Doubleday, Doran & Co., 1938.

Rowland, Eron Opha. *Andrew Jackson's Campaign Against the British, or the Mississippi Territory in the War of 1812 . . . .*

Freeport, N.Y.: Books for Libraries Press, 1971 reprint of 1926 edition.
Rush, Benjamin. *Observations on the Cause and Cure of the Tetanus.* Philadelphia, 1787.
Saffell, W. T. R. *Records of the Revolutionary War . . . .* New York: Pudney & Russell, 1859.
Saffron, Morris H. *Surgeon to Washington: Dr. John Cochran (1730–1807).* New York: Columbia University Press, 1977.
St. Clair Papers. *See under* Washington, D.C., Library of Congress, Manuscript Division.
Sanders, Jennings Bryan. *Evolution of Executive Departments of the Continental Congress.* Gloucester, Mass.: Peter Smith, 1971 reprint of 1935 edition.
Sanford, William. *A Few Practical Remarks on the Medicinal Effects of Wine and Spirits.* London: J. Tombs, 1799.
Sargent, Winthrop. "Winthrop Sargent's Diary While With General Arthur St. Clair's Expedition Against the Indians." *Ohio Archaeological and Historical Quarterly* 33 (1924): 237–73.
Schuyler, Philip John. "Proceedings of a General Court Martial . . . ." *Collections of the New York Historical Society for the Year 1879.*
Scott, Winfield. *Memoirs of Lieut.-General Scott, LL.D.* 2 vols. New York: Sheldon & Co., 1864.
Senn, Nicholas. "The Evolution of the Military Surgeon." *Surgery, Gynecology, & Obstetrics* 8 (1909): 393–400.
Sewall, Henry. "Letters." *Historical Magazine*, 2d ser. 2 (1867): 608.
Seymour, William. "Journal of the Southern Expedition, 1780–1783, by William Seymour, Sergeant-Major of the Delaware Regiment." *Pennsylvania Magazine of History and Biography* 7 (1883): 286–98, 377–94.
Shaw, John. "Narrative of John Shaw: Dictated to Lyman C. Draper." *Wisconsin State Historical Society Publications* 2 (1855): 197–232.
Shippen, William. "Text of William Shippen's First Draft of a Plan for the Organization of the Military Hospital During the Revolution." *Annals of Medical History* 1 (1917–18): 174–76.
Shippen, Just Account. *See* Philadelphia, Pa., Historical Society of Pennsylvania, Manuscript Department, Society Miscellaneous Collection.
Shreve, Lt Col Israel, to Mary Shreve, letter, 18 July 1776, Shreve copybook in the family collection of Mr. and Mrs. Charles J. Simpson, Potomac, Md.
Shryock, Richard Harrison. *American Medical Research: Past and Present.* New York: Commonwealth Fund, 1947.
———. *The Development of Modern Medicine: An Interpretation of the Social and Scientific Factors Involved.* New York: Alfred A. Knopf, 1947.
———. *Eighteenth Century Medicine in America.* Worcester, Mass.: American Antiquarian Society, 1950.
———. *Medical Licensing in America, 1650–1965.* Baltimore: Johns Hopkins Press, 1967.
———. "Medical Practice in the Old South." *South Atlantic Quarterly* 29 (1930): 160–78.
———. "The Medical Reputation of Benjamin Rush: Contrasts Over Two Centuries." *Bulletin of the History of Medicine* 45 (1971): 507–52.
———. *Medicine and Society in America, 1660–1860.* Ithaca, N.Y.: Cornell University Press, 1960.
———. "Public Relations of the Medical Profession in Great Britain and the United States: 1600–1870." *Annals of Medical History*, n.s. 2 (1930): 308–39.
Shute, Daniel. "The Journal of Dr. Daniel Shute, Surgeon in the Revolution 1781–1782." *New England Genealogical Register* 84 (1930): 383–89.
"Sickness in the Army at New Orleans, in 1809." *Medical Repository* 14 (1811): 85–87.
Simpson, Stephen, to George Simpson, 9 January 1815. *American Historical Review* 2 (1896): 268.
Slocum, Charles E. "Some Errors Corrected: Fort Winchester, at Defiance, Ohio." *Ohio Archeological and Historical Quarterly* 10 (1901-2): 483.
Smart, Charles. *The Connection of the Army Medical Department With the Development of Meteorology in the United States.* U.S. Department of Agriculture, Weather

Bureau. Report of the International Meteorological Congress Held at Chicago, Ill., 21–24 August 1893. Bulletin No. 11, 1895.

———. "Medical Department, U.S. Army." *Journal of Military Service Institute* 14 (1893): 692–708.

Smillie, Wilson G. *Public Health: Its Promise for the Future: A Chronicle of the Development of Public Health in the United States, 1607–1914.* New York: Macmillan Co., 1955.

Smith, Dwight L., ed. "From Greene Ville to Fallen Timbers." *Indiana Historical Society Publications* 16 (1951–52): 239–333.

Smith, Helen Burr. "Surgeon Jonathan Potts Planned Innoculation [sic] at the Winter Camp." *Picket Post* 16 (1947): 16–21.

Smith, Louis. *American Democracy and Military Power: A Study of Civil Control of Military Power in the United States.* Chicago: University of Chicago Press, 1951.

Smith, William Henry, ed. *The St. Clair Papers. The Life and Public Service of Arthur St. Clair, Soldier of the Revolutionary War; President of the Continental Congress; and Governor of the North-Western Territory, With His Correspondence and Other Papers.* 2 vols. Cincinnati: Robert Clarke, 1882.

Sparks, Jared, ed. *Correspondence of the American Revolution; Being Letters of Eminent Men to George Washington, From the Time of His Taking Command of the Army to the End of His Presidency.* 4 vols. Boston: Little, Brown and Co., 1853.

Spaulding, Oliver Lyman. *The United States Army in War and Peace.* New York: G. P. Putnam's Sons, 1937.

Sproat, James. "Extracts From the Journal of Rev. James Sproat, Hospital Chaplain of the Middle Department, 1778." Edited by John W. Jordan. *Pennsylvania Magazine of History and Biography* 27 (1903): 441–45.

Stahl, John M. *The Invasion of the City of Washington, A Disagreeable Study in and of Military Unpreparedness.* Argos, Ind.: Van Trump Co., 1918.

Steiner, Walter. "Dr. James Thacher of Plymouth, Mass., an Erudite Physician of Revolutionary and Post-Revolutionary Fame." *Bulletin of the Institute of the History of Medicine* 1 (1933): 157–73.

Stevens, James. "Revolutionary Journal." *Essex Institute Historical Collections* 48 (1912): 41–70.

Stille, Charles J. *Major-General Anthony Wayne and the Pennsylvania Line in the Continental Army.* Philadelphia: J. B. Lippincott Co., 1893.

Stookey, Byron Polk. *A History of Colonial Medical Education: In the Province of New York, With Its Subsequent Development (1767–1830).* Springfield, Ill.: Charles C Thomas, 1962.

Sullivan, John. *Letters and Papers of Major General John Sullivan, 1771–1777.* Collections of New Hampshire Historical Society, vols. 13–15. Concord: New Hampshire Historical Society, 1930.

Tarleton, Banastre. *A History of the Campaigns of 1780 and 1781 in the Southern Provinces of North America.* London: T. Cadell, 1787.

Tatum, Howell. *Major Howell Tatum's Journal, While Acting Topographical Engineer (1814) to General Jackson, Commanding the Seventh Military District.* Edited by John Spencer Bassett. Northampton, Mass.: Smith College Studies in History, 1922.

Temkin, Owsei. "The Role of Surgery in the Rise of Modern Medical Thought." *Bulletin of the History of Medicine* 25 (1951): 248–59.

Thacher, James. *American Medical Biography . . . .* Boston: Richardson & Lord and Cottons & Barnard, 1828.

———. *American Modern Practice; Or, a Simple Method of Prevention and Cure of Diseases According to the Latest Improvements and Discoveries, Comprising a Practical System Adapted to the Use of Medical Practitioners of the United States.* Boston: Ezra Read, 1817.

———. *A Miliary Journal During the American Revolutionary War, From 1775 to 1783: Describing Interesting Events and Transactions of This Period: With Numerous Historical Facts and Anecdotes, From the Original Manuscript.* 2d ed. Boston: Cottons & Barnard, 1827.

Thayer, Theodore G. *Nathanael Greene, Strategist of the American Revolution.* New York: Twayne Publishers, 1960.

———. "The War in New Jersey; Battles,

Alarums, and the Men of the Revolution." *New Jersey Historical Society Proceedings,* n.s. 71 (1953): 83–110.

Thomas, Robert. *The Modern Practice of Physic: Exhibiting the Characters, Causes, Symptoms, Prognostic, Morbid Appearances, and Improved Method of Treating the Diseases of All Climates.* 3d American ed. New York: Collin & Co., 1815.

Thoms, Herbert. "Albigence Waldo, Surgeon: His Diary Written at Valley Forge." *Annals of Medical History* 10 (1928): 486–97.

Tilden, John Bell. "Extracts From the Journal of Lieutenant John Bell Tilden, Second Pennsylvania Line, 1781–82." *Pennsylvania Magazine of History and Biography* 19 (1895): 51–63, 208–33.

Tilton, James. *Economical Observations on Military Hospitals and the Prevention and Cure of Diseases Incident to an Army. In Three Parts: Addressed I. To Ministers of State and Legislatures, II. To Commanding Officers, III. To the Medical Staff.* Wilmington, Del.: J. Wilson, 1813.

Tobey, James Abner. *The Medical Department of the Army.* Baltimore: Johns Hopkins University Press, 1927.

Tompkins, Daniel D. *Public Papers of Daniel D. Tompkins, Governor of New York, 1807–1817: Military.* 3 vols. New York: State of New York, 1898.

Toner, Joseph Meredith. *The Medical Men of the Revolution With a Brief History of the Medical Department of the Continental Army.* Philadelphia: Collins, 1876.

———. "A Sketch of the Life and Character of James Craik (1730–1814)." *Transactions of the Medical Society of the State of Virginia* 3 (1879): 95–105.

Torres-Reyes, Ricardo. *Morristown National Historical Park: 1779–1780 Encampment: A Study of Medical Services.* Washington: Office of History and Historic Architecture, Eastern Service Center, April 1971.

Trevelyan, George Otto. *Saratoga and Brandywine, Valley Forge, England and France at War. The American Revolution,* vol 4. London: Longmans Green and Co., 1929.

Trumbull, John. *Autobiography, Reminiscences and Letters of John Trumbull, From 1756 to 1841.* New Haven: B. L. Hamlen, 1841.

Underwood, Thomas Taylor. *Journal March 26, 1792, to March 18, 1800: An Old Soldier in Wayne's Army.* Cincinnati: Society of Colonial Wars in the State of Ohio, 1945.

Upton, Emory. *Military Policy of the United States.* Washington: Government Printing Office, 1904.

Urdang, George. "Portraits of Pharmacists." *American Professional Pharmacist* 22 (1956): 801.

U.S. Congress. *American State Papers: Documents, Legislative and Executive of the Congress of the United States. Class V. Military Affairs. Class IX. Claims.* Washington: Gales and Seaton, 1832–61.

———. *Journal of the Executive Proceedings of the Senate of the United States, 1789–1901.* 32 vols. Washington: Government Printing Office, 1828–1909.

U.S. War Department. *Subject Index, 1809–1860, General Orders, Adjutant General's Department, Subject Index of the General Orders of the War Department From 1 Jan. 1809 to 31 Dec. 1860.* Compiled under direction of Brig Gen Richard C. Drum by Jeremiah C. Allen. Washington: Government Printing Office, 1886.

Vail, R. W., ed. *The Revolutionary Diary of Lieut. Obadiah Gore, Jr.* New York: The New York Public Library, 1929.

Van Doren, Carl. *Secret History of the American Revolution* . . . . New York: Viking Press, 1941.

Van Swieten, Gerhard. *The Diseases Incident to Armies, With the Method of Cure . . . To Which Are Added: The Nature and Treatment of Gunshot Wounds, by John Ranby, Esquire, Surgeon General to the British Army* . . . . Philadelphia: R. Bell, 1776.

Van Tyne, Claude Halstead. *The War of Independence.* 2 vols. Boston: Houghton Mifflin Co., 1929.

Viets, Henry R. *A Brief History of Medicine in Massachusetts.* New York: Houghton Co., 1930.

Wain, Harry. *A History of Preventive Medicine.* Springfield, Ill.: Charles C Thomas, 1970.

Waldenmaier, Nellie Protsman. *Some of the*

Earliest Oaths of Allegiance to the United States of America. Lancaster, Pa., 1944.

Waldo, Albigence. "Valley Forge, 1777–1778. Diary of Surgeon Albigence Waldo, of the Connecticut Line." *Pennsylvania Magazine of History and Biography* 21 (1897): 299–323.

Walker, Adam. *A Journal of Two Campaigns of the Fourth Regiment of U.S. Infantry in the Michigan and Indiana Territories, Under the Command of Col. John P. Boyd and Lt. Col. James Miller, During the Years of 1811–1812.* Keene, N.H.: privately printed, 1816.

Walker, Alexander. *Jackson and New Orleans. An Authentic Narrative of the Memorable Achievements of the American Army, Under Andrew Jackson, Before New Orleans, in the Winter of 1814, '15.* New York: J. C. Derby, 1856.

Walsh, James Joseph. *History of Medicine in New York, Three Centuries of Medical Progress.* 5 vols. New York: National Americana Society, 1919.

Walters, Raymond. *Bethlehem Long Ago and To-Day.* Bethlehem, Pa.: Carey Printing Co., 1923.

Wangensteen, Owen H.; Smith, Jacqueline; and Wangensteen, Sarah D. "Some Highlights in the History of Amputation Reflecting Lessons in Wound Healing." *Bulletin of the History of Medicine* 41 (1967): 97–131.

Ward, Christopher. *The War of the Revolution.* Edited by John R. Alden. 2 vols. New York: Macmillan Co., 1952.

Ward, Harry M. *The Department of War, 1781–1795.* Pittsburgh: University of Pittsburgh Press, 1962.

Warren, Edward. *The Life of John Warren, M.D., Surgeon-General During the War of the Revolution: First Professor of Anatomy and Surgery in Harvard College; President of the Massachusetts Medical Society, etc.* Boston: Noyes, Holmes, & Co., 1874.

Warren, John. *A View of the Mercurial Practice in Febrile Diseases.* Boston: T. B. Wait and Co., 1813.

Warren, John; Dexter, A.; Jackson, James; and Warren, John C. *Report on Vaccination*, n.p., 1 June 1808.

Warren-Adams Letters, Being Chiefly a Correspondence Among John Adams, Samuel Adams, and James Warren. Massachusetts Historical Society Collections, 5th ser. 72 (1917); 73 (1925).

Washington, D.C. Library of Congress. Manuscript Division. Papers of George Washington.

———. Papers of Isaac Foster.

———. Papers of Jonathan Potts, 1776–80.

———. Papers of Peter Turner, 1778–1812.

———. Papers of William Eustis, II-33-N.H.

———. Papers of William Henry Harrison, microfilm series 1, roll 1.

———. Peter Force Collection, Arthur St. Clair Papers, series 7E, box 60, folders 1782 Ag24–1793 Jul6.

Washington, D.C. National Archives. List of Officers of the Medical Department U.S. Army 1775 to Present Date, Record Group 112, entries 83, 84, in room 201.

———. Post Revolutionary War Records, Record Group 98.

———. *Preliminary Inventories: War Department Collection of Revolutionary War Records.* Washington: National Archives and Records Service, General Services Administration, 1970.

———. Records of the Adjutant General's Office, 1780s–1917, Record Group 94, Letters Received by the Adjutant General 1805–1821, Microfilm Publication M566.

———. Records of the Adjutant General's Office, 1780s–1917, Record Group 94, Letters Sent by the Office of the Adjutant General, Main Series, 1800-90, Microfilm Publication M565.

———. Records of the Continental and Confederation Congresses and the Constitutional Convention, Record Group 360, Papers of the Continental Congress, 1774–89, Microfilm Publication M247.

———. Records of the Office of the Secretary of War, Record Group 107, Copies of War Department Correspondence and Reports, 1791–96, Microfilm Publication T982.

———. Records of the Office of the Secretary of War, Record Group 107, Letters Received by the Secretary of War, Main Series, 1801–70, Microfilm Publication M221.

———. Records of the Office of the Secretary of War, Record Group 107, Letters Received by the Secretary of War, Unregistered Series, 1789–1861, Microfilm Publication M222.

——. Records of the Office of the Secretary of War, Record Group 107, Letters Sent by the Secretary of War to the President by the Secretary of War, 1800–63, Microfilm Publication M127.

——. Records of the Office of the Secretary of War, Record Group 107, Letters Sent by the Secretary of War Relating to Military Affairs, 1800–89, Microfilm Publication M6.

——. Records of the Office of the Secretary of War, Record Group 107, Miscellaneous Letters Sent by the Secretary of War, 1800–1809, Microfilm Publication M370.

——. Records of the Office of the Secretary of War, Record Group 107, Registers of the Letters Received by the Office of the Secretary of War, Main Series, 1800–70, Microfilm Publication M22.

——. Records of the Office of the Secretary of War, Record Group 107, Reports to Congress From the Secretary of War, 1803–70, Microfilm Publication M220.

——. War Department Collection of Revolutionary War Records, Record Group 93, Miscellaneous Numbered Records, 1775–84, series 6, Microfilm Publication M859.

——. War Department Collection of Revolutionary War Records, Record Group 93, Names Index to Series 5, 6, and 9, series 4, Microfilm Publication M847.

——. War Department Collection of Revolutionary War Records, Record Group 93, Numbered Record Books, 1775–98, series 5, Microfilm Publication M853.

——. War Department Collection of Revolutionary War Records, Record Group 93, Revolutionary War Rolls, 1775–83, Microfilm Publication M246, Miscellaneous, Hospital Department, roll 135, folders 3–1 through 3–3.

——. War Department Collection of Revolutionary War Records, Record Group 93, Subject Index to Series 5, 6, and 9.

Washington Papers. *See under* Washington, D.C., Library of Congress, Manuscript Division.

Waterhouse, Benjamin. *Circular Letter From Dr. Benjamin Waterhouse to the Surgeons of the Different Posts in the Second Military Department*. Cambridge, Mass., 1817.

——. *The Rise, Progress, and Present State of Medicine. A Discourse, Delivered at Concord, July 6th, 1791, Before the Middlesex Medical Association*. Boston: Thomas and John Fleet, 1792.

Wayne, Anthony. "General Wayne's Orderly Book." *Michigan Pioneer and Historical Society Collections* 34 (1904): 341–733.

Webb, James Watson, ed. *Reminiscences of Gen'l Samuel B. Webb . . . .* 2 vols. New York: privately printed, 1882.

Weedon, George. *Valley Forge Orderly Book of General George Weedon of the Continental Army Under Command of Gen. George Washington, in the Campaign of 1777–8.* New York: The New York Times & Arno Press, 1971 reprint of 1902 edition.

Weigley, Russell F. *History of the United States Army*. New York: Macmillan Co., 1967.

Welch, William Henry. "Influence of English Medicine Upon American Medicine in Its Formative Period." In *Papers and Addresses*, vol. 3, edited by Walter C. Burket. Baltimore: Johns Hopkins Press, 1920.

Wells, Lloyd Allan. "Aneurysm and Physiologic Surgery." *Bulletin of the History of Medicine* 44 (1970): 411–24.

Wheaton, Joseph. *Appeal to the Senate and House of Representatives of the United States of America*. Washington, D.C., 1820.

Whipple, Allen O. *The Evolution of Surgery in the United States*. Springfield, Ill.: Charles C Thomas, 1963.

——. *The Story of Wound Healing and Wound Repair*. Springfield, Ill.: Charles C Thomas, 1963.

White, Leonard Dupee. *The Federalists: A Study in Administrative History, 1789–1801*. New York: Macmillan Co., 1948.

——. *The Jeffersonians: A Study in Administrative History, 1801–1829*. New York: Macmillan Co., 1959.

"A Whitemarsh Orderly Book." *Pennsylvania Magazine of History and Biography* 45 (1921): 205, 219.

Whittlesey, Charles. "General Wadsworth's

Division, War of 1812." *Western Reserve and Northern Ohio Historical Society Tracts* 2 (1879): 115–23.

Wickes, Stephen. *History of Medicine in New Jersey, and of Its Medical Men From the Settlement of the Province to A.D. 1800.* Newark: Dennis, 1879.

Wilkinson, James. *Memoirs of My Own Times.* 3 vols. Philadelphia: Abraham Small, 1816.

Williams, John S. *The Invasion and Capture of Washington.* New York: Harper & Bros., 1857.

Williamsburg, Va. The College of William and Mary in Virginia. Earl Gregg Swem Library. Special Collections Division. Tucker-Coleman Papers, 1780–82, microfilm roll M–13.

Wilson, Frazer Ells. *Arthur St. Clair.* Richmond, Va.: Garrett and Massie, 1944.

———. *Fort Jefferson: The Frontier Post of the Upper Miami Valley: A Fascinating Tale of Border Life Gleaned From Authentic Sources and Retold by Frazer Ells Wilson.* Lancaster, Pa., 1950.

Wilson, Frazer Ells, ed. *Journal of Capt. Daniel Bradley: An Epic of the Ohio Frontier.* Greenville, Ohio: Frank H. Jobes & Son, 1935.

Wilson, Leonard G. "The Clinical Definition of Scurvy and the Discovery of Vitamin C." *Journal of the History of Medicine and Allied Sciences* 30 (1975): 40–60.

Wiltse, Charles Maurice. *The New Nation, 1800–1845.* London: Macmillan & Co., 1965.

Winchester, James. "Papers and Orderly Book of Brigadier General James Winchester." *Michigan Pioneer and Historical Society Collections* 31 (1901): 253–313.

Winslow, Charles-Edward Amory. "The Colonial Era and the First Years of the Republic (1607–1799)—The Pestilence That Walketh in Darkness." In *The History of American Epidemiology*, by Winslow, C.-E. A.; Smillie, Wilson G.; Doull, James A.; and Gordon, John E.; edited by Franklin H. Top. St. Louis: C. V. Mosby Co., 1952.

Wistar, Caspar. *Eulogium on Dr. William Shippen.* Philadelphia: Thomas Dobson and Son, 1818.

Wolfe, Edwin P. "The Genesis of the Medical Department of the United States Army." *Bulletin of the New York Academy of Medicine*, 2d ser. 5 (1929): 823–44.

Woodhouse, Henry. "Colonial Medical Practice." *Ciba Symposia* 1 (1940): 379–89.

Wright, Albert Hazen. *The Sullivan Expedition of 1779, The Losses.* Studies in History No. 33 of New York Historical Source Studies, 1965.

Yost, Robert. "His Book." *Ohio Archaeological and Historical Quarterly* 23 (1914): 150–61.

Index

Ackland (Acland), Maj. John Dyke, 96
Adams, John, 28–29, 35, 37, 39, 60, 82
Adams, Samuel, 28, 35, 44, 60, 62, 82
Adams, Samuel, Jr., 51, 52, 66, 72, 74, 92
Adjutant General, 81, 152, 155, 230
Alabama, 181
Albany, N.Y., 48, 57, 63–64, 94–97, 106, 114, 127, 133, 144, 148–49, 155, 190–91
Alcoholic beverages. *See* Wine and spirits.
Alexandria, Va., 75, 84, 120
Alison, Francis, 107, 112
Allentown, Pa., 70–71, 81, 91
Allison, Richard, 133, 134, 136–37
Amboy, N.J., 69, 77
Ambulances, 167
Amputations, 7, 15–18, 84, 138, 151, 195–96
Andrews, Joseph Gardner, 139–40
Annapolis, Md., 148
Anthrax, 151
Apothecaries, 8, 33. *See also* Hospital Department; Medical Department.
Armstrong, John, 148
Army, Revolutionary War. *See* Continental Army.
Army, 1783–1812. *See also* Regiments.
  coastal and interior forts, 138–40
  Indian campaigns, 131, 133–38
  Louisiana Territory operations, 140–43
  organization of, 129–32, 134–35, 137–38, 140, 144
Army, War of 1812
  Military Districts, 150–51, 154, 166–67, 172, 177–85, 190, 195–96
  Northern operations, 148, 157, 159–71, 172–78
  organization and strength, 148–49, 153, 157, 159, 161–63, 172, 178, 180–81, 184–85
  Southern operations, 164, 178–85
Army, post-War of 1812, 186–87, 190
Army medical organization, 197. *See also* Hospital Department; Medical Department; Medical personnel.
Arnold, Maj. Gen. Benedict, 59–60, 64, 96
Articles of Capitulation, 123
Ashley, S.C., 124
Aspinwall, William, 51
Asthma, 65, 96, 111
Auenbrugger, Leopold, 3
Autopsies, 19, 140, 194–95

Backus, Christopher, 184
Baltimore, Md., 70, 75, 110, 172, 178, 180, 188
Bard, John, 15
Bard, Samuel, 8
Bartlett, John, 38, 95
Barton, William, 196, 266
Basking Ridge, N.J., 103, 111, 243, 245
Beaumont, William, 160, 167, 170
Beaverdam, Va., 120
Bedford, N.Y., 112–13
Bell, Whitfield Jenks, Jr., 29, 42
Benedict, Md., 178
Bennington, Vt., 94–95
Bethlehem, Pa., 42, 70–71, 80–83, 88–89, 91, 238
Bettering House (Philadelphia), 70, 109
Binney, Barnabas, 29, 44, 48, 67
Black Rock, N.Y., 165, 169
Bladensburg, Md., 180
Blaine, Ephraim, 83
Bleeding, 1–2, 14–18, 159–60, 193–95
Blistering, 1, 5, 7, 17–18, 159–60, 192, 194
Blood, Hosea, 175
Bloomfield, Moses, 44
Board of Treasury, 31, 40, 43
Board of War, 25, 45, 48, 118, 230
Boerhaave, Hermann, 1
Bond, Nathaniel, 75
Bond, Thomas, Jr., 40, 42–44, 46, 82, 109–10, 228
Bordentown, N.J., 72, 81
Boston, Mass., 26–28, 30, 48, 50–57, 74, 114, 144, 152, 154, 188, 193
Boswell, James, 29
Boulden, Nathan, 177
Bound Brook, N.J., 102
Brandywine Creek, 79–80, 90
Bristol, Pa., 79, 81
British Army, 3–4. *See also* Prisoners of war.
  commanders, 28, 40, 47, 80, 94–95, 120–21
  Medical Department, 8, 20–21, 36–37, 46–47, 82, 95
  in Revolutionary War, 33, 50, 56–57, 59, 67, 71–73, 77–80, 92, 94, 97, 99, 109, 117–19, 120–25
  in War of 1812, 148, 153, 161–62, 164–65, 168, 172–73, 177–81
British Navy, 57, 64, 77, 181
Brocklesby, Richard, 4, 6, 20

Brodhead, Col. Daniel, 106, 108, 110
Brookline, Mass., 51
Brown, Maj. Gen. Jacob, 172, 175
Brown, William, 69, 82, 89, 102, 239
Browne, James, 118
Brownville, N.Y., 175, 188, 190, 196
Brunswick, N.J., 69, 77, 99, 102, 110
Buckingham, Pa., 81
Buffalo, N.Y., 152, 161, 164–65, 169, 175
Bull, E. W., 177
Burgoyne, Maj. Gen. John, 40, 94–95
Burlington, N.J., 81
Burlington, Vt., 156, 157, 161, 167, 172–74, 188, 190, 194, 197
Burnet, William, 38, 44, 67, 98, 99, 102
Burr, Aaron, 140

Calhoun, John, 186–87
Cambridge, Mass., 22, 27, 29, 51, 52–53
Camden, S.C., 117
Canada
  Revolutionary War, 20, 32–33, 50, 57, 59–60
  War of 1812, 148, 153, 157, 159–67, 170, 172
Canajoharie, N.Y., 106
Capitol Hill hospital, D.C., 180
Carleton, Sir Guy, 47
Carlisle, Pa., 84
Carmichael, John F., 135–36, 139
Carolinas, 75, 103, 115, 120, 185
Casualties
  Indian campaigns, 134, 136, 138
  ratio of disease vs. wounds, 3, 8, 39, 108
  Revolutionary War, 67, 69, 71–72, 108, 119, 121–23
  War of 1812, 163–65, 168, 170, 172, 175, 177, 180
Catlett, Hanson, 180, 194, 262
Chadd's Ford, Pa., 79
Charleston, S.C., 115, 117–19, 121, 123–24, 152
Charlotte, N.C., 118–19, 123
Charlottesville, Va., 120
Cheraw, S.C., 118
Cherry Valley, N.Y., 106
Chesapeake Bay, 79
Cheselden, William, 15
Chesterfield Court House, Va., 120
Chippewa, battle of, 175, 177
Chippewa River, 172
Cholera, 96
Church, Benjamin, 26–28, 30, 35, 38, 46, 51, 52, 56
Cincinnati, Ohio, 134, 136–37
Claiborne, Governor, 183
Clark, James, 17
Clinton, Brig. Gen. James, 106, 108, 114
Clothier General, 40, 83
Clothing, 9–10, 40, 66, 73, 160, 191–92

Clothing shortage, 3, 22, 30, 39, 62, 77, 82–83, 85, 88, 92, 99, 103, 109, 114, 124, 134, 169–70
Cochran, John, 14
  Director General of Hospital Department, 44–48, 105–6, 112, 121, 125–27
  and Hospital Department reform, 36–37
  Physician and Surgeon General, Middle Department, 38, 40, 42, 71–72, 74
  Physician and Surgeon General of the Army, 43–44, 77–79, 82, 84–87, 92, 102, 105, 120, 236
Colchester, Va., 75, 120
College of William and Mary, 120, 122
Committee of Correspondence (Boston), 26
Committees of Safety, 26
Conanicut Island, R.I., 115
Congress, Revolutionary War, 82
  and Hospital Department funding, 30, 39–41, 44, 119
  Hospital Department legislation and regulation, 22, 25–41, 43, 45, 48, 74–75, 109, 115–18, 127, 228
  and Hospital Department staff, 34–35, 41–44, 46–49, 59–60, 64, 69
  Medical Committee, 14, 25, 35, 37, 40, 43–45, 72, 75, 77, 105, 110, 114
  Secret Committee, 224
  and supply problems, 39–40, 42, 46, 57, 59, 62–65, 83
Congress, 1783-1812, 131, 135
Congress, War of 1812, 149, 156
Congress, 1815-1816, 187
Connecticut, 57, 103, 113, 150. See also Hospital patients.
Connecticut Provincial Congress, 28, 56
Continental Army. See also Hospital Department; Washington, George.
  Boston operations, 50, 56–57
  commanders, 37, 50, 57, 59–60, 67, 98, 119–20
  desertions, 59, 91, 111, 119
  disbandment of, 48, 99, 133
  enlistment problems, 27, 33, 59, 74–75, 84
  mutinies, 31, 46, 103, 105, 124
  New Jersey and Pennsylvania operations, 39, 50, 67–72, 92, 103, 110
  New York area operations, 45, 50, 57, 65–67, 69, 72–74, 99
  Northern Army operations, 50, 57, 59–60, 98, 108
  smallpox and inoculation, 56, 62, 74–75, 84
  strength of, 33, 50, 59–60, 65, 70, 75, 77, 87, 95, 106, 121, 124
  at Valley Forge, 81–82, 84–87, 92
  Yorktown operations, 46, 112, 120–23, 127
Coosa River, 181
Cornwallis, Lt. Gen. Charles, 121

Council of War, 28
Crab Island, N.Y., 174
Craigie, Andrew, 44, 60, 63, 82-84
Craik, James, 40, 43-44, 82, 87, 92, 105, 115, 121-22, 126
Crawford, William H., 187
Creek Indians, 164, 181
Croton River, 73
Crown Point, N.Y., 60
Cullen, William, 1-2, 19, 54
Cunningham, Cornelius, 165
Cupping, 194
Cutbush, Edward, 11, 220
Cutbush, James, 156
Cutter, Ammi Ruhamah, 38, 98
Cutting, John Brown, 67, 82-84, 237
Cuyahoga, 162

Danbury, Conn., 98, 102, 112-13
Dartmouth medical school, 20
Dayton, Ohio, 162
Dearborn, Maj. Gen. Henry, 129, 148, 157, 161, 165, 167
Delaware, 91-92, 125, 150
Delaware Indians, 140
Delaware River, 73, 92
Detroit, Mich., 137, 148, 162-63, 165, 190, 194
Diarrhea, 5, 7-8, 73, 96, 111, 114, 122, 125, 127, 139, 142-43, 157, 167-70, 173, 178, 192-93, 195, 254, 260
Dimsdale, Baron, 56
Diphtheria, 4
Director General and Chief Physician, Hospital Department. *See also* Church, Benjamin; Cochran, John; Foster, Isaac; Morgan, John; Shippen, William, Jr.
  appointments and dismissals, 26, 28-29, 35-37, 43-44, 75, 77
  authority of, 22, 23, 27, 29, 32, 36-37, 41, 45, 98, 115, 117
  supply powers, 37, 39-40, 43
Disease. *See also* Casualties; Disease rates; Diseases.
  diagnosis of, 1, 3-6
  theories of cause and spread, 1-4, 77, 141, 186, 192-93
  treatment of, 1, 5-11, 14, 159-60, 191-95
Disease rates
  Indian campaigns, 132, 134-37
  Louisiana Territory, 141-43
  Northwest Territory forts, 139-40
  Revolutionary War, 59-60, 63, 70-75, 77, 84, 88-92, 94-97, 102-3, 105-6, 108, 128, 230, 240-41
  War of 1812, 157, 159-62, 165, 170, 173
Diseases, 7-8, 10, 65, 96, 114, 127-28, 140-42, 160, 192, 254. *See also* Fevers; and specific name of disease.

District of Columbia, 178
Doctors' Mob riot, 19
Downingtown, Pa., 109
Draper, George, 44
Dropsy, 7, 96, 193, 195
Drugs, 29, 57, 187-88. *See also* Medical and hospital supply; Medicine chests; Medicines.
  imported and purchased, 26, 39-40, 46, 82
  lists of requirements, 6-7, 63
  shortages, 22, 25-26, 30, 56, 60, 62-64, 82-84
Dumfries, Va., 75, 120
Dunkards, 90-91
Dunkerstown, Pa., 90
Dysentery, 3-5, 7, 9, 11, 56, 60, 63, 84, 96, 108, 111, 113-15, 123, 125, 139, 142-43, 157, 159-61, 168, 170, 173, 178, 184, 192-93, 195, 260

Eastern Department (Hospital Department)
  hospitals, 48, 50, 53, 57, 66-67, 72-76, 97-98, 108, 114, 125-26
  medical staff, 36-38, 40, 69, 74, 97-98, 99, 102, 112, 230
  supply, 56, 66-67, 70-73, 81, 98, 99
Easton, Pa., 70-71, 81-82, 91, 106-8
Edwards, Abraham, 162
Elizabeth, N.J., 69
Elliott, John, 133, 134
Ephrata, Pa., 81, 90-91
Epilepsy, 194
Erie, N.Y., 152
Ettwein, John, 70, 81, 88, 91
Eustis, William, 44, 72-73, 113, 126, 129, 134, 141-42, 144, 148-50, 243, 246
Eutaw Springs, S.C., 119, 123
Evacuation of patients, 21, 87-89
  land transport, 72, 77, 81, 118, 136, 167, 169
  water transport, 67, 94, 102, 108, 123, 125, 138, 142, 162, 167, 170, 173-75
Evansburg, Pa., 81
Ewell, James, 180

Fallen Timbers, battle of, 131, 136
Faulkner Swamp, Pa., 81
Fayssoux, Peter, 45, 118-19, 123
Fever
  causes and diagnosis of, 2, 4, 7, 193
  incidence of, 52, 60, 76, 96, 190, 192
  treatment of, 2, 7-8, 63, 194
Fevers, by type
  autumnal, 56, 137
  bilious, 3, 63, 96, 111, 120, 126-27, 137, 142-43
  bilious putrid, 112-13, 127
  camp, 69
  hospital, 4, 218
  inflammatory, 125, 127, 143, 193-94
  intermittent, 4, 63, 96, 103, 106, 111, 113-14,

Fevers, by type—Continued
  120, 122, 125–26, 138–40, 142–43, 157, 159–60, 167–68, 178, 193–94
  jail, 4, 218
  malignant, 4
  pernicious, 184
  putrid, 4, 61, 77, 79, 81, 84–85, 88, 90–91, 95–96, 103, 113, 126–27, 137, 218
  remittent, 4, 63, 106, 113–14, 120, 122, 125–26, 140, 142–43, 193
  scarlet, 4
  spotted, 159
  typhoid, 4–5, 84, 143, 160, 193, 218, 265
  typhus, 4–5, 7, 21, 84, 110, 140, 157, 159, 163, 168–70, 173, 193–94, 218, 265
  yellow, 3–4, 7, 143, 193
Fishkill, N.Y., 73–75, 97–98, 102, 112
Flood, (Doctor), 184
Florida, West, 164, 181
Food shortages, 3, 22, 39–40, 42, 46, 63–64, 71, 82–83, 91, 99, 103, 105, 114, 117, 124, 134
Food supply
  barley, 7, 159
  bread, 63, 77, 83, 103, 137, 159, 165, 168
  chocolate, 7, 83, 142, 155, 159, 170
  coffee, 7, 83, 114
  cornmeal, 63, 83, 149
  flour, 83, 103, 141, 170
  fruit, 8, 11, 14, 97, 193
  meat, 11, 63, 65, 83, 91, 115, 126, 137, 159–61, 193
  milk, 91, 108, 160, 169, 193
  molasses, 7, 63, 85, 114, 124, 159
  rice, 7, 63, 83, 114, 159
  salt, 6, 83
  sugar, 7, 11, 42, 64, 83, 114, 124, 140, 142, 159
  tea, 83, 114, 124, 142, 159
  vegetables, 11, 14, 39, 64–65, 77, 92, 94, 113, 115, 136–37, 193
  vinegar, 7, 39, 77, 83, 149
Forgue, Francis, 38, 233
Fort Adams, Miss., 139, 141–42
Fort Anne, N.Y., 94
Fort Constitution, 166
Fort Dearborn, Ill., 162–63
Fort Defiance, Ohio, 136–37, 139–40, 163
Fort Erie, 177
Fort Fayette, Pa., 162
Fort George, N.Y., 59–60, 62–65, 94, 165, 168–69
Fort Harrison, Ind., 138
Fort Independence, 166
Fort Jay, N.Y., 138
Fort Jefferson, Ohio, 134, 140
Fort Knox, 138
Fort Lee, N.Y., 69, 73
Fort Malden (Canada), 162–64

Fort McHenry, Md., 180
Fort McNair, D.C., 180
Fort Meigs, Ohio, 6, 164–65
Fort Nelson, Va., 185
Fort Niagara, 161–62, 165, 168
Fort Pitt, Pa., 106, 110, 133
Fort Preble, 166
Fort Schlosser, N.Y., 169
Fort Seammel, 166
Fort Stephenson, Ohio, 177
Fort Stoddert, Ala., 181
Fort Strother, Ala., 181
Fort Sullivan, N.Y., 108, 110, 166
Fort Sumner, 166
Fort Washington, N.Y., 72–73
Fort Washington, Ohio, 134, 136–37, 139
Fort Wayne, Ind., 133, 139
Forts and garrisons
  coastal, 138
  Northwest Territory, 131, 136, 139
Foster (Forster), Isaac, 28, 38, 46, 51, 57, 66–67, 74–75, 97–98, 99, 102, 112
Foster, Josiah, 137–38, 162
France. See also French forces.
  fear of war with (1791), 131, 138, 148
  funds and supply from (Revolutionary War), 26, 30, 46, 49
Franklin, Benjamin, 6–7, 54, 192
Fraser, Brig. Gen. Simon, 95
Fredericksburg, Va., 120, 194
French and Indian War, 20, 44, 64, 75
French Creek, Pa., 109
French forces, 40, 46, 106, 115, 121–23
French Mills, N.Y., 156, 166, 170, 174
Frenchtown, Mich., 163
Frostbite, 84, 163, 167
Frothingham, Ensign, 140

Gage, General Thomas, 28
Gangrene, 16
Gates, Maj. Gen. Horatio, 54, 60, 62–65, 95–97, 117, 227, 240–41
Genesee, N.Y., 106, 108
Georgia, 43, 115, 117, 150, 185
Germantown, Pa., 79, 81–82
Gould, David, 120
Governors Island, N.Y., 138
Grasse, Rear Admiral de, 106
Grasson, Victor, 134, 251
Great Britain, fear of war with (1791), 131, 138, 140
Green Spring, Va., 121
Greenbush, N.Y., 157, 159–61, 169, 171, 175, 188
Greene, Maj. Gen. Nathanael, 66–67, 81, 83, 118–19, 123–24
Greenleaf's Point, D.C., 180

Greenville, Ohio, 134, 137
Gregg, Captain, 114
Hackensack, N.J., 69, 72
Hagan, Francis, 44, 94
Hampton, Maj. Gen. Wade, 142, 166, 170
Hancock, John, 82
Hanover, Va., 120–21, 123
Harmar, Brig. Gen. Josiah, 131–33
Harrison, Maj. Gen. William Henry, 6, 131, 137–38, 152, 156, 163–65, 177
Hartford, Conn., 98, 113
Harvard medical school, 20
Hays, Adam, 177
Hayward, Lemuel, 51
Hayward, Nathan, 133, 136
Head of Elk, Md., 125
Heath, Maj. Gen. William, 47, 73–74, 103
Heerman, Lewis, 184
Henry, Patrick, 54, 75
Hessian troops, 71–72, 94–96
Heustis, Jabez, 143, 192–93
Heyward, Thomas, Jr., 33
High Hills of Santee, S.C., 199, 123
Highlands of the Hudson, N.Y., 103
Hillsboro, N.C., 118
Horner, W. E., 196
Hosack, David, 3
Hospital Department. *See also* Director General and Chief Physician; Eastern Department; Middle Department; Northern Department; Southern Department.
  Apothecary General, 30, 40, 44–45, 67
  Apothecaries General, 37, 60, 65, 69, 82, 84, 237
  British system as model for, 20, 36
  close of, 48, 99, 127, 133
  conflict with regimental system, 8, 26–27, 29–32, 40, 45, 48, 72
  Deputy and Assistant Directors General, 36–40, 43, 45, 65, 82, 97, 112, 114, 118, 120, 233
  internal staff disputes, 19–21, 26, 29, 32–35, 38–39, 41–43, 48–49, 62, 67, 69–70, 112
  legislation and reform, 22–41, 43, 48, 74–75, 77, 109, 115, 117–18, 127
  Physician and Surgeon General, 43–45, 77, 82, 236
  Physicians and Surgeons General, 36–37, 40, 43–45, 60, 65, 69, 82, 89, 95, 97–98, 102, 108, 114, 118
  Purveyor, 39–40, 43–46, 82, 118
  staff education and experience, 1–2, 9, 19–21, 22, 38
  staff pay and allowances, 27, 41, 43, 45–49
  staff selection and promotion, 22–26, 43, 45, 47, 60
Hospital patients. *See also* Evacuation.
  care of, 9, 15–18, 151

Hospital patients—Continued
  civilian, 91, 97, 106, 112, 114–15, 125, 127, 139, 177
  diet, 2, 11, 15, 66, 85, 119, 141, 159–60, 170, 193
  new recruits, 3, 10, 69, 102, 159, 168, 178
  prisoners of war, 80, 94–96, 110, 113, 121, 127, 153, 164, 175, 177, 180–81, 184–85, 190
  segregation and isolation of, 9, 37, 51, 56, 64–65, 74–75, 106, 109, 120, 123, 197
Hospital patients, Revolutionary War
  Connecticut, 72–73, 98, 113
  Delaware, 91, 125
  Maryland, 125
  Massachusetts, 22, 26, 27, 51, 52–57, 98, 114
  New Jersey, 67, 69, 71–72, 75, 81, 99, 102–3, 126–27
  New York City and Long Island, 66–67, 74
  New York State, 57, 59–60, 62–65, 72–74, 92, 94–98, 102–3, 105–6, 108, 110, 112–14, 125–27
  Pennsylvania, 69–71, 76, 77, 80–84, 86, 88–92, 106–12, 127
  Rhode Island, 98, 115
  South Carolina, 117–19, 123–24
  Vermont, 94–95
  Virginia, 84–85, 120–23
Hospital patients, 1783-1812
  Louisiana Territory, 141–43
  Northwest Territory, 133, 134–40
Hospital patients, War of 1812
  District of Columbia, 180
  Louisiana, 183–84
  Massachusetts, 190
  New York State, 157, 159–62, 167–71, 173–75, 178
  Northwest Territory, 162–65, 177–78, 194
  Vermont, 167, 172–74, 178
  Virginia, 185
Hospitals. *See also* Medical personnel.
  closings of, 48, 64, 91, 94, 108–9, 113, 123, 127, 133
  convalescent and invalid, 51, 52–53, 88, 133, 188
  design and siting of, 9, 65, 86, 87, 115, 126, 154, 167–69, 175, 196–97
  discipline, 9, 39, 50–52, 54, 66, 81, 87, 91, 102, 105, 109–11, 129, 136, 154, 178, 180, 190–91
  European, 8, 48
  funds for, 30–31, 35, 39–41, 44, 110, 114, 119, 155
  guards, 9, 20, 52, 69–70, 122, 138, 159
  huts and tents, 86, 92, 94, 102–3, 106, 111–12, 135, 137, 141, 157, 163, 166, 168–70, 175, 195–97, 243
  inspector general, 9, 36–37
  management of, 8–9, 66–67, 128, 171, 185, 197

Hospitals—Continued
  matrons, 45, 135
  nurses, 8, 31, 45, 64, 66–67, 70–71, 91–92, 94–96, 109, 117, 119, 121, 135, 150, 154, 159, 183, 185, 197
  in public and private buildings, 48, 65, 70–72, 81, 86, 94, 96–97, 99, 102, 112, 115, 120–24, 163, 165, 167, 174, 183
  reporting requirements, 31, 41, 53, 66, 77, 81, 87, 105–6, 125, 151, 154, 172, 175–77, 184–85, 197, 230
  sanitation, 3, 8–10, 20, 73, 92, 120, 122, 151, 154, 167–68, 173, 196–97
  for smallpox and inoculation, 56, 64, 74–75, 106, 120, 123
  stewards, 31, 40, 45, 65, 149, 159
  storekeepers, 31, 39, 66
  wardmasters, 40, 151, 159
Hospitals, flying, 8, 34, 44, 69–70, 85–87, 92, 95, 99, 102, 105–8, 112, 119–21, 125–26, 169, 177, 230, 243, 245
Hospitals, general, Louisiana Territory, 140
Hospitals, general, Revolutionary War, 8, 26–27, 31, 36–37, 43, 64–67, 86–88, 91–92, 95, 102, 106–8, 111, 114, 117, 120–21, 126, 230, 245
Hospitals, general, War of 1812, 150, 153–54, 164, 167–69, 172–75, 177, 180
Hospitals, regimental, Revolutionary War, 8, 22–27, 31, 35–37, 40, 43, 45, 63–64, 85–86, 102, 105–6, 125, 230
Hospitals, regimental, War of 1812, 170, 172–74, 177
Howe, General William, 77, 80
Hudson River, 34–36, 73–75, 77, 96–97, 103, 105–6, 112–13, 126, 138, 160
Hull, Brig. Gen. William, 148, 162–63, 165
Hunter, John, 5, 7, 14–19, 54
Hunter, William, 15, 19
Huntt, Henry, 172, 190, 195
Hygiene, personal, 9–11, 22, 50, 82, 154, 191

Indian-Loyalist forces, 106, 108, 114
Indiana Territory, 137
Indians, 106, 108, 110, 114, 129, 131, 133–38, 140, 148, 162–65, 181, 190, 197
Infection. *See also* Hospital patients; Hospitals, 3, 8, 17–18, 109, 167, 186
Inoculation, 14, 23, 32, 56, 59, 62–64, 74–75, 84–85, 97–98, 102, 115, 120, 125–27, 135
Invalid Corps, 127, 133
Izard, Maj. Gen. George, 172–73, 175, 191

Jackson, Maj. Gen. Andrew, 164, 181, 183–84
Jackson, David, 44
Jaundice, 21, 63, 96, 168, 178

Jenner, Edward, 14
Jockey Hollow, N.J., 103, 243
Johnston, Robert, 97, 114
Johonot, William, 44
Jones, John, 10–11, 14–20
Jones, Walter, 38
Jones, William, 180
Journal de Médicine Militaire, 20

Kalb, Baron de, 84
Kennedy, Samuel, 87–89
Kentucky, 150
Kerr, David, 183–84
Kerr, John, 184
King's College medical school, 20, 65
King's Mountain, battle of, 118
Kingsbridge, N.Y., 73
Knox, Brig. Gen. Henry, 47, 111

Lafayette, Marquis de, 112, 115, 121
Lafayette, Ind., 138
Lake Champlain, 37, 64, 94, 157, 166, 172, 174, 190
Lake Erie, 161–62, 164–65
Lake George, 59, 63
Lake Ontario, 161, 174, 190
Lancaster, Pa., 81
Larrey, Dominique, 196
Latimer, Henry, 44, 89, 125
LeBaron, Francis, 144, 148–49, 152, 155–56, 187–88, 190–91
Le Dran, Henri François, 20
Ledgard, Isaac, 44
Lee, Maj. Gen. Charles, 51, 57, 73
Lee, Richard Henry, 35–36, 70, 72, 82
Leeches, 194
Leesburg, Va., 121
Lewis and Clark Expedition, 133
Lewiston, N.Y., 161, 168–70, 175, 195
Lexington, battle of, 28
Lincoln, Maj Gen. Benjamin, 45, 117, 120
Lind, James, 11
Lititz, Pa., 81, 83, 89–91, 109, 239
Lockjaw, 165
London, 19, 26, 38
Long Island, N.Y., 65–67, 69
Louisiana, 140, 150, 181. *See also* Hospital patients.
Lovell, Joseph, 161, 167, 187, 190–92, 194, 197, 260
Lower Sandusky, Ohio, 177
Lundy's Lane, battle of, 172, 175

MacKenzie, Samuel, 70, 75, 95
Madison, James, 149
Maggots, 60, 96, 119
Malaria, 3–5, 122–25, 137, 142, 194, 254

Malone, N.Y., 167, 169–70, 174
Manheim, Pa., 83–84
Mann, James, 157, 159–61, 167–69, 171–74, 187, 190, 192–97
Martin, John R., 152–53
Maryland, 31, 70, 72, 74–75, 125, 150. *See also* Hospital patients.
Massachusetts, 26–28, 48, 50–51, 74, 150, 166. *See also* Hospital patients.
Massachusetts Provincial Congress, 26–28, 56
Maumee River, 162–64
McClurg, James, 120
McCrea, Doctor, 108
McDowell, Ephraim, 15
McHenry, James, 52, 60, 62, 129, 137
McIntosh, Brig. Gen. Lachlan, 91–92
McKnight, Charles, 43–44, 51, 52, 66, 72, 74, 81, 112
Mease, James, 144
Measles, 65, 96, 126, 159–61
Medical Department, 1783–1812, 129–33, 155, 157
Medical Department, War of 1812, 149–50, 153, 156–57, 159, 174–75, 177–78, 181, 184–86, 191
  Apothecary General, 149–50, 152, 155–56, 174
  Physician and Surgeon General, 149–52, 170–71, 186
Medical Department, post-1812
  Apothecary General, 184, 186–88, 190–91
  permanent department, 186–88, 190–91, 198
  Surgeon General, 187
Medical and hospital supply, Revolutionary War. *See also* Drugs; Medicine chests; Medicines.
  Commissary General, 40, 65–66, 83, 233
  imported, 26, 30, 40, 46, 49, 75
  purveyors, 8, 36–37, 39–40, 43–46, 82, 118
  shortages, 25, 29–32, 38–42, 44–46, 48, 56–57, 59–60, 62–64, 66–67, 70–73, 82–84, 88, 94–96, 98, 99, 103, 109, 113–14, 117–19, 121–23, 125–26, 197
  sources, 25–26, 30, 39–40, 46, 49, 56–57, 69, 75, 82–83, 110
Medical and hospital supply, 1783–1812
  attempts to improve, 144
  depots, 139, 144, 148
  forts and garrisons, 139–40
  Indian campaigns, 132, 134–37
  Louisiana Territory, 141–42
  purveyor, 129, 144
Medical and hospital supply, 1812–1816
  Apothecary General, 152, 155, 187
  Commissary General, 150, 155
  depots, 148, 155–56, 159, 188
  purchasing of, 149–50, 154–55
  purveyor and inspector, 148
  reform, 188, 190

Medical and hospital supply, 1812–1816—Continued
  shortages, 155, 162–65, 170, 172, 174, 184, 197
Medical literature, 20, 186, 191, 196
Medical personnel, 1, 129, 144, 170–72, 185, 186, 190–98. *See also* Hospital Department; Hospitals; Medical Department; Physicians; Surgeons.
  Army surgeons and mates, Revolutionary War, 27, 32–33, 36, 44–45, 65–66, 72, 90, 92, 95, 108, 114
  garrison surgeons and mates, 1783-1812, 131, 138–39
  garrison surgeons and mates, War of 1812, 151–53, 166, 177–78, 181, 185–87
  hospital surgeons and mates, Revolutionary War, 27, 30–33, 40, 43–44, 47, 59, 66–67, 69, 87, 92
  hospital surgeons and mates, 1783-1812, 133, 140, 148
  hospital surgeons and mates, War of 1812, 150–52, 159, 170, 174, 177–78, 180–81, 185–87
  and line officers, 37, 41, 47, 49, 79, 129, 133, 159, 173, 228
  militia surgeons and mates, 137, 148, 153, 164
  pay and allowances, 27, 32, 36–37, 41, 46–48, 64–67, 109, 133, 150–54
  regimental surgeons and mates, Revolutionary War, 26–27, 30–32, 37, 40–41, 45, 59–60, 63–64, 66–67, 69, 72, 77–79, 80–81, 94–95, 98–99, 102–3, 106–8, 117, 125
  regimental surgeons and mates, 1783-1812, 129, 131–35, 140
  regimental surgeons and mates, War of 1812, 148, 150–51, 153, 164, 169–70, 172–74, 177, 180–81, 186
Medical Sketches (Mann), 197
Medical societies, 20
Medical training, 1, 102, 151, 164, 198–99
  American medical colleges, 18–20
  by apprenticeship, 19, 38, 44
  European, 15, 18–20, 26, 38
  examination boards, 26, 45, 47, 129, 150, 154
Medicine, 1, 128, 186, 197. *See also* Medical personnel.
Medicine chests, 30–31, 57, 83–84, 135, 148–49, 155–56
Medicines, 234. *See also* Drugs.
  antimony, 6, 14, 169, 195
  arsenic, 57, 194
  bark, 6, 9, 16–17, 57, 62–63, 119, 124, 137, 144, 160, 194, 254
  calomel, 2, 6–7, 17, 159–60, 192, 195
  camphor, 6, 9, 63
  castor oil, 7, 192
  corrosive sublimate, 6–7
  cream of tartar, 57
  digitalis, 160

Medicines—Continued
  emetics, 5–6, 124, 160, 192
  ipecac, 6, 57, 63, 192
  jalap, 2, 6, 62–63, 160, 192
  manna and senna, 6, 192
  mercury, 6–7, 14, 18, 143, 194–95, 254
  nitrate of silver, 194
  nitre, 6, 63
  opium, 5–6, 8, 16–18, 62, 122, 137, 159–60, 192–93, 195, 254
  purgatives, 6–7, 159–61, 192–93
  quinine, 3, 16
  rhubarb, 6, 192
  salts, 7, 62, 192
  sugar of lead, 193, 195
  sulfur, 6, 83–84
  tartar emetic, 6, 63, 192
  vegetable remedies, 63, 66, 143, 144
Mercer, Brig. Gen. Hugh, 33, 34, 69, 72
Miami Indians, 134, 163
Michilimackinac, Mich., 190
Middle Department (Hospital Department)
  hospitals, 67, 69–72, 74, 77, 79–92, 97–99, 108, 110
  medical staff, 36–37, 39–40, 44, 82, 84, 89, 102, 108, 112, 115, 237
  supply, 67, 70–72, 81–84, 98, 99, 109–10, 114
Middlebrook, N.J., 102, 110–11
Middleton, Peter, 9
Military Journal (Thacher), 114
Mississippi River, 141–42
Mississippi Territory, 150, 164, 181
Mobile, Ala., 164
Mohawk River, 106, 188
Monmouth, N.J., 92, 99, 110
Monro, Donald, 4, 6, 8, 11, 54, 80
Monroe, Mich., 163
Montgomery, Brig. Gen. Richard, 59
Montreal, 59–60, 157, 159, 165, 170
Montresor's Island, N.Y., 66, 74
Moravian Order, Bethlehem, Pa., 70–71, 80–83, 88–91
Morgan, John, 20, 44
  as Director General, Hospital Department, 29–32, 36, 38–39, 51, 54–57, 60, 62, 66–67, 69–70, 72–74, 83
  dismissed, 29, 74–75
  feud with Shippen, 19–20, 29, 33–35, 42–43, 67, 224
  power struggle with Stringer, 32–33, 62
Morris, Robert, 45–46, 110
Morristown, N.J., 50, 69, 71, 75, 99, 103, 111–12, 243
Mortality rate
  Louisiana Territory, 141–43
  Revolutionary War, 3, 48, 53, 57, 82, 86, 88, 91, 95, 99, 103, 124

Mortality rate—Continued
  from smallpox and inoculation, 14, 75, 115
  from surgery, 17–18, 196
  War of 1812, 161–63, 169–70, 172–75, 184
Mosquitoes and nets, 4, 124, 139, 142–43
Mount Holly, N.J., 81
Mount Independence, N.Y., 64–65, 92
Mumps, 194

Napoleonic Wars, 21, 167
Narragansett Bay, 115
Natchez, Miss., 139, 141–43
Natchitoches, La., 181
Navy, American, 129, 155, 164, 170, 172, 174
Negroes, 117, 125
New Boston, N.Y., 126
New England, 37, 50, 72, 113, 122, 138, 166
New Hackensack, N.Y., 113
New Hampshire, 56, 106, 150, 166
New Jersey, 34, 50, 67, 69–73, 75, 77, 79, 108, 110–11, 150. *See also* Hospital patients.
New London, Conn., 98, 113, 152
New Orleans, La., 140–42, 152, 155–56, 172, 181, 183–84, 188, 263
New Windsor, N.Y., 103, 112–13, 125–26
New York City, 33–34, 50, 56–57, 60, 65–67, 72–73, 99, 106, 113, 138, 144, 152, 188
New York State, 47, 72, 105–6, 121, 150, 164–66. *See also* Hospital patients.
Newark, N.J., 67, 69
Newark, N.Y., 169–70
Newport, Del., 92
Newport, R.I., 98, 102, 115
Newtown, Pa., 71, 74, 108
Niagara, N.Y., 148, 157, 159, 190
Niagara River, 162, 165, 169, 172, 175, 177, 194
Norfolk, Va., 152, 185
North Anna River, Va., 121
North Carolina, 43, 115, 117–19, 150
North Castle, N.Y., 72
Northampton, Pa., 81
Northern Department (Hospital Department)
  hospitals, 59–60, 62–65, 94–97, 108, 114
  medical staff, 27, 32–34, 36–38, 40, 57, 59–60, 62–65, 81–82, 95, 97, 102, 114, 233
  supply, 22–26, 30, 57, 59–60, 62–64, 83–84, 94–96
Northwest Territory, 133–38, 150, 157, 163–66, 170, 177. *See also* Hospital patients.
Norwalk, Conn., 72–73
Nottingham Meeting House, Del., 92

Ohio, 137, 150, 152, 162–63
Oliphant, David, 45, 117–19
Ophthalmia, 96, 111
Otterkill, N.Y., 113
Otto, Bodo, 44, 69–70, 75, 79, 87, 92, 109

Otto, Frederick, 79, 87
Otto, John Augustus, 79, 87

Paoli, Pa., 79
Paralysis, 96, 170
Paramus, N.J., 102, 111
Paris, 19
Patuxent River, 178
Peekskill, N.Y., 73–74, 98, 102
Pennsylvania, 20, 47, 64, 70, 75, 77–92, 103, 108–11, 121, 125, 150. *See also* Hospital patients.
Pennsylvania Evening Post, 38
Pennsylvania Packet, 43
Pennypacker Mills, Pa., 81
Perkins, Elisha, 51
Perry, Commander Oliver Hazard, 164
Petersburg, Va., 120
Petit, Jean Louis, 16, 20
Pharmacopoeia, 89, 239
Philadelphia, 105
  hospitals, 70–71, 74–76, 80, 89, 91, 109–10, 125, 127, 133
  medical supply from, 30, 57, 60, 67, 69, 144, 149, 152, 188
  military operations, 77–79, 80, 92, 99, 109
Philadelphia Hospital, 109–10, 127
Physicians, 1, 8–10, 15, 18–20, 37. *See also* Medical personnel; Surgeons.
Pike, Brig. Gen. Zebulon, 167
Pittsburgh, Pa., 134, 148, 152, 156, 162
Pittsfield, Mass., 159, 190
Plague, 115, 143, 193
Plattsburg, N.Y., 157, 159, 161, 166–67, 173–74, 190
Plattsburg Bay, battle of, 172–74
Pleurisy, 6–7, 96, 160, 194
Pluckemin, N.J., 103, 111
Pneumonia, 6–7, 159, 161, 167, 169–70, 174, 195
Potomac River, 36, 180
Potts, Jonathan, 32, 38–40, 59–60, 62–65, 70, 72, 81–85, 94–97, 109, 233
Pottsgrove, Pa., 81
Poundridge, N.Y., 112–13
President, U.S., 129, 131, 149–50
Preventive medicine, 10, 14, 160, 191–92
Princeton, N.J., 71–72, 79–81, 91–92, 99, 110
Princeton College, 72, 81
Pringle, Sir John, 3, 11, 19–20, 54, 80, 217, 218
Prisoners of war
  American, 80, 113, 117, 119, 121, 153, 164, 170, 180
  British, 47, 94–96, 110, 119, 127, 175, 177, 180–81, 184–85, 190
  Hessian, 94–95
Providence, R.I., 98, 114, 115
Purging, 1–2, 5–6, 14–15, 18
Purveyors. *See* Medical and hospital supply.

Putnam, Maj. Gen. Israel, 51, 52, 56, 98

Quartermaster, 40, 66, 73, 83, 135, 149, 155, 175, 185
Quebec, 59
Queenston, Canada, 161

Ramsay, David, 7
Ranby, John, 16
Rand, Isaac, 56
Ravaton, Hugues, 8
Read, Willliam, 118–19
Reading, Pa., 81, 91, 109
Reamstown (Rheimstown), Pa., 81, 91
Regiments, 133, 140
  1st, 180, 262
  2d, 134
  4th, 137
  5th, 142
  7th, 142
  14th, 162
  17th, 163
  18th, 153
  28th, 177
  39th, 181
  54th, 163
Regulations for the Order and Discipline of the Troops of the United States, 82
Reporting and data collection, 154, 186, 193–94, 198
Respiratory illness, 4, 6, 8, 65, 96, 136, 160, 167, 192, 194
Reynolds, James, 162
Rheims, 19
Rheumatism, 7, 96, 106, 111–12, 114, 120, 139, 152, 157, 159
Rhode Island, 56, 98, 114, 115, 150
Rhode Island College (Brown University), 115
Richmond, Va., 121, 185, 188
Rickman, William, 33, 41, 84–85, 117, 119–20, 122, 227, 228
Robinson, Col. Beverly, 97
Robinson's House, 97, 105–6, 112, 243
Rochambeau, Comte de, 115
Roxbury, Mass., 51, 53
Rush, Benjamin, 2–3, 6–7, 17–20, 124, 144
  member of Medical Committee, 23, 35–37, 72, 75–76, 79
  Physician and Surgeon General in Middle Department, 37–39, 72, 80–82, 98
  and Shippen controversy, 39, 41–43, 69–70, 224

Sackett, J.H., 187
Sackett's Harbor, N.Y., 152, 156, 164–68, 173–75, 177, 190
St. Clair, Maj. Gen. Arthur, 123–24, 131–34
St. Johns, Canada, 59–60

St. Lawrence River, 157, 166, 174
Salisbury, N.C., 118–19
Sandusky, Ohio, 163
Sanitation, 3–4, 9–11, 50, 77, 102, 129
Saratoga, N.Y., 75, 83, 95–96
Scabies, 3–4, 6, 84, 96, 197
Scalping, by Indians, 96, 114, 134–35
Schaefferstown, Pa., 91, 109
Schenectady, N.Y., 65, 96–97
Schuyler, Maj. Gen. Philip, 32, 57, 59, 63–65, 92, 94
Schuylkill River, 79, 81
Scott, Brig. Gen. Charles, 120
Scott, Daniel, 52
Scott, John M., 133
Scott, Moses, 44
Scott, Brig. Gen. Winfield, 172, 175
Scurvy, 4, 11, 14, 63, 84, 96, 115, 142–43, 254
Secretary of the Army (1815), 187
Secretary of War, 45, 124, 126, 129, 133, 137, 139, 141–42, 144, 148, 154–55, 180–81, 186–88, 190
Senter, Isaac, 59
Seven Years' War, 6, 8
Shawnee Indians, 131, 137–38
Shippen, William, Jr., 54, 65, 233
   acquitted in court-martial, 42–43
   and Army hospitals, 34, 69–71, 80–81, 84, 88, 91–92, 97, 108, 110, 113, 120
   Director General, Hospital Department, 37–39, 41–44, 105
   and Hospital Department reform, 35–37, 77
   medical training and teaching, 19–20, 38, 44, 114
   and rivalry with Morgan and Rush, 19–20, 29, 33–35, 38, 42–43, 67, 70, 224
Skenesboro, N.Y., 94
Skippack, Pa., 81
Smallpox, 3–4, 7, 14, 62–63, 65, 92, 115, 125–27, 135, 195. *See also* Inoculation.
   epidemics, 53–56, 59–60, 74–75, 98, 122, 191
   hospitals, 56, 74, 106, 120, 123
Smallwood, Brig. Gen. William, 31, 91–92
Smith, Captain, 134
Sorel, Canada, 59
South Carolina, 115, 117–19, 150. *See also* Hospital patients.
Southern Department (Hospital Department) hospitals, 117–25
   medical staff, 36, 45, 47, 99, 115, 117–18, 120–21, 227
   supply, 117–19, 121
Spencer, Oliver, 181, 184
Springfield, Mass., 112
Springfield, N.J., 99
Sproat, James, 109
Stamford, Conn., 72–73, 98

Steuben, Baron von, 82
Stringer, Samuel, 27, 32–35, 57, 59–60, 62–65
Sullivan, Maj. Gen. John, 27, 60, 67, 79, 106–8, 110, 114
Sunbury, Pa., 107, 110–11, 114
Superintendent of Finance, 45
Supply. *See* Medical and hospital supply.
Surgeon General, 161, 187
Surgeons, 14–17, 197–98. *See also* Hospital Department; Medical Department; Medical personnel; Physicians.
   British, 3–6, 8, 15, 20, 174, 196
   French, 8, 15, 19, 196
   Hessian, 72, 94, 96
Surgery, 1, 14–18, 96, 170, 174, 191, 196. *See also* Amputations.
Surgical instruments, 7, 29–31, 46, 67, 72, 82–83, 121, 162, 188
Susquehanna River, 106–7
Swieten, Gerhard van, 4–6, 11, 16–18, 20

Tarleton, Lt. Col. Banastre, 119
Tarrytown, N.Y., 102
Tecumseh, 131, 137–38, 165
Tennessee, 150, 164, 181
Terre aux Boeufs, La., 141–43
Terre Haute, Ind., 138
Tetanus, 17–18
Thacher, James, 56, 94, 96–97, 114, 123, 126
Thames River, battle of, 165
Thomas, Maj. Gen. John, 60
Thomas, Robert, 17
Three Oaks mansion, New Orleans, 183–84
Thruston, Alfred, 142
Ticonderoga, N.Y., 59–60, 63–65, 92, 94
Tillotson, Thomas, 102
Tilton, James, 245
   hospital hut design, 103, 111, 196–97, 243
   Physician and Surgeon General of the Army (1813), 152–54, 170–71, 175, 177–78, 180, 184–85, 187, 191–92, 256
   as surgeon in Revolutionary War, 44, 47, 75, 80–81, 122–23, 249
Tioga, Pa., 106, 108, 110
Tippecanoe River, 138
Toledo, Ohio, 136–37
Toronto, 165, 167–68, 170
Townshend, David, 44, 125–26
Trappe, Pa., 81
Treason, 27–28, 46
Treat, Malachi, 38, 43–44, 65, 95, 111–12, 114, 123, 249
Treaty of Ghent, 181
Treaty of Paris, 48, 99, 128, 133
Trenton, N.J., 69–73, 74–75, 79–81, 87, 99, 110–11, 125–27
Trepanning, 7, 18, 96

Trumbull, Jonathan, 63, 73
Tuberculosis, 7, 159
Tucker, Thomas Tudor, 118, 121
Turner, (Doctor), 152
Turner, Philip, 38, 44, 72–73, 98, 114
Typhoid. *See* Fevers.
Typhus. *See* Fevers.

Ulcers, 125
University of Edinburgh, 2, 15, 19, 38
University of Pennsylvania Medical School, 19–20, 137
Upshaw, William, 142
Ursuline convent, New Orleans, 183

Vaccination, 14, 191
Valley Forge, Pa., 75, 81–89, 92, 98, 102, 239
Van Ingen, Dirk, 65, 96
Van Voorhis, Isaac, 163
Venereal disease, 3–6, 8–9, 39, 96, 106, 111–12, 125, 135, 190, 195, 197
Vermont, 150, 166. *See also* Hospital patients.
Vincennes, Ind., 137–38
Vineyard Hospital, Va., 120
Virginia, 33, 41, 75, 84, 103, 106, 115, 119–21, 150, 178, 227. See also Hospital patients.

Wabash River, 138
War Department, 129, 135, 137, 144
War Office, 45
Ward, Maj. Gen. Artemas, 53, 74
Warren, James, 28
Warren, John, 7, 44, 48, 51, 52, 56–57, 66–67, 69, 114, 193
Warwick, Pa., 81
Washington, George, 37, 50, 85, 126. *See also* Continental Army.
 and Army medical organization, 22, 36, 38, 133
 and Boston hospitals, 53, 56–57, 127
 and general vs. regimental hospitals, 27–28, 31–32, 40–41
 and Hospital Department senior staff, 28–29, 32, 34–37, 42–43, 60, 63, 69, 102, 133
 and hospital reporting requirements, 40–41, 53, 77–79, 87, 105, 230
 and medical personnel, 40–41, 47, 51, 67, 77–80, 87, 92, 102
 and medical supply, 30, 39, 46, 56–57, 84, 114
 and Middle Department hospitals, 72–74, 81, 91, 99, 115, 125
 New York area operations, 57, 67, 69, 72–73, 75–76, 77, 99, 102, 106

Washington, George—Continued
 at Philadelphia, 70, 77–79, 92
 and smallpox inoculation, 56, 62, 74–75, 84
 at Valley Forge, 77, 83, 86–87, 92
 Yorktown operations, 112, 120–21, 123, 125
Washington, D.C., 152–53, 172, 178, 180
Waterhouse, Benjamin, 153–54, 187–88, 191–93, 195
Watertown, Mass., 51
Watertown, N.Y., 167
Watkins, Tobias, 187
Wayne, Maj. Gen. Anthony, 79, 121, 123–24, 131, 135–37
Weather, climate, and terrain, 154, 157, 168, 191, 193, 195
 cold, 4, 10–11, 38, 84, 94, 103, 139, 159, 163, 165, 167, 170, 173–74, 192, 194
 heat, 4–5, 10–11, 99, 118–19, 124, 142–43, 184, 192, 196–97
 swamps and stagnant water, 3–5, 10–11, 124, 141, 177, 183, 192
West, (Doctor), 156
West Indies, 26, 28, 40
West Point, N.Y., 73, 97, 102, 105, 112–13, 126, 133, 138
Wheaton, Joseph, 185
Wheaton, Walter W., 167, 173
White Plains, N.Y., 69, 72–73, 99, 113
Whitridge, Joshua, 169
Whooping cough, 96
Wilkinson, Maj. Gen. James, 96, 140–43, 156, 164–65, 167, 169–70, 172, 181, 190, 253, 254
Williamsburg, Va., 33, 120–23, 249
Williamson, Hugh, 117–18
Williamsville, N.Y., 152, 169, 175, 188, 249
Wilmington, Del., 80, 85, 92, 125, 152
Wilson, Goodwin, 120
Winchester, Brig. Gen. James, 163–64
Winder, Brig. Gen. William H., 178, 180
Wines and spirits
 medicinal purposes, 6–8, 11, 17–18, 114, 159–60, 170, 193–94
 shortage of, 41–42, 57, 83, 88, 114, 134
 supply of, 64, 136–37, 139–42, 155
Wolcott, Oliver, 33
Wooster, Brig. Gen. David, 59
Wounds, 3, 15–18, 138, 175, 177, 196. *See also* Amputations; Casualties.
Wyoming, Pa., 106–8.

Yellow Springs, Pa., 48, 84, 87, 89, 92, 109
Yorktown, Va., 4, 46–48, 99, 106, 109, 112, 120–23, 125, 127

www.ingramcontent.com/pod-product-compliance
Lightning Source LLC
Chambersburg PA
CBHW080532170426
43195CB00016B/2537